UNDERSTANDING
THE
HEART

—/\—

UNDERSTANDING
THE
HEART

—∿—

SURPRISING INSIGHTS INTO
THE EVOLUTIONARY ORIGINS
OF HEART DISEASE
—AND WHY IT MATTERS

DR. STEPHEN HUSSEY, MS, DC

Chelsea Green Publishing
White River Junction, Vermont
London, UK

Figures 6.1, 6.2, 6.3, and 7.1 adapted from illustrations in *The Fourth Phase of Water*, used with permission from Dr. Gerald Pollack, PhD.

Originally published in 2021 by Stephen Hussey as *Understanding the Heart*.

This edition published by Chelsea Green Publishing, March 2022.

Project Manager: Patricia Stone
Developmental Editor: Brianne Goodspeed
Copy Editor: Deborah Heimann
Proofreader: Diane Durrett
Indexer: Shana Milkie
Designer: Melissa Jacobson
Page Layout: Abrah Griggs

Printed in the United States of America.
First printing March 2022.
10 9 8 7 6 5 4 3 2 1   22 23 24 25 26

Library of Congress Cataloging-in-Publication Data
Names: Hussey, Stephen, 1986– author.
Title: Understanding the heart : surprising insights into the evolutionary origins of heart disease-and why it matters / Dr. Stephen Hussey.
Description: White River Junction, Vermont : Chelsea Green Publishing, [2022] | Includes bibliographical references and index.
Identifiers: LCCN 2022003453 (print) | LCCN 2022003454 (ebook) |
  ISBN 9781645021308 (paperback) | ISBN 9781645021315 (ebook)
Subjects: MESH: Heart Diseases | Heart—physiopathology | Complementary Therapies | Biological Evolution | Healthy Lifestyle
Classification: LCC RC682 (print) | LCC RC682 (ebook) | NLM WG 200 |
  DDC 616.1/2—dc23/eng/20220209
LC record available at https://lccn.loc.gov/2022003453
LC ebook record available at https://lccn.loc.gov/2022003454

Chelsea Green Publishing
85 North Main Street, Suite 120
White River Junction, Vermont USA

Somerset House
London, UK

www.chelseagreen.com

Contents

Introduction

It happened shortly before noon on January 5, 2021. I was in my kitchen making lunch when I turned to get something out of the refrigerator, and felt a sudden pain in my chest. At first, I thought my pec muscle was tightening up after the workout I'd done forty-five minutes prior. But then the pain intensified, and soon it was so bad I couldn't continue cooking. I turned off the stove, stood still for a moment in the kitchen, and then—feeling flushed and hot—walked outside, into the backyard, to sit for a minute and cool off.

Outside, the pain continued to intensify. I realized that whatever was happening to me wasn't normal, and that I needed to get help immediately. I thought for a moment about driving myself to the hospital, but the mounting intensity in my chest convinced me to call 911 instead. When the EMTs arrived, I walked a few steps to the stretcher and off I went in the back of an ambulance.

Inside the ambulance, the pain ratcheted so much that I couldn't keep a lid on it. I felt sorry for the EMT riding with me, who had to listen to my wails. When we arrived at the hospital he wheeled me into the ER and handed the doctor a printout. The doctor looked at it and instructed her team: "Possible STEMI, prep the cath lab."

An ST-elevation myocardial infarction, or STEMI, is a heart attack in which one of the three major arteries gets blocked. When a STEMI occurs in the left anterior descending (LAD) coronary artery, as mine did, it is known as a "widowmaker" because only 12 percent of people who experience them outside of a hospital setting survive.

The medical team wheeled me into a room, cut off my shirt, took off my pants and underwear. I felt like there were a million hands on me inserting IVs and prepping for the cardiac catheterization. Nurses bombarded me with questions about my health and how long I had been feeling this pain. I remember asking them not to call my parents just yet; I didn't want to burden them. Eventually, the nurses wheeled me out of the room and into an elevator, and up we went to the lab.

Once in the catheterization lab, there were more hands, everywhere. At first, they tried to go in through the radial artery in my wrist, before abandoning that for the femoral artery. There was a sudden cold sensation on my groin as they sterilized the site. A male voice next to my left ear told me I was doing great and that it was going to be okay, but someone put defibrillator pads on me "just in case." I heard the welcome instruction to administer morphine and from there it got hazy, but the pain eased as people worked diligently all around me. When I started shivering, someone covered me with warm blankets.

At the end of the procedure, the interventional cardiologist stood at my side and told me that although he'd found minimal atherosclerosis, a major acute clot had formed in the LAD artery, the largest coronary artery. He performed a balloon angioplasty, placed a stent, and told me it went in beautifully. I uttered an exhausted "thank you" before the man who saved my life turned and walked away.

———

I make my living as a chiropractor, so though I'm not an MD, I have enough training in anatomy, physiology, pathology, neurology, nutrition, and clinical diagnosis to understand the gravity of what I was experiencing that January afternoon, even while it was playing out.

More importantly, I've lived with autoimmune type 1 diabetes since the age of nine. Even as a child, I understood that being diabetic increased my risk of other health conditions, including poor eyesight, weak circulation, and damaged kidneys—and that the diet and lifestyle choices I make to control my diabetes would have a major impact on how long, and how well, I'll live. Because I've never been able to take my health for granted, I've always kept tight control of my blood sugars through diet and exercise, and dedicated myself to learning as much as I could about my own health, in order to avoid becoming a statistic.

I've also understood from a young age that having type 1 diabetes heavily predisposes me to oxidative stress, insulin resistance, and an imbalanced stress response (all topics I'll discuss in this book). These predispositions double, or even quadruple, my risk of heart disease. But I'm hardly alone in facing that terrifying prospect. The occurrence of heart disease has reached epic proportions. In 2018, there were approximately 720 thousand first-time heart attacks and 335 thousand recurrent heart attacks in the United States. By 2035, it is estimated that more than 130 million people in the United States will have some form of cardiovascular disease. The annual direct and indirect cost of heart disease and stroke in the United States is estimated at approximately $329.7 billion.[1] The cardiovascular system is the human body's most commonly diseased system, and despite all the latest technology, drugs, and surgeries, it's getting sicker and sicker, in more and more people.

The medical orthodoxy about heart disease is that saturated fat and cholesterol clog up our arteries, leading to coronary atherosclerosis and heart attacks. It is also thought that measuring cholesterol, especially low-density lipoprotein (LDL) cholesterol, is the best indicator of heart attack risk. As a young adult, when I asked my doctors why people with type 1 diabetes were at particular risk, they offered various explanations of how high blood sugars damage arteries. But I always sensed there was more to the story. Every time I heard something about cardiovascular disease, no matter how far out there it seemed, my ears perked up and I soaked in as much as I could. Through my own health journey and experimentation, my formal medical and nutrition educations, and my relentless independent research, I have tried to learn everything I could about how to prevent this disease.

What I've learned about the heart over the years has often surprised me and differed in many ways from what I had been taught and told. For example, the evolutionary origins of the nervous system helps explain current rampant rates of heart disease in the Western world; special characteristics of heart tissue make heart cancer one of the rarest cancer diagnoses a person can receive; a body of research suggests that the heart is not actually the main mover of blood in the body; and the research-based critiques of the widely accepted idea that saturated fat and cholesterol lead to atherosclerosis, or clogging of the arteries, are quite convincing. As a result, my own diet is actually high, not low, in saturated fat, replete with animal proteins, animal fats, and organic vegetables.

My interest in the heart is so deep, in fact, that I wrote a book about it— a first edition of the book you hold in your hands—which I was intending to self-publish within a matter of weeks when I experienced the STEMI. Needless to say, as I lay there in the cath lab, having suffered a major heart attack at the age of thirty-four, I began to doubt that I had any knowledge or authority on the subject to share. I knew my doctors would draw a connection between the heart attack and my high-fat diet and elevated LDL. And they did. One by one, the doctors looked at my chart, saw elevated LDL, and explained that it was the cause of my heart attack. Despite the large amount of evidence presented that LDL does not cause heart attacks, as I lay there on the table, having suffered a major heart attack, with credentialed experts explaining to me the reasons why, I had to ask myself: Why should anyone listen to me?

What happened in the hospital over the next few days changed my mind. Although I was extremely grateful to the people who saved my life, doubts began to surface about my care as early as that first night in the cardiac ICU as a nurse relayed the plan for managing my diabetes during my hospital stay. It was nothing like what I do at home. When I told the nurse my typical protocols, she said she would have to run it by the doctors in the morning. For that night, I would have to take the doses and type of insulin they recommended, not the amounts and types of insulin I use at home. Despite having had nothing to eat for the past twenty-four hours, the stress and inflammation from the heart attack had significantly increased my blood sugar. (Point in fact: When I entered the cardiac ICU, my blood sugar was over 300. Normal for me is below 150. Earlier that day making the lunch I never ate, it was about 87.) The doses they gave me didn't bring it down, and in my experience, if blood sugar doesn't come down within a few hours with a given dose of insulin, you get more aggressive. In the hospital, no matter how high my blood sugar tested between meals, they would only administer insulin at mealtimes.

The following day I requested to speak with the doctor. When the resident cardiologist and a pharmacist came in, I told them that I had been managing type 1 diabetes for twenty-five years. They had seen how good my A1c was, so they knew that I could do this on my own. I asked if they would permit me to manage it the way I usually do. But they didn't budge. They stuck to their plan. And I was stuck with high blood sugars.

All told, they wanted me to take eleven different medications not including my insulin, some of which I was familiar with, many of which I was not.

As I watched ESPN, messages kept popping up on the screen telling me I had a new medication, and a moment later, a nurse would come in to try and administer it, but the only doctor I'd spoken to about medication was the cardiologist and that was specifically about insulin. I was uncomfortable taking the other medications until I had an opportunity to speak with a doctor and understand what I was being prescribed, and why. I wasn't necessarily opposed to taking medication—I get it: I had just had a heart attack—I just didn't want to take medication I didn't understand until I had an opportunity to speak with someone who did.

The attending cardiologist arrived for rounds with a handful of interns and residents mid-morning. He began by telling me I needed to take a blood thinner for a year and a baby aspirin every day for the rest of my life to prevent a clot from forming around the stent. This made some sense to me. I had never had a stent in my body. There was no telling how my body would respond to it. However, I also had some concerns about the long-term use of blood thinners and baby aspirin. I was aware that chronic aspirin use has been shown to increase the likelihood of gastrointestinal bleeds and kidney failure (which I'll cover in chapter 17). As a type 1 diabetic, I already had increased risk of kidney failure. When I asked the doctor's opinion about the baby aspirin, he told me there is old research suggesting a connection to kidney failure, but that it wasn't a real concern. I agreed to disagree and moved on to the blood thinner. I told him the few doses of the blood thinner I had taken was giving me bloody noses. He replied that the hospital air is dry, and many patients experienced this.

"What about magnesium?" I asked.

"What about it?" he said. "I know that if you test it in the blood and it's low you should take it."

I clarified, "I mean, use it as a blood thinner?"

"Magnesium is not a blood thinner," the attending cardiologist replied.

I knew that wasn't true. Magnesium has been shown to decrease viscosity of the blood, especially in combination with vitamin E, and prevent clotting.[2] Granted, I didn't know if it would have the same effect as a medication in preventing a clot after a stent. I was hoping to discuss that. No luck. The doctor told me he was not going to comment further on magnesium because he was only familiar with allopathic treatments, an answer I could respect. However, the doctor then promptly left the room before I had the opportunity to ask any additional questions about the other medications I was being prescribed.

Of course, I'm not an MD, and certainly not a cardiologist. I'm speaking as a well-educated patient: Not having the opportunity to even ask these sorts of questions made me feel like the doctors were treating my disease, a heart attack, instead of assessing me as a patient—and a person. Trying not to be rude with my concerns was starting to become difficult, and yet I also felt it was essential for me to understand the medications I was taking and why. "Informed consent" is supposed to be the hallmark of good medicine, but I felt that I had not been informed about what I was consenting to, or why. How does one navigate this, especially as one is lying in a hospital bed, exhausted and vulnerable, having just suffered a near fatal experience?

That evening I was well enough to move from the cardiac ICU to a room on the cardiology floor. Of the eleven medications that my doctors expected me to take, I had only taken the blood thinner and one of the blood pressure medications, a beta-blocker called metoprolol (aside from the insulin). Metoprolol has been shown to decrease insulin sensitivity over time, so while I don't think it contributed to the struggles I had regulating my blood sugar that night—I had only had two doses of metoprolol by that point, and my blood sugar struggles probably had more to do with the poor management of my diabetes by the doctors than metoprolol—I later felt surprised that as a type 1 diabetic, I'd been prescribed metoprolol for long-term use, especially as opposed to other beta-blockers, which have been shown to increase insulin sensitivity.

The doctor had also recommended a second blood pressure medication, an ACE inhibitor, but since my blood pressure is normally on the lower end, I decided to take only the metoprolol. I think that was a good decision. In the middle of the night, a nurse came in to take my blood pressure. It had dropped to 98/50, which is very low, even for me. After she left, I realized I was hot. I sat up in bed—slowly—and eventually stood up to turn down the thermostat. Halfway to the thermostat, I got very lightheaded and reached for the wall so I wouldn't fall over. I steadied myself, turned down the thermostat, and got back in bed, grateful I hadn't agreed to the additional blood pressure medication.

The next day I persuaded one of the resident physicians to show me the images of my echocardiogram and explain to me what they were trying to accomplish with each of the eleven recommended medications. Many doctors and nurses had already told me that, based on my echocardiogram, the ejection fraction of my heart had dropped to about 35–40 percent. (The ejection fraction is the amount of blood that leaves the left ventricle with each contraction.) A normal ejection fraction is 50–70 percent. The damage done to my heart was in the septum, the heart muscle tissue between the two ventricles. The resident explained that the purpose of the two blood pressure medications was to decrease the workload on the heart by decreasing the signals that tell it to increase pressure or beat faster. This would prevent what is called cardiac remodeling, which is where weakened areas of the heart can change shape, while my heart tissue healed. If my heart did remodel, it could lead to the development of chronic heart failure. I agreed with him that this was important, but expressed my concern with dropping my blood pressure. He said that my body would get used to the medications and that would stop happening.

However, I also know that his recommendations—and the standard of care for cardiac events—are based on the conventional wisdom that the heart is the main mover of the blood in the body. In fact—and I realize this may be hard to accept—there is a good body of evidence, which I discuss in chapter 6, that the heart is *not* actually the main mover of blood in the body. There is also a body of evidence suggesting there are other methods besides blood pressure medications to upregulate the flow of blood, thereby preventing cardiac remodeling, including a fascinating medicine called ouabain (see chapter 17) and the use of infrared sauna (see chapter 6).

After talking with the resident physician, of the eleven I had been prescribed, I concluded that there were only four medications worth consideration. He thought I should definitely be on the aspirin and blood thinner, as well as the two blood pressure medications.

Later in the day, the cardiac rehab nurse came in. She was very sweet and gave me lots of good information. She said the approach to recovering as much of my heart function as possible was time, rest, and medications. Later in the day a different nurse, the heart failure nurse, came in to educate me on how best to prevent the development of heart failure, which is common after a heart attack. She explained that since my ejection fraction was low, there was a risk of blood getting backed up and that fluid could start to pool in my lungs and other areas of my body. She echoed what the cardiac rehab nurse told me: Time, rest, and medications were the best prevention.

What she said next shocked me. She outlined the recommended diet to prevent heart failure. She told me, first off, that I needed to drastically restrict my salt intake because too much would cause fluid retention. (I will debunk that idea, and other nutrition fallacies, in chapters 10 and 11 and show how it might even be harmful to restrict sodium.) Then we moved on to diet. While the vegetables, fruits, and lean meats on the list were acceptable because they are whole foods, my jaw dropped at the other foods recommended as "heart healthy." They included canned fruit, fruit juices, instant breakfast, margarine, mayonnaise, tofu, breads and cereals, cornstarch, sherbet, sugar, jellies and jams, graham and animal crackers, and cookies and fig bars. I could not believe she was recommending a diet so high in processed foods, especially the processed grains, sugars, and vegetable oils. I knew, right then and there, that I would not be following the recommended diet. It looked, to me, like a one-way ticket right back into the hospital, and to chronic poor health.

That evening, my nurse told me I might be discharged in the morning. I was relieved. I couldn't wait to get home and start my own carefully planned heart-healing routine. In the morning, I spoke again with one of the resident physicians and we had a good conversation about my situation. She still thought I should do everything they were telling me to do, like take all the medications, but she also acknowledged that it was obvious I was putting a lot of thought into my decisions.

Then I met a different attending physician for the first time. I told him I had been feeling better every day, and doing very well under the circumstances. He said that was great. Then he said he was not going to have a discussion with me about medication. He'd heard that I'd made up my mind, and he didn't want to discuss it. I was discharged from the hospital later that morning.

A few days later I was reviewing my medical records, which I had requested be sent to me from the hospital. Aside from it being more information on my care than I had received from anyone in the hospital, one thing struck me as odd. My first night in the cardiac ICU, I had some chest pain, which I was told was normal after the heart attack and stent procedure. One of the nurses called in the resident physician who tried to troubleshoot it. She asked me a lot of questions, and I remember answering one with a lengthy explanation of the stress I had been under. Her response was to prescribe me a Xanax. Nowhere in the medical records did anyone report that conversation. Perhaps they didn't think my stress was clinically relevant? In fact, as we'll see in chapters 2 and 8, there is a massive amount of evidence that chronic imbalance in our autonomic nervous system—essentially, our stress response—is a main contributor to heart disease and heart attacks, and that in many ways the diseases of modern society—including heart disease—are a direct result of the massive lifestyle changes humans have undergone in an evolutionarily short amount of time.

I'm not criticizing my care because I'm angry. I understand the strengths and weaknesses of modern medicine—I think most of us do—and I remain incredibly grateful to the people and the medical advances that saved my life. I describe all this to illustrate the dilemma we all must grapple with: that modern medicine has two very different faces. In my case, the production of synthetic insulin and the development of a stent procedure are modern medical miracles that saved my life. I will be forever in debt to those who made those discoveries and perfected those advancements, as well as to those who used them with such skill and care. The flip side is that modern medicine is incredibly lacking. It's shockingly unenlightened about what actually fosters good health in humans, as well as about managing care following events such as the one I had in a way that will put a patient on the true road to recovery and back in the land of good health.

During my first night in the ICU, I had all but decided there was no way I could release this book. I was filled with self-doubt. But by the time I returned home, I had come to understand that many people have faced—or will face—the sorts of decisions and dilemmas I faced in the hospital. I believe the information in this book is critical for them, and no less relevant or correct because I had a heart attack. It is my hope that the information found in this book can ignite the open conversation about heart disease that is needed to inspire progress and change in our care and understanding of the heart. And while it's true that I don't have an MD and I'm not a cardiologist, and I'm cognizant that in our credential-driven world some will write me off entirely on that basis, my credentials are different—and I believe stronger. Aside from having a medical background, I'm a *patient*. And this is *my health*. There is not a person in the world for whom the stakes are higher than the patient. It's not a person's career on the line. It's a person's life on the line.

That said, my goal in writing and publishing this book is not to be right, or to prove anyone else wrong, so much as it is to seek the truth, wherever it may lie. I know we can't do that without open-minded, honest, and unbiased discourse. I was deeply disturbed in the hospital by the shutdown of conversation about alternative ideas and therapies. As soon as I started to question my doctors' recommendations and approaches, I felt immediately branded as noncompliant and cast out of conversation—*about my own care*. All I really wanted was to have a discussion about my treatment options. I was taking the recommendations and my recovery seriously. I valued the doctors' expertise and opinions and wanted as much information as possible. What in the world is going on with medical care that that's so threatening? How did we get so far off course?

As soon as I was discharged from the hospital, I began a routine to restore the health of my heart. The rationale behind my approach is laid out in the pages of this book. I was told that if I didn't restrict salt, eat the recommended diet, or take the aspirin, ACE inhibitor, beta-blocker, and statin, my heart would not fully recover. I did not follow these recommendations.

Instead, I sought the advice of a cardiologist who treats *the whole person* and who helped me decide what medications to take on a short-term basis, and what ones to avoid altogether. I started by taking two medications, the blood thinner and the ACE inhibitor, for a month, then just the blood thinner for the next six months. After six months, I stopped taking any prescription medications. I've also relied on a nutrient-dense diet and supplements like magnesium, taurine, L-arginine, and carnitine, as well as ouabain, and I have procured an infrared sauna and use it often. I make it a top priority to manage stress and expose my body to environments that help it be more resilient in the face of stress. This proved difficult at first because a new stress emerged following my heart attack: My confidence in my health was shaken. At times during my recovery, it felt almost as if my relationship with my heart was strained, like my heart had lost my trust and vice versa. As I healed, recovered, and slowly returned to normal activity, my emotional relationship with my heart recovered as well.

How's it working out for me? So far so good. At my three-month follow-up, my echocardiogram report indicated that my interventricular septum (the middle part of the heart muscle that was damaged) had gone from "severely akinetic" to only "mildly hypokinetic." This indicates that the signal conduction of that area of heart tissue was just shy of being normal. My left ventricular ejection fraction had improved from the 35–40 percent to 50–55 percent, the lower end of normal. There was no sign of anything suggesting heart failure.

All this said, I want to be clear. If you have heart disease or any symptoms of heart disease, you should be under the care of your physician or cardiologist. I hope that your doctor's goal is to find the underlying causes of your disease and get you to the healthiest state possible as well as keep you off of medications, if practical. If this is not their goal, it may be time to find a new doctor. Many of the ideas presented in this book are very different from what you will find within the medical practice of cardiology, a field of medicine that is proving unsuccessful at preventing heart disease and fostering good heart health. Instead, this book presents information about the heart, what it is, why it is there, the ways it can malfunction, and how we can keep it healthy. It is my hope that being under the care of the correct doctor and being armed with the information in this book will empower people to take back control of their health, to prevent—and even reverse—heart disease.

PART I

HEART DISEASE: BILLIONS OF YEARS IN THE MAKING

CHAPTER I

Order and Energy

The Purpose of Life

To find the true cause of heart disease, we must go back—way back. All the way back to the origins of life, at least 3.8 billion years ago, and the famous primordial soup of various molecules, including ammonia, hydrogen, methane, and carbon dioxide. There was no order to these molecules ... yet ... and little to no oxygen ... yet.[1] Both of those things were to come: oxygen and order both being basic requirements of life as we know it. So how did we get from that primordial soup to oxygen and order—and life as we know it today?

One of the most compelling explanations of how order arose has come from a physicist named Jeremy England at MIT. Dr. England has theorized that the beginnings of life were nothing special—more like an inevitable event given the laws of thermodynamics. In thermodynamics, entropy is the tendency of things to move from order to disorder, meaning that systems don't like concentrated energy to be concentrated for very long. Any system, including the Earth, will find ways to dissipate energy. England is aiming to prove that living things—be they insects, birds, whales, humans—are the best way that the Earth has "found" to dissipate concentrated sources of energy from an outside source—that is, the Sun.

Essentially, Dr. England says that if we had a bunch of molecules (primordial soup) in an environment with energy constantly pouring in (sunlight), then life eventually emerges as an efficient way for the system to concentrate and then disperse built up energy.[2] At first, the Earth was concentrating the Sun's energy within itself until, at some tipping point, it required temporary storage tanks for the energy and—voila!—life sprung forth: energy-needy storage tanks. If Dr. England is on the right track, this theory has huge implications for our ability to sustain health. Let's look more into the formation of life and how it connects to avoiding disease.

At first, life was simple. Blob-like gels of molecules, *protobionts* or *protocells*, were the precursors to the first single-celled organisms. (*Proto* means "first.") The environment was hostile and unpredictable, and protobionts, which could efficiently use the only consistent form of energy around, the Sun, had a survival advantage. The better a protobiont could harvest energy from the Sun in the form of adenosine triphosphate (ATP)—the same molecule of energy currency our bodies use today—the better it could survive. That survival advantage was the beginnings of natural selection. Eventually, the protobionts developed the internal processes to create ATP on their own rather than having to harvest it from the Sun.[3] This happened 1.5 billion years ago and set things up for evolutionary advances that led to the first single-celled organisms, prokaryotes (bacterial cells), and eventually to eukaryotes (plant and animal cells).

These single-celled organisms made energy by photosynthesis, and released oxygen into the atmosphere as a by-product. Around the same time, the Earth's volcanic activity started to decline. These two circumstances led to a shift in the composition of the gases in the atmosphere. There was a decline in the hydrogen, methane, and carbon dioxide gases from the volcanic activity and an increase in atmospheric oxygen from protobionts' photosynthesis. This dramatic change in the composition of atmospheric gases was disadvantageous to the single-celled organisms that had grown accustomed to an atmosphere heavy in hydrogen, methane, and carbon dioxide. On the other hand, it was highly *advantageous* to other primitive bacteria, which adapted to use oxygen to make ATP. These opportunistic bacteria flourished on what was becoming an oxygen-rich Earth.

This is amazing if you pause to think about it. But then, something even more amazing happened. Somewhere along the way, one of those primitive oxygen-adapted bacteria took up residence in another larger bacterium that had not yet learned how to use oxygen. It started making energy for the larger bacterium. Both parties apparently decided it was an agreeable arrangement and thus consummated one of the most exciting partnerships in the history of life on Earth: the symbiotic origins of mitochondria in animal cells, including humans (and of chloroplasts in plants).[4] These bacteria held on to their DNA and their original cell membrane even as they evolved into our mitochondria—the "powerhouse of the cell" that everyone learned about in middle school biology.

The evidence for this is that they have their own DNA, separate from the DNA found in the nucleus of our cells. Further, they have also been found in the bloodstream on their own, doing their job without the need of a cell to keep them alive.[5] These structures are also the only ones in our cells with an inner and outer membrane. This suggests that these once independent entities had a new membrane formed around them in order to become part of the larger bacteria as their energy producer. This relationship still exists today. These bacteria held on to their DNA and their original cell membrane even as they evolved into our mitochondria.

Mitochondria were first seen in modern science by Richard Altman in 1886 and by 1890 he determined they were organelles and dubbed them "bioblasts." Nearly a decade later, Carl Benda renamed them "mitochondria." With these bacteria now assuming the burden of energy production, the larger cell could focus on the processes that led to specialization of cells and the formation of multicellular life, about 600 million years ago. Photosynthesizing bacteria used energy from the Sun to build more highly ordered organisms: plants. Plants produced oxygen for the oxygen-hungry bacteria and life continued evolving into more and more complex forms, each one better at consuming and ordering energy than the last. With life, Earth solved its problem of energy buildup from the Sun.

While the symbiotic origins of mitochondria and chloroplasts are well accepted in the scientific community, Dr. England's thermodynamic theory is still being developed. He has published some promising preliminary studies that support his theory, but many of his peers consider him far from proving it. However, Rahul Sarpeshkar, a professor of engineering, physics, and microbiology at Dartmouth College, said, "What Jeremy is showing is that as long as you can harvest energy from your environment, order will spontaneously arise and self-tune."

This is an important statement. "Harvesting energy from your environment" is one way of thinking about human health, and warding off chronic disease. Let me explain. If what England is saying is true, the very function of life is to absorb energy that has been concentrated into a system, the Earth, and then disperse it. If we fail at "harvesting energy from our environment," we will not experience "order and self-tuning." One way of looking at health is through the lens of order and disorder: Health is order in the system and disease is disorder in that system. A healthy cell is ordered and efficient. A diseased cell is disordered and dysfunctional. In a sense, our ability to absorb energy from our environment influences the order or disorder in our bodies. This, order or disorder, in turn influences the state of our health.

How do we absorb energy from the environment and convert it into a form our bodies can use? That process is the job of our oxygen-using mitochondria. Without this energy-making process, humans would not exist. We would not be able to accomplish the basic tasks to sustain life; our bodies would tend toward disorder. Without our mitochondria making energy, our tissues fail, leading to disorder and death; if our mitochondria are only able to make some energy, we may sustain life but only in a semidisordered state, also known as chronic disease. Healthy mitochondria are imperative for us to continue absorbing energy to maintain the health, or order, in our body tissues.

How do mitochondria make energy? They use oxygen to make ATP—the energy currency of our body—mainly by passing electrons down the electron transport chain (ETC). The ETC is located on the inner mitochondrial membrane. In this process, with the help of the oxygen we breathe, certain molecules are oxidized, meaning they donate an electron. This electron donation is passed down the ETC, and it is this passing along that generates our energy.

Where do we get these molecules that donate electrons? Mainly from the food we eat. Your body can convert sugar into glucose or lactate, or it can burn fatty acids and ketones (the better option). Any of these molecules can be converted into acetyl-CoA, which then runs through the Krebs cycle where it is oxidized, creating more molecules that can donate more electrons down the ETC to make ATP.

Contrary to popular belief, however, food is only a small part of how our bodies get energy. While the mitochondria are the way we use food to create energy in the form of ATP, our bodies can also soak up lots of energy from the environment that surrounds us. This energy is in the form of electrons and has a direct effect on the water in every organ, tissue, and cell in our bodies. Energizing the water in these structures by harvesting electrons from the environment makes everything easier for mitochondria and all cellular processes. We are designed to soak up and dissipate energy. Our ability to do this keeps us in good health.

Our mitochondria are important, and not just so that we can continue to maintain equilibrium with the laws of thermodynamics. Aside from making our energy they are also responsible for cell-to-cell communication, regulating the cycle of cell growth and death, and cell differentiation. Losing these functions is a recipe for disorder and disease. But what causes the damage we see in our mitochondria?

We have been talking a lot about electrons and we are not going to stop now. Any time energy is produced, a waste product is also produced; think exhaust from burning gasoline or heat from burning wood. In the case of our mitochondria, when they burn a fuel source, one of the waste products they produce are free radicals. A free radical is a molecule with an unpaired electron. (Electrons like to travel in pairs and are unhappy when they don't have one.) If a molecule has an unpaired electron it will look around for one to steal, including from an antioxidant. Luckily, our body makes its own antioxidants, like glutathione and superoxide dismutase, that are good at neutralizing free radicals, something life has done (mitigate free radicals produced in the energy-making process) for billions of years.[6] Of course, we must give our bodies the right food to stimulate antioxidant production (see chapter 11).[7]

Life is all about harvesting energy in the form of electrons from our environment, and health is all about neutralizing the waste products created via this process. We all know that the more "wear and tear" we put on a car the shorter life it will have. This is the same for living things. We have to create enormous amounts of energy to maintain the order in our bodies and counteract the entropy that leads our bodies toward disorder. The problem is that the more energy we produce, the more wear and tear in the form of free radicals we get. This is inevitable, yet wear and tear can happen throughout our lives without us experiencing poor health. We must maintain a balance between the number of free radicals we produce and the ability of our bodies to negate those free radicals. When this balance is off, it will contribute to illness.

Unfortunately, living the way we do in our modern civilizations, we tend not to produce enough internal antioxidants to take care of these free radicals. Most people don't eat enough of the right nutrients for our body to make our own antioxidants, and they don't get enough contact with nature to absorb electrons. What's more is that these days, we are exposed to thousands of unnatural toxins (heavy metals, artificial fragrances, air pollution, etc.) that act as free radicals in our bodies.[8] All these free radicals can spell disaster for our mitochondria. Whenever those free radicals—whether produced by mitochondria or an external toxin—aren't neutralized, they will steal an electron from the nearest place they can. Due to proximity, this often ends up being the membranes of the very mitochondria that made them. When a free radical steals an electron from the mitochondrial membrane, it damages that membrane. If this happens enough, then the mitochondria cannot do their job of enabling us to use and dissipate energy. The breakdown in mitochondria results in chronic disease. When things get bad enough, free radicals can damage many tissues in the body, including the lining of an artery.[9]

Before we get into the role that mitochondrial damage plays in the heart, let's look at another consequence of poor mitochondrial health. In the 1920s, Otto Warburg and his team discovered that cancer cells stopped relying on oxidative phosphorylation, the main way our cells make energy, and instead relied on glycolysis and lactate fermentation.[10] This is called the Warburg effect and it won him the Nobel Prize in 1931. This effect basically means that instead of using oxygen to make energy, the cells found a way (or were forced to find a way) to make energy without using oxygen.

More recently, metabolic researcher Dominic D'Agostino and cancer researcher Dr. Thomas Seyfried have solidified the metabolic theory of cancer.[11] Cancer cells have some interesting characteristics. They are anaerobic (meaning they don't use oxygen), they are acidic, they are rapidly dividing, and they are undifferentiated.[12] So, we have cancer cells that display these unique characteristics. Why? Let's illustrate this another way.

When a human is conceived, the egg and sperm come together to form a zygote cell. That cell implants itself in the lining of the uterus. At this point, the cell has no blood supply and therefore no oxygen. Initially this cell grows into what is called a morula, and then a blastocyst, by rapidly dividing to start the process of growing a fetus. Interestingly, these early dividing cells are anaerobic, undifferentiated, and rapidly dividing. Sounds like cancer.[13] Once the blood supply from the placenta develops at around the two-week mark, the cells of the fetus start to use oxygen and become aerobic, they start to differentiate into different types of cells, and they have more controlled cell division. This is the normal, noncancerous way cells usually act. The key here is the presence of oxygen.

The question is: Why does a cell stop using oxygen and become cancerous? Remember that the mitochondria are the structures in our cells that allow us to use oxygen. When they become damaged, the cell cannot utilize oxygen anymore. This triggers the cell that contains this damaged mitochondria to turn on oncogenes (tumor cells) in the DNA in the nucleus of the cell, which instruct the cell to become anaerobic, undifferentiated, and rapidly dividing cancer cells, the only thing it knows how to do in order to survive. When faced with the inability to use oxygen, the cell must either die or become cancerous. It's sort of a survival mechanism. The cancer solution keeps the tissue alive short term. Obviously, it is not a good long-term solution.

There are many things that can cause the excess free radicals in our bodies that damage our mitochondria. One is the large amount of toxins our bodies are exposed to on a daily basis. According to Herbert Needleman, who spent his life studying the effect of chemicals on children, at least seventy thousand new chemical compounds have been invented and dispersed into our environment since 1950, and many of them can act as free radicals directly. Free radicals can also increase dramatically when our cells become too reliant on burning carbohydrates (in the form of glucose) for fuel instead of fatty acids and ketones.[14] This is what brings us to the heart.

The cardiac myocytes (muscle cells) are some of the most mitochondria-dense cells in the body;[15] this is because of the massive amount of energy the heart needs and the large amount of oxygen it uses. Most of our organs prefer to burn fat for fuel, but this is especially true of the heart.[16] When other organs are forced to burn predominantly glucose for long periods of time, cells can switch from oxidative phosphorylation to glycolysis, leading to cancer. If the *heart* is forced to burn predominantly glucose, something far worse and potentially fatal can happen: a heart attack.

Do you see the importance of these little bacteria that the cells of life adopted so long ago? Aside from helping us fulfill life's role on Earth, they keep us healthy by using oxygen to make fuel for our bodies. The breakdown of this energy-producing process can result in excess free radicals, a state called oxidative stress, and this is one of the imbalances that contributes to heart disease. (Luckily, there are ways to repair mitochondria or generate new ones, which we will discuss in part 3).

CHAPTER 2

The Stress of Becoming Mammals

One Christmas, my wife, Kinga, and I were coming to the end of a ten-day trip to visit her family in Europe. We had decided we were going to spend the last few days on our own and take a side trip to Turkey. I had never been that far east in Europe and didn't really know what to expect. I had not researched much about Turkey before we left.

Since this was the end of our trip and our travel budget was nearly spent, I was hoping that Turkey would be on the less expensive side as European countries go. As we flew into Istanbul Atatürk Airport, I was struck by the both architecturally elaborate and modern buildings in the vicinity. I started to get a little worried about that budget.

Walking through the airport, I noticed the fancy interior and impressive number of shops. We always try to figure out public transport when we travel, and I was now particularly interested in its cost-saving benefits. However, it wasn't the easiest and we were tired after the last ten days of travel, so we decided to take a cab to the hotel. At the curb, fancy looking cars pulled up. These were the cabs! We took off down the excellently built and maintained highway leading into Istanbul. It took us right past all the fancy hotels I had seen from the plane. Periodically, I glanced at the cab meter as it went up and up and up, along with my stress level. Ten euro, twenty euro, thirty euro.

As Kinga can tell you, I don't like to go over budget if I can avoid it. But the cab fare continued to climb. I asked the driver how much longer to the hotel, but he did not speak much English. Instead of answering, he just smiled and asked where we were from.

Ninety euros later, we got to the hotel. I was fuming. I made up my mind that we would just have to sit in the hotel these last few days because I didn't want to spend any more money on this trip, though I know that would have never been acceptable to my wife. I got out. The driver and I got the bags out of the trunk and then stood by the front door of the hotel. When Kinga handed the cab driver a one hundred euro bill, he looked confused and said something in Turkish. Not understanding what he said, we all just stared blankly.

About then the hotel receptionist came out to help with bags, and I guess he saw the confused looks on our faces. He asked the driver something in Turkish and then turned to us to translate: The driver was asking if we had any smaller bills. I explained that the fare was ninety euro and pointed into the cab to show him. The receptionist smiled and told me that it was ninety Turkish lira, not euro. I asked how much that was and he said about twelve euro. I felt a wave of relief. As we walked into the hotel, I saw Kinga roll her eyes. She knows me well enough to know I was freaking out about the fare.

My reaction is the perfect example of a trait unique to humans: We can think our way into a stress response. I misinterpreted the cab meter, as well as all the things in my environment that, I thought, suggested Turkey was going to be an expensive country for tourists. Nothing actually stressful was happening to me; my thoughts alone drove me into a full-body stress response. The development in this ability was a key step in human evolution. It started with mammals, and it plays a key role in our quest to understand heart health.

———————————

Sometime between 1.5 billion years ago and 600 million years ago, two single-celled organisms—one that could use the newfound oxygen in the atmosphere and one that could not—teamed up in a relationship that has stood the test of time. A lot has happened since then. Multicellular organisms appeared around 600 million years ago. Plants appeared on land around 465 million years ago. And evidence of the first reptiles appeared around 370 million years ago. Reptiles are the next stop on our journey to understand the evolutionary roots of heart disease.

Let's start by looking specifically at the origins of the reptilian stress response—a physiologic characteristic still present in many reptiles, one that is still buried deep down in humans, today. In both humans and reptiles, the autonomic nervous system (ANS) controls this response by delivering cues about safety or threats from the animal's environment to the animal's brain. In all animals, the nerve that communicates this information throughout the body is the vagus nerve—always has been, and still is. When the newly evolved reptiles sensed a threatening environment, they would have one of three reactions: fight, flight, or freeze. Fight and flight are fairly self-explanatory, but what does freeze mean exactly? In essence, it means to play dead.

Most people know that reptiles are cold-blooded. They lack the body heat that mammals have because they are not as metabolically active. In mammals, our metabolism produces heat as a by-product, making us "warm-blooded." Reptiles have a much lower body temperature; their less metabolically active bodies do not produce much heat. This is relevant to the freeze stress response: Reptiles are evolved to this slower metabolism, and their physiology does not need them to maintain body heat, so they can make their freeze response pretty darn convincing. They can literally shut down certain organs or organ systems without dying in order to convince a predator that they are dead. Anatomically, it is important to know that most reptiles have only one pathway in the vagus nerve that communicates the signal for this to happen. That pathway is the dorsal motor nucleus of the vagus nerve.

At 225 million years ago, there was evidence of the first mammals, which evolved from reptiles. Many characteristics had to change for some reptiles to evolve into mammals. The singular stress response pathway is one of them. In highly evolved reptiles such as turtles and crocodiles, the vagus nerve began to develop two pathways—the dorsal motor nucleus and a newly evolved nucleus ambiguous—though it remains only a partial split. With mammals, the dual pathways in the vagus nerve are fully split. This is one of the characteristics that distinguishes us from reptiles.[1]

This split was necessary because when mammals evolved, they were much more metabolically demanding than any other class of life that came before them. Mammals lost the ability to drastically slow their metabolism in exchange for being faster, stronger, warmer, and bigger, while maintaining the stress response system of our ANS. Unlike reptiles, getting into a "freeze" would cause great harm to mammals. We have body heat to maintain and energy-demanding organs, and we move around more quickly and for longer periods of time than reptiles do.

As I'll explain in further detail, this split in the vagus nerve allowed a full freeze response demanded by the dorsal motor nucleus pathway of the vagus nerve to be, in a way, downregulated by the other, the nucleus ambiguous. Without this adaptation, during an overstimulating stress response, the single tract dorsal motor nucleus would slow our metabolism and blood flow of the organ systems as in the reptiles and prereptile animals. This would create oxygen deprivation, or hypoxia, and metabolite deprivation. The organ systems of mammals cannot tolerate this, and it would likely cause organ shutdown and death.

There are a few nonreptilian species that we know of that seem to have held on to the ability to severely slow metabolism without inflicting damage. A look into their metabolic physiology clarifies what goes wrong with ours in chronic disease—especially with heart attacks, which we will discuss in depth in chapter 8.

One nonreptilian animal that can do this is the common goldfish. It has been observed that during the winter, when water temperatures are very cold, goldfish can survive several days without any oxygen at all. Without oxygen, the fish are forced to use anaerobic glycolysis to produce energy. Over long periods, anaerobic glycolysis usually produces an increase in lactic acid production, causing metabolic damage. How does the fish get around this? While the mechanisms are not fully understood, scientists believe that these fish may convert lactate into ethanol and excrete it through their gills.[2] Carp display similar metabolic characteristics. Scientists have observed that they can survive for at least six hours in an oxygen-free environment.[3] North American freshwater turtles also rely on anaerobic glycolysis in a low- or no-oxygen environment, though instead of converting lactic acid to ethanol, they balance the lactate's acidity by releasing alkaline calcium bicarbonate from their shells into their blood.[4]

All of these animals have evolved mechanisms that allow them to survive in low-oxygen conditions, but these are fish (and a reptile). What about mammals? There is one mammal we know of that carries this adaptation as well: the naked mole rat. In a 2017 study, scientists found that naked mole rats could tolerate an atmosphere of only 5 percent oxygen for five hours, whereas mice died of asphyxiation in under fifteen minutes. (Ambient air is considered 21 percent oxygen.) Under anoxic conditions (0 percent oxygen), mice and naked mole rats both lost consciousness. But whereas the mice could not be resuscitated even when reexposed to ambient air within a minute of anoxia exposure, the naked mole rats fully recovered from eighteen minutes of anoxia exposure.[5]

How do the mole rats do this? By severely depressing their metabolism to suppress lactate production,[6] as well as by using fructose for fuel instead of glucose like other mammals would in anaerobic glycolysis. This allows the mole rats to bypass metabolic steps that would normally signal an overload of lactate, disrupting cellular function (more on this in chapter 8).

You may be wondering, how does this information help us understand heart disease? Humans do not have the unique capabilities of the mole rat, but we also don't live in the low-oxygen subterranean dwellings that necessitated such an evolutionary adaptation. While most mammals don't experience organ stress resulting from excess lactic acid production, there are some situations where humans do. This is because something has changed in our modern-day environments that can force us to revert to the oxygen-depleted state of anaerobic glycolysis. It has to do with our stress response.

The ANS that controls our stress response (as well as our breath and heartbeat) is not under our conscious control. We cannot consciously turn on or off a stress response. It automatically activates or deactivates based on the information we received from our environment. Dr. Robert Sapolsky, a neuroendocrinologist at Stanford University, studies the stress response of mammals of the African savannah. His research illuminates what happens physiologically during the normal stress response of mammals in the wild. He found that when a mammal is not faced with a threatening situation, they have low levels of stress hormones in their system. If presented with a threat, such as a predator, stress response hormones are released, the signal is transmitted through the vagus nerve, and the appropriate fight or flight behavior happens. If the animal manages to fight off or flee the threat successfully, the signs of a physiologic stress response go away completely within minutes. This is the way a mammal is physiologically supposed to respond to a threat.[7]

Brilliantly, Dr. Sapolsky took this information and compared it to the stress responses of humans living in modern society. He found that humans, with our highly evolved brains, are the only species on Earth capable of *thinking our way into a stress response*. For mammals in the wild, when the threat is gone, their physiologies go back to normal, almost as if the threat never happened. Because we humans are so often bombarded with information that we interpret as threatening, the human body's stress response can be turned on all day long.[8]

Instead of threat by an animal higher up on the food chain, we live in a society with constant demands. Despite lack of daily life-threatening *situations*, Sapolsky has found that we regularly experience physiologically life-threatening *responses* due to these demands. In other words, humans are the only species with the ability to think our way into a stress response because that's what happens when you combine our highly evolved levels of thinking with a bombardment of demands.

When something stressful happens to us, instead of turning off the stress response after the stressor is gone, we may continue to think about it for the rest of the day, or longer, perpetuating that heightened state. We can also see something stressful happen to someone else or in a far-off place in the world and think ourselves into a stress response. We can even have an unnecessary stress response when we think things are not going as we had planned, like a cab fare seemingly rising to vacation-ending levels. As Sapolsky says, "If you're constantly but incorrectly being convinced you're about to be thrown out of balance, you're being an anxious, neurotic, paranoid, or hostile primate who is *psychologically* stressed."[9]

My experience shows how this can happen. Although I took great care with my health, I had also become "a psychologically stressed primate" in the year leading up to my heart attack. Many things in my life felt like they were out of my control and the unpredictability was getting hard to handle. We all know that 2020 was hard on everyone. For me, it was the second of two years that my wife and I were living apart due to her job. As travel became restricted, I lost control over when I would see her again. I had also worked hard to build a speaking career, only to see engagements cancelled throughout 2020. And I became angry that poor metabolic health was consistently not part of the public health discussion about preventing severe outcomes from COVID-19. Add to that the division taking place in the country around social injustice and the presidential election, and I ended up internalizing much of my frustration, becoming quite cynical about some of what was going on in the world instead of finding ways to properly mitigate my stress and view the world in a positive light. The end result was I felt chronically frustrated over things that I had no control over. This type of feeling is one of the biggest contributors to a chronic stress state and has been shown to increase risk of atherosclerosis and heart attacks.[10]

As the frustration mounted from all these stressors, I felt myself building up chronic tension to the point of what is called a "functional freeze." This left me vulnerable to more acute stress. Early in 2021, I received some unexpected stressful news about the situation of a close family member, someone I am very close to and care about deeply. As stressful as the news was, it was the inability to control or immediately help resolve the situation that made it worse. I received this news on Sunday evening and then barely slept Sunday night. My workday Monday was a blur because I was so tired and my thoughts were consumed by how I could possibly help resolve the situation, but no solution presented itself. I had another terrible night of sleep on Monday night. I got up Tuesday morning, did my usual workout, took a shower, and then had a heart attack while making my first meal of the day.

Obviously, I am not the only one who struggled in 2020—and heart attacks represent a confluence of medical events; I'm not suggesting stress alone gave me a heart attack. But it's incredibly important for us to look at this: A study released mid-2020 found that there was a "significant increase in the incidence of stress cardiomyopathy during the COVID-19 pandemic when compared with prepandemic periods."[11]

Of course, our higher-level thinking has given us a huge advantage. But within modern society, especially in a time like a pandemic, it has also created an imbalance in our stress response physiology. Our stress response is the same one that allowed mammals—and our higher metabolic activity—to evolve 225 million years ago. The constant, unnatural stressors of modern civilization have only been around for ten thousand to twelve thousand years at most. There simply has not been enough time for us humans to evolve a stress response adapted to this modern environment.

Putting ourselves in an environment (like modern society) that is not the environment that our stress response evolved within has some dangerous consequences. Our ANS, which is constantly monitoring our environment for threats, has two states: the sympathetic (reserved for stressful times) and the parasympathetic (for nonstress times). These two states act together, rather than one being stimulated and the other turned off.[12] Primarily, the parasympathetic system keeps the sympathetic system from getting out of control, and for good reason.

The more recently evolved nucleus ambiguous pathway of the vagus nerve is what communicates the parasympathetic signal. If we did not have the nucleus ambiguous during a sympathetic stress response, our ANS would only activate that older evolved dorsal motor nucleus pathway of the vagus nerve, which could result in oxygen depletion and organ shutdown. When our stress response is overstimulated, even falsely so, over time the nucleus ambiguous can lose the ability to communicate its signal. This is called decreased vagal tone. If we lose vagal tone of the nucleus ambiguous and then we have a stress response, the body can revert back to that older pathway, and may shut down our organs. This is a life-threatening state for mammals.

Can you see the connection between our environment, organ shutdown, and heart attack? Looking back through evolutionary time gives us answers about our modern-day physiology and the prevalence of heart disease. In chapter 1, we learned how we share the evolution of our energy metabolism with all life. In this chapter, we saw how we share our stress response with all mammals. There is a third aspect of our evolved physiology we must discuss when it comes to heart disease. It plays a vital role in differentiating us from our closest ancestors and making us human.

CHAPTER 3

Becoming Human

After I graduated from chiropractic school in 2013, I decided it was time for an adventure. I started looking for jobs and soon found one just outside of Dublin, Ireland, at a clinic with one other doctor. After a few months of waiting for a work visa, I was on my way.

In my first week, my colleague and his wife invited me to their house for dinner. The spread was incredible: Seated at the table in the dining nook of their kitchen I was staring at plenty of roasted vegetables, baked chicken, and quinoa soup. At the time, however, I had been a vegan for a few years. I had convinced myself it was the healthiest choice for me and, since I'd gone to chiropractic school in vegan-friendly Portland, Oregon, it was easy to maintain. Despite eating only whole foods, after a year or so, I always felt tired, got a cold every few months, and became deficient in a few B vitamins and minerals. Because of this, I started taking supplements and added eggs and cheese to my diet a few times a week.

In front of me now, though, was a great whole-food dinner with plenty of plant and animal fare. Given my diet, I mostly went for the plants. The soup, they said, was best with some Irish grass-fed butter in it. I was hesitant. I had convinced myself that saturated fat from animals was bad for me and that eating animals was bad for the environment, but since it wasn't meat, I went for it. After eating the soup, I found myself wanting more butter. I put a little more on the vegetables I was eating, but I didn't take as much as I truly wanted.

The next day was Saturday, and I needed to figure out the food situation around my apartment in Dublin City Centre. Not yet familiar with the local food scene or farmers markets, I headed off to the Tesco, a supermarket chain, put my usual vegetarian fare in my basket, and headed toward the checkout. On the way, I walked past some whole chickens in one of the warming displays. They smelled incredible. Because I didn't have all the food spots down yet for a nutrient-dense vegetarian diet, I decided to pick one up to eat little bits throughout the week.

When I got back to my apartment, I started preparing lunch. As it was cooking, I ate a little of the chicken. Then I ate some more, and then some more. By the time my meal was ready, I wasn't hungry for it . . . because I had eaten the entire chicken. I stored the food I had cooked for later and then started to read a book. But I couldn't concentrate. I decided to go back to Tesco and get another chicken. In fact, I bought two more whole chickens.

I continued to eat more and more meat while in Ireland. I learned that all the beef in Ireland is grass-fed and this led me down the rabbit hole of learning about regenerative agriculture with ruminant animals. I felt my energy return, and I especially noticed a difference when I played pickup soccer. I got sick less often and was able to control my blood sugars more easily. But the biggest difference I saw was something I hadn't even realized was an issue—my brain. I was able to read more quickly, grasp concepts better, and apply them to other material I was learning.

Once I gave myself permission to eat meat and animal fat again, my body couldn't get enough. I also saw the health benefits. I felt like my body was telling me what it needed, and it rewarded me when I finally listened. Knowing all that I know now, it makes sense that my body was telling me this. Animal foods played a key role in making us human, and one of the defining characteristics of humans is our very large brains.

From approximately 225 million years ago until about 65 million years ago, mammals were pretty small, averaging about 100 grams in body weight, about the size of a field mouse. Of course, the dominant animals up until about 65 million years ago were the dinosaurs. After the dinosaurs went extinct, there was a gradual increase in the size of mammals over the next 60 million years. They maxed out at an average of about 550 kilograms (around 1,200 pounds) about 2.5 million years ago. Those were some large mammals. At that time there were giant sloths, woolly mammoths, saber-toothed tigers, and cave bears that were all huge compared to modern-day mammals. Around 7 million years ago, a smaller group of mammals, early hominins, began to emerge.

Hominin is the word used to describe the species of mammals that eventually gave rise to modern humans. However, a lot happened between the first appearance of early hominins and the first signs of modern humans sometime between 200 to 300 thousand years ago. What happened during that time is important to our discussion of heart disease.

The first hominins to appear were species like *Sahelanthropus tchadensis*, *Orrorin tugenensis*, and *Ardipithecus ramidus*. These species would have looked much closer to modern-day chimps than modern-day humans, but they had some distinct differences that indicate they had started on the evolutionary path to becoming humans. Those differences include the ability to walk upright and slight changes in the sizes of some teeth. These hominins would have eaten a diet similar to what modern-day chimpanzees eat: lots of fruit, leaves, seeds, and the occasional small animal.

Around 4.5 million years ago, we see archaeological evidence of the next group of prehuman species, the australopiths. This group consisted of species such as *Australopithecus anamensis*, *Australopithecus afarensis*, and *Australopithecus africanus*. These prehumans were small bodied, small brained, and upright walkers. Archaeologists believe that this group of hominins was also eating a diet of mainly fruit, leaves, and various other edible parts of plants.

At about 2.5 million years ago, the australopiths split into two different genera, *Homo* and *Paranthropus*. *Paranthropus* are distinguished by massive teeth, cheeks, and skulls that made them capable of generating powerful chewing forces. Archaeologists think that this characteristic evolved to allow them to chew very thick and fibrous plants. *Paranthropus* went extinct around 1.3 million years ago.

In the other direction we have the genus known has *Homo*, which gave rise to modern humans. Our genus began with species such as *Homo habilis* and *Homo erectus*, then *Homo heidelbergensis* and *Homo neanderthalensis*, and eventually us, *Homo sapiens* (which include Cro-Magnons). The appearance of the first members of the *Homo* genus coincides with a die-off of the megafauna. (Anywhere humans show up, it seems, we also see this die-off.) These megafauna decreased from an average weight of 550 kilograms 2.5 million years ago to an average weight of 10 kilograms today.[1] Do we know for sure that this meant that our distant human ancestors were killing and eating those megafauna? Not with certainty, but the evidence is compelling.

Compared to the australopiths, humans have much larger brains and they also developed much bigger bodies. Considering that prehuman species ate fruit, nuts, leaves, and only small amounts of animals, it's likely that a shift in diet was an important factor in becoming human. Indeed, the first primitive tool making also occurred during this time. These were tools mainly used to butcher animals and gain access to different parts of an animal, like the brain and bone marrow.

In *The Origin of Our Species*, Dr. Chris Stringer, the lead researcher in human origins at the London Natural History Museum, described the diet of *Homo neanderthalensis* and early modern humans: "Over a dozen Neanderthals and even more Cro-Magnons have been analyzed, and clear patterns have emerged that confirm our view that the Neanderthals were heavily dependent on meat from large game such as reindeer, mammoth, bison, and horse. They were at the top of their food chains and their isotope signatures places them with wolves and lions as the dominant predators in their landscapes."[2] Stringer explained how scientists compared the stable isotopes of nitrogen in the bones of Neanderthals and early modern humans with known carnivores of that time. The results showed that the Neanderthals were more carnivorous than those carnivorous wolves and lions.[3]

As our *Homo* ancestors started eating meat, they evolved a digestive system to extract nutrients from meat. Compared to our closest living relatives, the chimpanzees, human stomach acid has a very low pH, like that of carnivorous animals. Like other carnivores, we also have a long small intestine and short large intestine made for direct absorption of animal foods rather than fermentation of plant foods.[4] Once our ancestors had these digestive adaptations, they could absorb many more nutrients and their brains started growing.[5] Then they controlled the use of fire and started cooking meat. This made the nutrients even easier to absorb, and our ancestor's brains and bodies saw another jump in growth.[6] Humans did not evolve to eat large quantities of animal fat and protein; we evolved *because* we ate large amounts of animal fat and protein. Animal foods played a major role in making us humans who we are today.

From about 2.5 million years ago, our ancestors ate a lot of red meat and animal fat and mastered the process of burning fat for fuel. How is it that something that provided such a profound evolutionary advantage is exactly the same diet that, today, we're told will give us heart disease? The truth is that it doesn't. A high-meat diet per se does not cause heart disease. Actually, the heart thrives on it.

In every single one of our cells we have mitochondria that allow us to use oxygen to harvest the energy we need to run our bodies. Because the heart uses a ton of oxygen and is one of the most metabolically active tissues in the body, it makes sense that heart tissue is dense with mitochondria. The efficiency of those mitochondria is important, and they are most efficient when they are allowed to burn fatty acids and/or ketones for fuel.[7] Our heart metabolism works best on these fatty acids because it evolved on high amounts of animal fats and very little carbohydrates and nonanimal sources of fat.

Many studies have demonstrated that the heart runs predominantly on fats and that it will "choose" to burn fat over anything else.[8] It has also been shown that the heart loves to burn ketones, which we make from fatty acids when we eat fat and restrict carbohydrates.[9] Certain ketones, such as beta-hydroxybutyrate, have been shown to regulate heart metabolism.[10] A recent review of research on the therapeutic potential of ketones for the heart stated, "evidence from both experimental and clinical research has uncovered a protective role for ketones in cardiovascular disease. Although ketones may provide supplemental fuel for the energy-starved heart, their cardiovascular effects appear to extend far beyond cardiac energetics. Indeed, ketone bodies have been shown to influence a variety of cellular processes including gene transcription, inflammation and oxidative stress, endothelial function, cardiac remodeling, and cardiovascular risk factors."[11]

The heart even has mechanisms to ensure there are enough fatty acids at its disposal. The fats we eat are packaged into what are called chylomicrons. Since chylomicrons are too big to be absorbed through the intestines, they are transported through our lymphatic system. The lymphatic system drains into the veins that lead directly to the heart. From there it only makes one stop, the lungs, before delivering the fatty acids to the heart. It's like this system was designed to give the heart first dibs on the fats we eat. The heart also has a signaling pathway that allows it to communicate directly with fat cells, which allows it to mobilize fats from those cells if it finds itself in need.[12]

The heart, and the body in general, is designed to burn fat and is more efficient when it does. However, humans can also survive on carbohydrates as a fuel source. Our ability to run on multiple fuels gave us a huge advantage and allowed us to survive during times when our optimal food source—animals—was not available. Today, we can choose to eat our optimal fuel source all the time and it would behoove us to do so. When our body is forced to burn primarily carbohydrates for fuel, it leads us down a path of disease.

CHAPTER 4

The Consequences of Defying Evolution

Midway through chiropractic school, I took a break and spent three and a half months traveling through Central America. Toward the end of my travels, I was in Guatemala and arranged for a trip to Semuc Champey, a series of stepped, turquoise waterfalls in the middle of the jungle. The morning of my departure, my driver showed up in a minivan. After picking up other travelers at a few other hostels, we set off toward our destination.

Our route took us through Guatemala City, where vehicles of all sorts sped and braked hard, paid minor attention to the lanes and changing traffic lights, and drove close enough to extend a handshake across open windows. It was also close to election time. Campaign signs were everywhere, and on this particular morning, multiple protests disrupted the traffic.

We eventually escaped the city and, a few hours later, arrived in a small mountain town. We stopped in front of a hostel and all the other travelers got out and walked up to the front door, but a look at the sign told me that this was not where I had arranged to stay. The driver grabbed my bag out of the van and put it into the back of a pickup truck parked across the road. He pointed at me and then the truck and said, "You wait." The driver then walked off down the street.

Almost an hour had passed when the driver returned and gestured for me to get in the bed of the truck. We drove through town and eventually made a stop on the other side, but I still saw no sign of a hostel. A bunch of locals climbed in, and we continued on into the jungle, the road just barely parting the dense foliage in places. Another little village, more locals climbed on. After a few more villages, the truck bed was so crowded that we all stood up next to each other, grasping metal bars that extended vertically from the sides, connecting horizontally over our heads. Then things got interesting.

We had been on dirt roads since the last two villages, but at this point the road got rough. It was a workout to stay upright. I felt like I was surfing. We drove on this road through dense jungle for about an hour and made many stops where people got off and walked toward little huts just off the road. Eventually the last person got off, and I was by myself in the truck again. We drove on for a few more minutes and, as the sun was setting, crossed a bridge that went over a large river. Once across, the driver pulled over and got out. He grabbed my bag and walked me down a path to a small building with a pavilion attached to it. On the side of the building was the sign for my hostel.

A couple sat under the pavilion, eating. A man came out with a plate of pulled chicken and rice that had been cooked over a fire, with tomato and avocado. I joined the couple, who were from Australia, and asked how they liked the hostel. They loved how secluded it was. I was the only other guest they had seen since they arrived two days ago. There was no electricity.

After dinner, the host led me by flashlight to one of four huts along the river. I couldn't see much, but I could hear the gentle flow of the water, smell the humid jungle air, and hear the nocturnal animals and insects begin to fill the night with sounds. Once inside my hut, I turned on my headlamp and looked around. Not wanting to venture out in the jungle at night, I lay in my cot and read by headlamp for a while. As I drifted off to sleep, I thought about how radically my environment had changed that day. I began in a major city, packed with people, the scent of car exhaust and modern conveniences on every corner. I ended it in the jungle, in a hut with no electricity, with probably only a handful of people within a mile or two of me. It got me thinking about the history of civilization and how drastic the change from living in the wild to living in big cities has been for humans. While the change was very slow in the eyes of us humans, from an evolutionary standpoint, it essentially happened like my trip in reverse: in the depths of a wilderness teeming with animal and plant life in one part of the day and in an asphalt- and concrete-laden city bursting with overstimulating human activity in the other.

———

From the time when our ancestors split from australopiths (approximately 1.8–2.5 million years ago) until ten to twelve thousand years ago, we have evidence that the genus *Homo* was hunting and eating animals in substantial amounts. Then something happened that substantially shifted the human way of life: agriculture.[1]

We may never know for sure why exactly this happened, but there are many theories. Some have suggested that as the planet warmed out of the Younger Dryas, it created a climate in which certain plants could thrive where they couldn't before, and humans took advantage of that. Another possibility is that humans overhunted the large megafauna they relied on for the previous 2 million years and were forced to resort to finding another food supply. Livestock domestication and farming were the solutions.

Whatever the impetus, agriculture led to the dawn of civilization. Not only did farming bail early humans out of the overhunting predicament, it also allowed them to stay in one place and grow in numbers. This made life easier, provided more reliable calories, and allowed early humans a way to step back from the brutality of the nature.

The advent of agriculture also brought about diseases of civilization. These started out as infectious disease due to domesticated animals being in close quarters with humans, sewage issues, and general human overcrowding, but agriculture and civilization also set the stage for the development of what we call chronic disease today. There is evidence of chronic disease, including heart disease, in the early agricultural civilizations. Perhaps the earliest known evidence of heart disease comes from ancient Egypt, where the practice of mummification has allowed scientists today to study preserved Egyptian bodies. In one study, CT scans showed that fifteen of twenty-two scanned mummies had atherosclerosis.[2]

Of course, the ancient Egyptians farmed the fertile banks of the Nile, and their diets were heavily based on emmer wheat and barley. Their artwork is full of depictions of Egyptians harvesting and processing grains. One study concluded that the amount of protein from animal foods in the Egyptian diet could be estimated at 29 percent, comparable to a lacto-ovo vegetarian of today.[3] I suspect that the atherosclerosis found in ancient Egyptians was in part caused by the shift in fatty acid ratio through their high consumption of grains. Wheat grains have more polyunsaturated fat than saturated fat, and as we will see in chapter 11, consumption of too much polyunsaturated fat can lead to insulin resistance in the body. Atherosclerosis is more likely to happen if the cells of the lining of the arteries are insulin resistant.

Not only is there evidence of atherosclerosis among ancient Egyptians, it's also likely they suffered from heart attacks. The Egyptian medical text *Ebers Papyrus*, dating to approximately 1550 BC, explained, "And if though examinst a man for illness in his cardia, and he has pains in his arm, in his breast, and in side of his cardia, and it is said of him: It is illness, then thou shalt say thereof: It is due to something entering the mouth it is death that threatens him." This statement describes a heart attack, and it suggests to me that the Egyptians understood the role of diet in its etiology.[4]

Heart disease also surfaced in ancient Arabia. In a story by seventh-century poet Qays ibn Al-Mulawah called "Majnoon Lila" (Crazy About Lila) a young man named Qais falls in love with a girl named Lila. She loves him back, but her father will not consent to their marriage. He forces Lila to marry some-one else, and the heartbroken Qais exiles himself to the desert. In despair, Qais loses interest in family, friends, and society and writes poems describing his sleeplessness, fainting episodes, lack of appetite, and heart palpitations, before he dies of a broken heart immediately after writing these words:

> *My heart is firmly seized*
> *By a bird's claws.*
> *My heart is tightly squeezed,*
> *When Lila's name flows.*
>
> *My body is tightly bound,*
> *When the wide world I found*
> *Is like a finger ring around*

Dr. H. A. Hajar Albinali is a modern-day cardiologist who translated the poem to English and authored the book, *Majnoon Lila: Between Medicine and Literature*. In it, Dr. Albinali claims that this is the first documented descrip-tion of angina in the history of medicine. He concludes, based on that poem and other documented symptoms from the story, that Qais had coronary artery disease and died from myocardial infarction.[5]

Various notable people throughout history took an interest in the identification and study of heart disease. Leonardo da Vinci, for example, made elegant drawings of human anatomy and was probably the first to describe the swirling of blood as it travels through the heart. In *De Motu Cordis*, William Harvey published the first description of how blood travels through the cardiovascular system in 1628. And in the 1800s, Rudolf Virchow and Ludvig Hektoen came forth with the idea that heart attacks are caused by blockages in the coronary arteries which, as we will see in chapter 8, may not always be the case.

While civilization was pushing forward and learning about what doctors would eventually describe as heart disease, people living *outside* of civilization seemed to have fewer health issues. In the early twentieth century, researchers began to study these populations as well. In 1906, Vilhjalmur Stefansson, a Harvard-trained anthropologist, lived with the Canadian Arctic Inuit people to see how they survive in the extreme cold. He tried to live exactly as they did, eating a diet almost exclusively of meat and fish for a year. Stefansson and his team estimated that the diet of the Inuit was 70–80 percent fat and yet, despite their harsh living conditions and high-fat diet, they saw no obesity or disease among these people. Stefansson stated that "they seemed to be the healthiest people I have ever lived with."[6]

Later in his career, Stefansson attempted to re-create this diet in an experiment. He and another man ate nothing but meat for an entire year. For the first few weeks they were monitored in a hospital, before returning to their homes to continue the experiment. At the end of the year, both men felt healthy. They initially lost weight, their blood pressure remained normal, they had no gastrointestinal issues or vitamin deficiencies, and testing revealed them to be in excellent health.[7]

In the 1930s, Dr. Weston A. Price, a dentist from Cleveland, Ohio, became curious about the diseases he was seeing among the patients in his practice. He decided to seek answers from those living outside of Western civilization and, for years, every summer, Dr. Price and his wife would travel to some place in the world to study a group of people that had little to no contact with the Western world. He studied groups of people in Switzerland, the Hebrides of the British Isles, Alaska, the southern Pacific islands, Africa, Australia, New Zealand, Peru, North America, and the Amazon basin.[8]

As a dentist, Dr. Price focused on the health of these peoples' teeth. Aside from noticing that they had far lower incidence of dental problems like cavities and underdeveloped dental arches, he also documented that these populations had little to none of the chronic diseases that were starting to run rampant within the Western world at that time. He noticed a theme among the many groups of people he studied: They all made adequate nutrition a priority. For all of the tribes, attaining a source of fat, and fat-soluble nutrients, was important. He noted that in many of the groups men and women who were set to marry had special diets months before the wedding. Pregnant women were also given special diets and given priority for valued nutrient-dense animal fats. This prioritization of nutrition ensured these people did not get the diseases that those in the West were suffering from.

The tribes that Price studied were living a more ancient lifestyle. Their lifestyles were not exactly like what humans and prehumans lived before the Agricultural Revolution, but they were closer. In our modern-day society we have made survival so much easier. We can be exposed to the toxins, unnatural stressors, and terrible foods and still survive. But we survive with poor health.

In his book *Good Calories, Bad Calories*, journalist Gary Taubes discussed the use of a low-carbohydrate diet by many physicians in the 1800s and early 1900s. He described a man named William Banting who sought advice from a doctor in 1862 about his weight, hearing, eyesight, and digestive issues. The doctor recommended Banting reduce his carbohydrate intake. He did. Banting lost 50 pounds and all his ailments subsided.

In an 1892 medical textbook, Sir William Osler of Johns Hopkins Hospital promoted a low-carbohydrate, high-fat diet.[9] In 1905, a physician named Nathaniel Yorke-Davies used the low-carbohydrate diet to help President William Taft lose 70 pounds. In 1919, a physician named Blake Donaldson stumbled upon this diet when hearing about the good health of the Alaskan Inuit from experts at the American Museum of Natural History. He decided to start trying this diet with his patients and got amazing results.[10] When Donaldson lectured about this experiment in 1944, a physician by the name of Alfred Pennington was in attendance. Pennington was a company doctor for DuPont. Frustrated with not being able to help his patients lose weight, he decided to try the diet with them. He reported that his patients stopped feeling hungry between meals and lost 7–10 pounds per week despite eating large quantities of food.[11]

While humans strayed from the animal-food diet that made us human, it seems that in the first half of the twentieth century, many were on the right track to discovering the more ancient diet that would save us from the highly processed plant foods of the Agricultural Revolution and subsequent Industrial Revolution. We were figuring out how to restore health and prevent heart disease. We were learning from the wisdom of those living more traditional lifestyles and seeing results within the Western medical system. Then, just as we were starting to figure things out, things took a turn for the worse in the 1950s.

CHAPTER 5

The Infamous Diet–Heart Hypothesis

During my senior year of college, my cousin, Luke, and a mutual friend, Caleb, decided to thru-hike the 2,200-mile Appalachian Trail. The trail, which runs from Georgia to Maine, passes close to Asheville, North Carolina, where I was an undergraduate at the University of North Carolina at Asheville. So when they neared Asheville, I joined them for three days as they hiked through the Great Smoky Mountains along the Appalachian Trail.

At the end of the third day, we reached Max Patch, one of the famous "balds" of the southeastern United States. Max Patch was cleared of trees long ago for grazing cattle, and hikers today enjoy the resulting 360-degree views. Unfortunately for us, on the day we approached the crest of the mountain, fog and rain obscured our view. It had been a rough three days for me. It rained most of the time, and fifty miles with a heavy pack had taken a toll on my body. I was not nearly as conditioned as Luke and Caleb were.

Our party of three crossed over the summit of Max Patch and hiked down into the trees to set up camp. Luke had a bivy tent that hung over a string tied between two trees, Caleb had a small one-man tent, and I had a two-man tent. Rather than set up three tents, Luke slept in his bivy, and Caleb slept in the two-man tent with me. When the rain and the wind picked up during the night, and Luke's bivy tent wouldn't stay put, he came a-knocking, too. All I can say is that three stinky guys in a small two-man tent is a tight squeeze.

After a sleepless night for all of us, Luke and Caleb continued on their trek north, and I set off to the south, back up and over Max Patch again to find the parking lot, where I had arranged for my girlfriend to pick me up. The wind had brought in even denser fog than the day before and I could only see ten feet in front of me. Just before I reached the summit, I encountered a sign I hadn't noticed the day before. It said "Appalachian Trail," and "Max Patch 0.1 mile." I continued to the top.

As I started down the other side of Max Patch, however, I became disoriented from the fog. There were no signs or trail junctions for the path down to the parking lot. I thought maybe I missed it. Ever more disoriented, I turned around and headed back the way I came. I passed back over the summit, past the spot where we'd camped, and slowly through the fog for another quarter mile. With increasing worry, I realized that didn't feel like the right direction either.

I decided to turn around once again. It was so foggy I figured I could have missed anything—a sign, a spur path—that was only a few feet off the trail, so I went extra slow and paid careful attention. I eventually got back to the sign. Frustrated at this point, I decided that I would just have to sit there and wait for the fog to lift so I could get my bearings. As I rested, I realized that it was odd for a sign to be placed so randomly on the trail. Usually, you encounter signs at trail junctions, but this one seemed randomly plunked in the middle of a trail.

Trying to make sense of this as I sat in the fog, a thought came to me. This sign wasn't randomly plunked in the middle of the trail. There must be another trail nearby; I just wasn't seeing it. Since Max Patch is bald, the trail is basically a narrow path through a grassy field; it could have been in any direction! With some anxiety, I walked off the trail and into the grass straight ahead. Sure enough, after about twenty feet, the grass started turning to dirt and a path emerged. But for the fog, it would have been easily visible from the trail. The fog lifted as I continued down the trail until a little wooden fence appeared and, on the other side, a small gravel parking lot. My frustration lifted.

I'm often reminded of being lost in the fog on top of Max Patch when I think about what it's like to navigate a heart-healthy lifestyle in today's world. We are all corralled toward a single path—low fat, low cholesterol—to such a degree that it obscures our ability to see the big picture, think clearly, and make intelligent judgments. In fact, the truth is just *off* that beaten path. In chapter 4, I explained how one of the major recommendations for heart health—eating a low-fat diet with small amounts of lean meat—doesn't make much sense. In this chapter, I'd like to examine *why* and *how* things got to be this way. The answer lies in the vexing history of federal nutrition guidelines and the influence of industry on research at academic institutions. This brings our timeline to the middle of the last century.

———

In the 1920s heart disease was rare in the United States. The American Heart Association was quite a small entity, and there were not many cardiologists because they simply weren't needed. Then, in the late 1940s and early 1950s, heart disease became a growing issue in the United States. Chest tightness and pain running down the arm became a common fear. The introduction and mass distribution of seed oils (canola oil, soy oil, corn oil, sunflower oil, etc.) in the early 1900s likely had a hand in this, as did the reduction of meat intake during and after World War II, but these factors were largely overlooked.[1] A University of Minnesota physiologist named Ancel Keys was determined to get to the bottom of exploding rates of heart disease.

Keys had traveled widely and encountered many ideas and experiences that piqued his curiosity about how the body worked. At the time, the idea that cholesterol-clogged arteries caused heart disease was beginning to take hold. It was thought that high cholesterol in the blood would eventually coat the lining of an artery. Keys was a proponent of this theory, even though his research proved experimentally that a high-cholesterol diet does not necessarily result in higher levels of cholesterol in the blood.[2] Nevertheless, Keys seemed determined to show that a high-fat diet was the cause of heart disease.

Keys began favoring an observational approach over an experimental one. He traveled to parts of the world where there were higher or lower rates of heart disease than what was considered normal at the time and measured the inhabitants' cholesterol. He was fascinated with the Mediterranean, where people had particularly low rates of heart disease. In a 1952 presentation at Mount Sinai Hospital in New York, Dr. Keys showed a graph that plotted fat consumption and rates of heart disease in six countries. The graph seemed to show a convincing correlation between dietary fat and heart disease. The more fat, the more heart disease. The data became known as the Six Countries Study, published in 1953. He followed up with a Seven Countries Study, which showed the same correlation.[3]

The type of epidemiological research Keys conducted is called epidemiology and is on the very bottom tier of the hierarchy of research. While it has its uses, it is incapable of yielding concrete conclusions. First, epidemiology can only indicate association, not causation. It can show that two things are happening at the same time—like a correlation between increased fat intake and higher rates of heart disease—but it cannot prove that one causes the other. Say, for example, we are standing on a sidewalk, witnessing a traffic jam on a cloudy day. We can say that the traffic jam and the clouds are associated with each other because we see them on the same day at the same time. We cannot, however, say that the clouds *caused* the traffic jam or that the traffic jam *caused* the clouds. No matter how many times we observe these two things occurring simultaneously, we cannot prove that one caused the other. We would have to conduct experiments for that. Epidemiology is useful for finding associations, but only insofar as they lead to follow-up clinical trials. On their own, we can only look at them as associations. Clinical trials were not conducted with Keys's Six Country Study, or the Seven Country Study—and yet his conclusions were adopted in the development of federal nutritional guidelines.

Another shortcoming of epidemiological studies is that they often use surveys to gather information. Researchers must rely on people's memories —for example, what they ate, sometimes months or years prior. No matter how truthful people may try to be (and not everyone is), research shows there is a risk in relying on the human memory for accurate data.[4] Epidemiological studies are also susceptible to what's known as healthy user bias. With healthy user bias, even if survey data are accurate, it is impossible to say that one variable, such as the consumption of animal fat, is the cause of disease, because there are many variables at play. For example, we may see lower reported animal-fat consumption and lower reported rates of disease—except that people who eat less animal fat are also more likely to engage in other recommended behaviors, such as exercising, not smoking, not drinking, reducing stress, and eating whole foods. Therefore, we can't determine if animal fat is the determining factor when so many other behaviors could be contributing factors.

Finally, many epidemiological studies report their results as relative risk rather than absolute risk. This can be extremely misleading. Relative risk uses a set of data to assess risk to a group of individuals with something in common, for example, females with high cholesterol. Absolute risk uses a set of data to assess risk to an individual based on his or her behaviors. If a study finds an association between eating animal foods and developing heart disease, the researchers can analyze that data in a way to tell them the increased risk to a certain group (relative risk), but they can also assess it in a way that tells them the increased risk to an individual either engaging or not engaging in that behavior (absolute risk). Understanding the absolute risk is more valuable to an individual looking to improve his or her health. However, researchers often look at relative risk.

Let's say, hypothetically, that the baseline risk of developing heart disease was 1 percent. If a study found that eating animal foods raised that risk to 1.5 percent, the absolute risk of developing heart disease by eating animal foods is a 0.5 percent increased risk. However, if we report this as relative risk, we could say that the risk of heart disease goes up 50 percent (from 1 to 1.5) when eating animal foods. Stating research results in terms of relative risk can render those results more dramatic and more likely to grab the headlines—even if the findings are negligible. This is a common practice in epidemiological research.

On top of the shortcomings of epidemiological research, Keys did something troubling. At the time he was conducting his research, data on fat consumption from twenty-two countries was available. Yet his study only included six, and later seven, countries. It appears that Keys handpicked the data to prove his theory. In 1957, two scientists—a New York State commissioner of health and a UC Berkeley statistician—repeated Keys's research using data from all twenty-two countries. They found no correlation between fat consumption and heart disease.[5]

Unfortunately, Keys's faulty science has had a lot of influence on federal nutrition guidelines, even those we have today, as well as on public perception of what a healthy diet looks like. In 1955, after President Eisenhower suffered a heart attack, his personal doctor urged Americans to stop smoking, reduce stress, and reduce intake of saturated fat and cholesterol. The President's doctor mentioned Keys by name and from that point forward, Keys's theory became prominent in the media. This has led to the generally accepted idea that dietary saturated fat and cholesterol cause heart disease. This idea, which combines weak science with great marketing, led to the standard of care in cardiology today. It is a world full of cholesterol-lowering statins, one of the most commonly prescribed drugs today, as well as surgeries to install bypasses and stents.

Around the same time as the widespread uptake of Keys's studies, however, contrary research cast doubt on Keys's diet–heart hypothesis, including the data coming in from around the world about people living traditional lifestyles with high-fat diets and no heart disease. For example, Dr. George Mann, a Johns Hopkins–trained medical doctor who spent time teaching nutrition and medicine at Harvard and Vanderbilt during his career, studied the Maasai in Africa and found that their diet was almost entirely meat, blood, and milk from cattle. Yet none of them died of heart disease.[6] Meanwhile, an Italian pathologist named Giorgio Baroldi was studying autopsied hearts when he discovered that his findings did not match up with Keys's diet–heart hypothesis or the idea that cholesterol is the driver of atherosclerosis and heart attacks. Baroldi found significant clots in some people who did not have heart disease, as well as no clots among some who died of heart attacks. His work was largely ignored and is still not well known today, but I'll discuss the importance of his findings in chapter 8.

A couple of large studies were also conducted in the late 1960s and early 1970s that yielded surprising results on the cause of heart disease and heart attacks. Between 1968 and 1973, the Minnesota Coronary Experiment studied the effects of replacing saturated fat with vegetable oil high in unsaturated fat among 9,423 men and women. Likely because it didn't reach the conclusions the researchers—who, yet again, included Ancel Keys—were expecting or hoping for, the paper wasn't published until over a decade later and, even then, left out critical data. When it was reassessed and updated in 2016, it became clear that while switching from saturated to unsaturated fat lowered cholesterol in the study participants, there was a 22 percent increased risk of death for every 30 milligrams per deciliter (mg/dL) drop in cholesterol.[7] Then, from 1966 to 1973, the Sydney Diet Heart Study found that "substituting dietary linoleic acid in place of saturated fats increased the rates of death from all causes, coronary heart disease, and cardiovascular disease."[8] Shockingly, although the study ended in 1973, the results weren't published until 2013. Again, this was because the results were not what the researchers were looking for.

More recently, in June 2020, a study published in the *Journal of the American College of Cardiology* assessed all the available evidence on saturated fat and heart disease and stated that "the recommendation to limit dietary saturated fatty acid (SFA) intake has persisted despite mounting evidence to the contrary. Most recent meta-analyses of randomized trials and observational studies found no beneficial effects of reducing SFA intake on cardiovascular disease (CVD) and total mortality, and instead found protective effects against stroke."[9]

There was an innocent bystander in the war against saturated fat: red meat. But recent research exonerates it as well. As I'll discuss much more in the coming pages, poor metabolic health (insulin resistance) and markers of inflammation are the best indicators of heart disease risk. One recent meta-analysis of randomized controlled trials looked at red meat intake and risk of heart disease using these markers. The authors expected to see a correlation between red meat consumption and glycemic control and inflammation, but instead found that eating red meat improved insulin resistance and reduced inflammation.[10]

If saturated fat and red meat have been incorrectly blamed for rising rates of heart disease, what explains the rising rates? For starters, there's an important nuance. Higher levels of certain saturated fatty acids (palmitoleic acid) in the blood have been shown to increase risk of diabetes, atherosclerosis, and heart attack. But *consuming* saturated fat does not necessarily *affect* the levels of saturated fat in the blood.[11] I will discuss how high amounts of palmitoleic acid, also called lipokine, can end up in the blood in chapter 11.

Despite abundant evidence to the contrary, the idea that saturated fat and cholesterol cause heart disease is so engrained in society that it almost seems like the only factor when it comes to heart disease. This is the power of the media, industry influence, and effective marketing, but by the end of this book I hope you will see that heart disease is far more complicated and multifactorial than the messages we've been inundated with.

How can humans, who have been shaped in so many different evolutionary ways, be so susceptible to one thing: a diet high in saturated fat? The truth is, we aren't. Cholesterol is the wrong focus, and although diet can be a major player, preventing heart disease is about so much more than diet. In fact, as I argue in this book, Western medicine fundamentally misunderstands the role of the heart altogether.

PART II

THE HEART AND ITS MALFUNCTIONS

CHAPTER 6

The True Function of the Heart

During my first year in chiropractic school, a group of classmates and I spent a weekend camping. I enjoy the outdoors, and the Pacific Northwest offered a different natural environment for me to explore. The six of us found a perfect campsite by a river, hung out there for the afternoon, and then set up tents and prepared a fire for dinner. It was close to dusk when a man approached and politely asked if he could "shoot down by the river." We nodded, no problem. I figured he was staying at one of the other campsites we'd passed on our short hike into our own.

Then, oddly, the man turned and went back up the trail from the direction he'd come from. A few minutes later, as darkness continued to fall, he returned with a big gun in his hand. My heart skipped a beat, but he smiled and headed off toward the river. I could tell by the look on my friends' faces that it never occurred to any of us that he literally wanted to "shoot"—as in with a gun—down by the river. We had assumed he meant that he wanted to hang out by the river, and the easiest access was through our campsite.

I don't think I would have minded if it had been a regular hunting gun, but a few minutes later, he started to shoot what was clearly a loud, rapid-fire weapon. The sound was deafening and filled the forest. We all got fearful looks on our faces—even my friend who was used to guns and had been a hunter most of his life. We were very close to the river, but we couldn't see the man shooting—or the direction he was shooting in—because of the dense trees.

Now uncomfortable, and having to yell to carry on our conversation, we started discussing whether one of us should go and tell him we would like him to stop. He seemed like a nice guy, but none of us was keen to approach an unknown man with such a powerful gun. We decided to keep our heads down and hope that it wouldn't last long. After about thirty minutes the gunfire stopped. The man walked back by, gave a polite nod, and thanked us.

Relieved that it was over without anyone getting hurt, we settled back to talking. Many things were shared. One of my friends said that her heart was racing the whole time he was shooting. Another remarked how amazing it is that the heart never stops pumping for our entire lives. We marveled at its ability to keep blood moving while sustaining huge pressure from the flow of that blood. Even as we were talking about this around the fire, I thought to myself how interesting it is that the body evolved in a way that made us so dependent on a single organ for blood flow. Years later, I discovered that this isn't exactly true, and that what the physiology textbooks tell us about the circulation of the blood through the body isn't entirely accurate either.

———————

If we want to understand heart disease, we have to understand the role of the heart. Most of us think that the heart pumps blood, and this pumping is the way blood moves through the body. It is thought that with some help from one-way valves in our veins and the contraction of skeletal muscle, the human heart can contract with enough force to pump blood through our arteries, all the way to the tips of our toes, back through the veins, and to our heart again. This is the conventional wisdom, and it is taught in medical schools all over the world. But what if it's not correct?

To my knowledge, William Harvey was the first person to describe the systemic circulation of blood through our vascular system in his 1628 publication *De Motu Cordis*. However, in a letter to a colleague, Harvey expressed doubt that the heart does all the pumping. "I do not believe the heart is the fashioner of the blood," he wrote, "neither do I imagine that the blood has powers, properties, motion, or heat as the gift of the heart."[1] He clearly struggled with the idea that the blood was moved all over the body entirely by the heart. We will see shortly that the second part of his statement, about the blood having powers, was slightly inaccurate as the blood does indeed have its own kind of power. In the mid-1800s, a German physician and researcher named Johann Thudichum doubted the ability of the heart to move the blood through the entire body, and declared, "If there were no other force promoting circulation than the heart, the heart of a whale would be required in the human chest, to affect even a very slow and languid circulation."[2] Another German physician, named E. H. Weber, constructed a model of the vascular system using a section of small intestines and a pressure-propulsion pump for a heart. He found that no matter how forcefully the pump operated, he could not maintain pressure in the venous side of his model. He concluded that "the mean pressure does not depend on the action of the heart, but on the amount of fluid in the model."[3]

In addition to these early doubters, some modern research also questions our understanding of the heart as the main mover of the blood through the body. For example, in 2003, researchers studied the efficiency of heart cardiac muscle. When they examined how much energy heart muscle cells use compared to the amount of pumping the heart actually does, they found that the heart is about 30 percent effective as a pressure-propulsion pump.[4] If the heart's evolutionary role is as pressure propulsion to pump blood, why did evolution select for something that was only 30 percent effective? Is it possible that the heart's role in the body is not—or not only, or not primarily —as a pump?

Indeed, some research shows that a functioning heart is not necessary for blood flow. In the 1940s, researchers used artificial ventilation to provoke "mechanical circulation" in a dead dog. After the dog died and oxygen levels dropped, the researchers injected a tracer into the femoral artery. Then they induced breathing with an artificial ventilator. Not only did the trace substance make its way to other parts of the body, the oxygen saturation of the blood increased throughout the body as blood continued to cycle through the lungs.[5] The researchers concluded that the movement of the lungs was sufficient to create blood flow, and indeed it has been shown that when someone suffers a collapsed lung, cardiac output drops 66 percent, bronchial blood flow drops 84 percent, and right pulmonary artery flow drops 80 percent.[6]

In the 1960s, however, the experiments were repeated with results suggestive of a more complex mechanism at play. A Polish surgeon named Leon Manteuffel-Szoege dedicated his career to investigating blood flow in the cardiovascular system, and he repeated the dog experiments with a twist. First, he replicated the original experiment and found that postmortem mechanical ventilation eventually produced oxygen saturation of 100 percent. Next, he insufflated (blew) oxygen rather than mechanically ventilating the lungs, which removed the variable of lung expansion and contraction as a possible mechanism of blood flow. In this experiment, the blood's oxygen saturation increased from 20–30 percent to 85 percent. Finally, Manteuffel-Szoege administered no oxygen in any way. Instead, he simply injected a tracer. He found that the blood continued moving for up to two hours after the heart stopped beating. Manteuffel-Szoege concluded that the blood had its "own motor energy."[7]

Before you write this off as impossible, consider our environment. Think about plants, especially very tall trees. They have no pump, yet somehow, water travels from the Earth all the way to the tips of the leaves on the highest branch. How is this possible? That answer—which also explains the postmortem blood flow in the dog experiments—has to do with some unique and little-understood properties of water.

The Fourth Phase of Water

Water is all around us. It is the most abundant molecule on Earth, and it is up to 70 percent of what makes up humans. In school, most people learn that water—H_2O—has three phases: solid (ice), liquid (water), and gas (water vapor), depending on temperature. But researchers—notably, Dr. Gilbert Ling and Dr. Gerald Pollack—have actually found a *fourth* phase, and this fourth phase can help us understand phenomena we see around us every day, including the way the blood moves through the body.

Let me explain: Water has the ability to hold energy—radiant energy, to be specific. It gets this energy from the Sun, from the Earth, even from living organisms, such as humans. When water is next to a hydrophilic (water loving) surface, and radiant energy is applied, the energy breaks one of the oxygen–hydrogen (O–H) bonds and cleaves off a hydrogen. The O–H molecules then combine to form a hexagonal structure, link up with other hexagonal structures, and form a flat lattice-like plane. These planes stack themselves neatly next to the hydrophilic surface.[8] (See figure 6.1.)

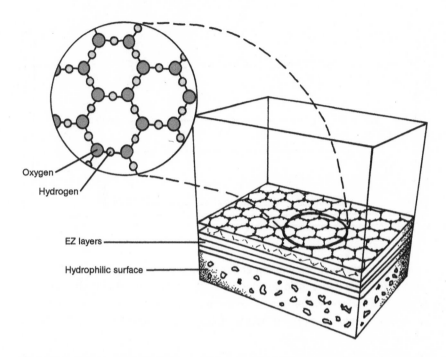

Oxygen

Hydrogen

EZ layers

Hydrophilic surface

Figure 6.1. The formation of structured water on a hydrophilic surface. Planes of structured water stack on top of one another creating thicker and thicker areas of structured water. Adapted from *The Fourth Phase of Water*.

This structured water is neither solid like ice nor liquid like water. It is more of a gel, like Jell-O. It has a few different names: structured water, exclusion zone (EZ) water, and fourth phase water. While Dr. Pollack has artificially created this in his lab, he also found it happening naturally. In *The Fourth Phase of Water*, he wrote, "We also found exclusion zones next to natural biological surfaces; they included vascular endothelia, regions of plant roots, and muscle."[9] That's right, vascular endothelia! Our arteries are a hydrophilic surface, and because our blood is about half water, this phenomenon occurs on the lining of our arteries.

It gets even more interesting. Dr. Pollack also found that the formation of structured water on the inner surface of a tube *can create flow on its own*. When he placed a tube made of hydrophilic material in a tub of water and applied radiant energy, the water began to move through the tube without any other outside force. (See figure 6.2.) Why? Because of an energy gradient.

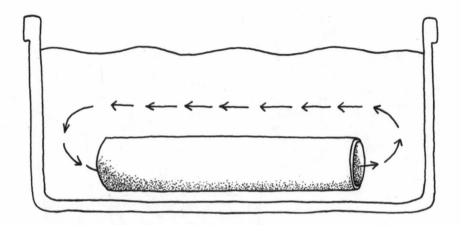

Figure 6.2. Illustration of an experiment on structured water by Dr. Gerald Pollack. A tube made of a hydrophilic substance is placed in water. As structured water forms on the surface, water begins to flow through the tube and will continue to flow provided radiant energy is applied to the water. Adapted from *The Fourth Phase of Water*.

The O–H molecules that form the lattice are negatively charged (because the negatively charged oxygen is a bigger molecule than the positively charged hydrogen it is still attached to), but the hydrogens that get cleaved off make the fluid in the tube hold a positive charge.

When enough lattice-like layers of structured water form on the lining of the tube, the space in the middle gets cramped. Since the hydrogens are all positively charged, and like charges repel each other, they start to move, creating flow. (See figure 6.3.) Dr. Pollack found that "flow of this nature could persist indefinitely if the protons and water were continually replenished. . . . sustained water flow occurs inevitably in almost any scenario involving EZ's and radiant energy."[10]

Could this be the mechanism by which Manteuffel-Szoege observed blood moving through the arteries of dead dogs after their hearts stopped pumping? Recent work by a graduate student in Pollack's lab named Zheng Li suggests that the answer is yes. After stopping the heart in chick embryos, Li discovered that blood can flow independently. "When the heart was stopped, blood continued to flow, albeit at a lower velocity.

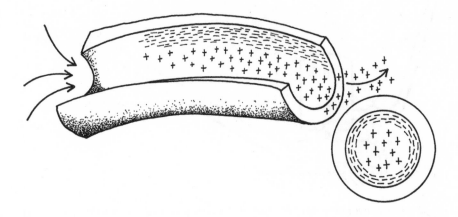

Figure 6.3. Depiction of fourth phase water forming on the lining of an artery and inducing flow. Studies have shown that blood moves through arteries via this mechanism without the aid of a contracting heart. Adapted from *The Fourth Phase of Water*.

When IR [infrared] was introduced, flow increased, by ~300%."[11] While there are multiple mechanisms that assist in the movement of blood in the body, including the heart pumping and contraction of skeletal muscles, the work coming out of Pollack's lab strongly suggest that the primary way blood moves through the body (or water travels upward to the tops of trees) is due to the energy gradient that is created with the formation of fourth phase water following exposure to radiant energy. The implications of this research are huge, and we will discuss more of them in the coming chapters. Now, let's use this information to help us figure out the purpose of the heart.

The Heart: A Vortex-Creating Hydraulic Ram

We have seen evidence that the heart is not a very effective pressure-propulsion pump. Nor does the heart have to be an effective pressure-propulsion pump in order for blood to circulate through the body. If that's the case, what *is* the heart? Why is it there?

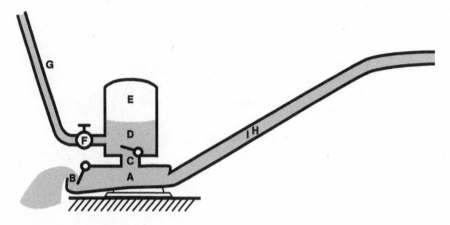

Figure 6.4. A hydraulic ram, labeled with structures analogous to the heart. (A) first chamber, (B) spill valve, (C) one-way valve, (D) second chamber, (E) air that creates interchamber pressure as chamber fills with fluid, (F) flow valve, (G) fluid exit pipe, (H, I) fluid delivery pipe.

The work of Dr. Manteuffel-Szoege offers some insight. Manteuffel-Szoege made great efforts during his career to, as he described, "put the heart in its place." In one paper he wrote, "A pump sucks in fluid from a reservoir, which is a hydrostatic system and not a hydrodynamic one. The heart is a mechanism inserted into the blood circuit, and so it is a very peculiar kind of pump."[12] What he means is that a pressure-propulsion pump is one that takes water from a standstill, like a lake or reservoir, and forcefully pumps it to another location.

Since we've established that the blood moves on its own and it is therefore not at a standstill, a more accurate description is that the heart is situated in the midst of a system in which liquid is already flowing. Instead of comparing the heart to a pressure-propulsion pump, it's more accurate to think of a "pump" system that works when liquid flows into it on its own. And there is such a system like that.

Rudolf Steiner, the late-nineteenth-century Austrian philosopher, argued throughout his life that the heart actually serves as a "damming" organ whose function could be compared to a flow-activated hydraulic ram. What does that mean? If you refer to figure 6.4 and figure 6.5, you'll see that water flows into the ram under the force of gravity through the pipe (I, H). The first chamber (A) catches the water. Some of the water spills out of the spill valve (B). Once

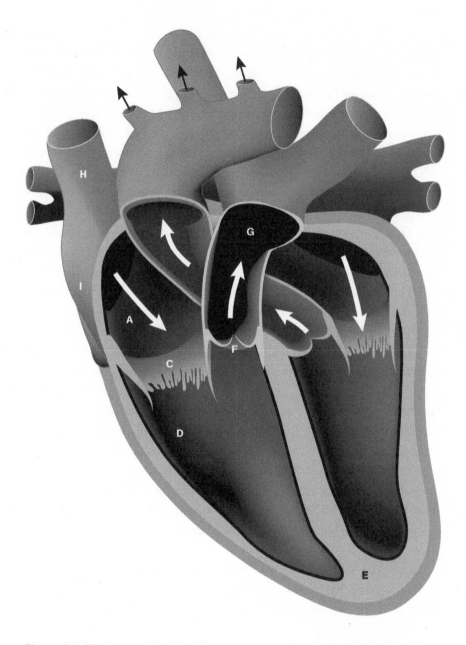

Figure 6.5. The heart, labeled with structures analogous to the hydraulic ram. (A) right atrium, (C) atrioventricular, or tricuspid, valve, (D) right ventricle, (E) muscular ventricle wall, (F) pulmonary, or semilunar, valve, (G) pulmonary artery, (H, I) superior and inferior vena cava.

enough water fills the chamber and pressure builds, the spill valve closes. Water then pushes up through the one-way valve (C) at the top. Water flowing through there ends up in a second chamber (D), compresses the air and building pressure. Once the pressure builds up enough, it pushes the water back down, closing the one-way valve (C). Since the water can't go back the way it came, it goes out through the pipe (G). Once it flows out, pressure drops through the system and new water flows in to the first chamber (A), restarting the process.

The hydraulic ram is a good analogy for the heart, with two slight exceptions. The building of EZ water and hydrogen ions drive the flow of blood through the veins toward the heart, much like gravity does in the hydraulic ram. Once it arrives, it flows into the right atrium (A); this is similar to the first chamber in the hydraulic ram. Here is the first difference. In the heart, there is technically no spill valve ("B" on the hydraulic ram); instead pressure builds in the atrium (A) as blood flows in until there is enough pressure to open the atrioventricular, or tricuspid, valve (C). This is a one-way valve, just like in the hydraulic ram. Once this is open the blood flows into the right ventricle (D), mostly on its own, but it does get a little push from the slight contraction of the atrium. Here is the second difference. In the ram we had air in the second chamber (D). There is no air in the right ventricle to build up pressure and eventually push the blood out. Instead we have muscle in the ventricle wall (E) that contracts to help push the blood out of the ventricle. Since the tricuspid valve (C) is a one-way valve, when the ventricle contracts the valve shuts and the blood goes out through another one-way valve, the pulmonary or semilunar valve (F), into the pulmonary artery (G). The same thing happens on the left side when blood is flowing back to the heart after going through the lungs. Perhaps the most accurate analogy is that the heart is like two side-by-side hydraulic rams.

You may be thinking that this sounds like a pump, except that as a pressure-propulsion pump, the heart is only 30 percent efficient. While the chambers of the heart do contract and move blood through, they only do so enough to help blood navigate through the heart, not enough to propel blood through the whole body. A pressure-propulsion pump would be forcefully sucking blood in one side and forcefully pushing it out the other. This is not what the heart does.

We have answered our first question: What is the heart? Now we have to answer why it is there. If the blood moves mainly on its own, then why do we even need this contracting muscular organ right in the middle of the whole system? The answer presents itself when we observe people during exercise. In fact, one purpose of the heart is to *restrain*—rather than pump—the flow of blood.

In his recent book, *The Heart and Circulation*, Dr. Branko Furst of Albany Medical College stated, "The existence of muscle pump serves the same purpose as the heart, namely, to 'restrain' the massive increase in venous return, with venous valves protecting against the backflow and peripheral congestion. Performance of the heart during exercise is perhaps the best example of the fact that the heart sets itself against the flow of the blood and impedes rather than propels it."[13]

When we exercise, the body needs more blood flow to meet tissue demands for oxygen and nutrients. If we think of the heart as a pressure-propulsion pump, then the heart beating more quickly is what would forcefully push that essential flow. But that is *not* what increases blood flow. Blood flow increases because when we exercise, the tissues' increased demand causes our fourth phase blood flow to kick into overdrive. The increase in heart rate is the heart *reacting* to the increase in flow, not causing it.

During exercise, the blood is needed in the tissues so that our body can perform—or get away from a threat, in evolutionary terms. However, when there is that much metabolic demand in the tissues, blood rushes to the arterial side of the system to deliver; at least, that's what would happen if the heart wasn't there. If all the blood went to the arterial side of the system, the venous side would collapse, causing a system-wide breakdown. The heart's placement directly between the arterial and venous systems prevents this breakdown by slowing the flow of blood, or damming it up, in Steiner's words. Remember E. H. Weber, who designed a cardiovascular system and tried to run it with a pressure-propulsion pump? No matter what he did, the venous side kept collapsing. What he didn't understand is that the heart helps maintain equal pressure, in the same way a hydraulic ram has the ability to slow flow and direct fluid.

Here's another analogy: Think of a pitcher, catcher, and batter in baseball. The pitcher throws a strike that the batter swings at and misses. The catcher is the heart and the pitcher throwing the ball (the blood) is the blood flow. The ball from the pitcher (blood flow) is coming into the heart forcefully, especially during exercise, and the catcher (the heart) stops that momentum.

But the catcher doesn't just catch it and keep it, he stands up and throws the ball *with much less force* back to the pitcher, just like the heart dams up the blood, and then tosses it back into circulation with much less force than it came in. The batter swinging and missing the ball (the blood) is the vortexing the heart does as the blood passes through (which we will discuss soon). But it doesn't just make sense theoretically; research also confirms it.

In 2004, the study of heart hemodynamics during exercise led a group of researchers to conclude that "the combined maximal vascular conductance of arms and legs outweighs the maximal pumping capacity of the heart, implying that the muscular vasodilatory response [widening of the blood vessels] during maximal exercise must be restrained to maintain perfusion pressure."[14] Translation? This means that the blood flow created by exercise surpasses any pumping capacity the heart could create. Instead, the heart moderates blood flow to make sure the system can maintain pressure and not collapse. Another research group found that during exercise, the increase of cardiac output of blood flow they observed was a result of increased venous return to the heart. No matter how much they tried to manipulate heart rate, they could not affect the flow of blood. Venous return was the only variable that increased heart rate.[15]

Endurance athletes are known to have larger, more muscular hearts. You might think that this is because the heart pumps harder and more often for these well-trained individuals, but a study of professional soccer players found that they had a reduced angle of left ventricular twist and torsion velocities at rest, suggesting that the larger hearts of these athletes had more inertia, interrupting the flow of blood more efficiently.[16] This finding means that these athletes have more muscle in their hearts not because the heart needs to be more forceful due to their exertion, but because extended durations of exercise demand the heart to be effective at slowing the flow of blood in order to maintain pressure in the cardiovascular system. Larger heart musculature allows this to happen.

Dr. Furst summed it up: "Only when seen as an organ of impedance can the heart place itself effectively against the 'runaway train' of oncoming blood to generate only moderately increased mean arterial pressure even during maximal exercise. . . . this mechanism allows the heart to maintain normal dimensions and protect it from overdistention in the face of greatly increased blood flow ('cardiac throughput')."

The Vortexing Heart

Regulating pressure is only one of the heart's jobs. In fact, in a way, the heart may be responsible for much of the flow of blood after all—just not in the way most of us think, as a pump.

If you look at the shape of the heart, the side that contains all the muscle is shaped like one end of a football. A football is best thrown in a tight spiral; it is more efficient and travels farther. If we look at the way the heart contracts, it does so in a spiral-like fashion. This is because the heart consists of a band of muscle called the "ventricular band," that is wrapped around itself in a sort of spiral knot. This band was discovered by a Spanish cardiologist named Francisco Torrent-Guasp. When a contraction signal is sent to the heart, it starts at one end of the band and travels through the heart in a linear fashion. Because of the wrapping around of the muscle on itself, when this contraction signal is sent, the heart contracts in a twisting motion.[17] This spiral orientation is seen throughout nature: pinecones, rams' horns, weather patterns, even the solar system.

This orientation of the heart is billions of years in the making. It has been theorized that the structure in which the blood circulated in early blood-containing life forms over a billion years ago, looked like little more than a worm. There was no pump. Through the fourth phase water energy gradient and a little help from the peristaltic contractions of the muscular tube, the blood moved through on its own. These organisms would have gotten plenty of energy from their environment to energize the blood and ensure its flow. As life evolved more complexity, this structure started to change. The wormlike muscle started to fold on itself, and we see the first fish heart with a small contracting chamber. With more folding, the fish heart evolved into an amphibian/reptilian heart. Still more folding, and eventually we ended up with a mammalian heart. If you trace the development of the heart in a mammalian embryo, you will witness stages of folding as it develops.[18]

To understand the implications of this structure, let's revisit the lab of Dr. Gerald Pollack. Remember that Dr. Pollack found that water can hold energy and when it does, it forms fourth phase water. He has also found that there are many ways that water can acquire that energy. Any type of radiant light, like from the Sun or a lamp, would do it. Energy given off from the Earth can also energize water. He also discovered that vortexing (or swirling) water in the presence of oxygen (air) can energize it.

This kind of process happens all the time in nature. Have you ever been at a river and watched water flow past a rock? On the other side of the rock, the water eddies, creating vortices. This process energizes the water. It is no coincidence that when the heart contracts it does so in a way that spirals the blood. As more complex life began to evolve, the body evolved an internal mechanism of keeping the water in the blood energized. The heart began to fold on itself to vortex blood in the presence of oxygen and keep it energized. As long ago as the Renaissance, Leonardo da Vinci was one of the first to notice the spiral of blood as it flows through the heart.[19]

The blood, in fact, gets swirled many times as it moves through the chambers of the heart. First, when the blood flows from the superior and inferior vena cava (see figure 6.5: H, I), the separate flows do not collide but flow past one another, creating a vortex. Then, as the blood flows through the tricuspid valve (C), vortexes form on either side. Once the ventricle (D) is full, the muscles (E) contract it in a spiral formation, further vortexing the blood. Last, a small about of vortexing happens as the blood goes through the pulmonary valve (F), exiting the ventricle.

Since the blood is never fully depleted of oxygen, even in venous blood, the blood is always spiraled when oxygen is present. This spiraling energizes the water in the blood so that it can become structured on the lining of our arteries. In this sense, I suppose you could say that the heart is responsible for the movement of blood . . . just not as a pump. Once we understand the heart through this lens, we have a much better foundation for understanding one type of heart disease.

Heart Failure

According to the Mayo Clinic, heart failure happens when the "heart muscle doesn't pump blood as well as it should."[20] Do you now see the flaw in that statement? The heart is not the mover of the blood. Heart failure is characterized by many symptoms, but two of the most prominent ones are an expansion in the shape of the heart and pooling of blood or fluid in the extremities. Let's discuss how these inefficiencies develop and contribute to heart failure in the context of the heart's real function in the body.

If the heart is not the main mover of the blood through the body, we can't "blame" the heart for failing to pump well when blood and fluid pools up in the body. It would be more accurate to say that there is insufficient energy in the system and that the water in the body is not energized enough to build structured water and keep blood, lymphatic fluid, and other fluids moving. Further, inadequate blood flow forces the heart to take on a role (a pump) that it is not really built for.

In a healthy body, blood flows through the heart more or less on its own, with the heart chambers contracting and vortexing the blood as it flows through. In an unhealthy body, the blood doesn't flow through as it should. It collects in the chambers more than it should and the contracting chambers have to pump more forcefully than they are designed to. This slow transit of blood through the heart creates excessive pressure in the chambers. Over time, this distends them into the characteristic round shape of a heart in heart failure (see figure 6.6).

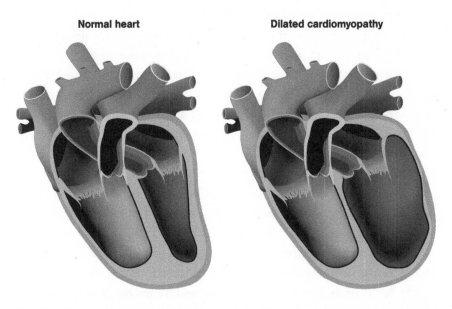

Normal heart   **Dilated cardiomyopathy**

Figure 6.6. The size of a normal heart versus the size of a heart with cardiomyopathy.

There are a few things that can predispose someone with inadequate blood flow to heart failure. One is scarring. An individual who has already had a heart attack is more likely to develop heart failure because the heart tissue is damaged and scarred. (I cover this in more detail in chapter 8.) Scar tissue will never perform as well as the original healthy tissue, leading to an inefficient heart that responds poorly to increased pressure caused by inadequate blood flow. It's important to know that things besides a heart attack can cause scarring of heart tissue, and to understand what causes poor blood flow.

Aside from a heart attack, there is evidence that a poor fuel source (i.e., food) can contribute to scarring. This scarring can be seen in studies of endurance exercisers. One study compared the hearts of older, lifelong endurance athletes to age-matched, nonendurance athletes, as well as younger endurance athletes. The older endurance athletes were the only group that had intense scarring of their hearts.[21] During endurance exercise the heart is forced to burn more glucose, which results in the buildup of lactic acid and hydrogen ions in the heart tissue. This buildup can damage the heart muscle and lead to scar tissue. The now-less-functional heart tissue in turn predisposes us to heart failure by weakening the heart's ability to vortex water. This weakened state then leads to inadequate blood flow and increased pressure in the heart chambers, eventually contributing to heart failure.

There is evidence that the preferred fuel source of the failing heart is ketones.[22] Ketones are made in the liver from fatty acids when there is less glucose available. The heart can burn multiple fuel sources, but it prefers fatty acids and ketones. In fact, infants born with glucose storage diseases cannot store carbohydrates as fat and have severely limited availability of fatty acids. One treatment is a diet of high-carbohydrate meals. Infants with one of these diseases who are placed on this diet, however, often develop heart failure. One case study showed that when these vulnerable infants were switched to a ketogenic diet, the intervention improved the metabolic function of the heart and therefore reduced their risk of heart failure.[23] Another study done on two siblings with a glucose storage disease also showed improvements with a switch to a ketogenic diet.[24] Another study found that an impaired ability to use fat for fuel is associated with cardiac dysfunction and heart failure. In the study's mice, cardiac dilation and contractile dysfunction "was completely reversed by a high-fat, low-carbohydrate ketogenic diet."[25] All this research suggests that if the heart does not have to burn an unhealthy level of glucose, it may help prevent scarring and predisposal to heart failure.

Heart failure has also been correlated with chronic obstructive pulmonary disorder (COPD).[26] One study found that the risk ratio of developing heart failure among COPD patients is 4.5 times higher than that of control individuals without the disease, after adjusting for age and other cardiovascular risk factors.[27] Any decline in lung function is obviously going to decrease the availability of oxygen in the blood. Remember that in order for the heart to energize the water in blood through vortexing, it needs to do so in the presence of oxygen. With less oxygen this process doesn't happen as well, and structured water cannot form in the arteries as well as it should.

All of these issues—scarring, a poor fuel source, and low blood oxygen—are different mechanisms that predispose someone to a decreased ability to energize the water in the blood and maintain blood flow. Importantly, Dr. Pollack has found that infrared light, especially the 3,000 nanometer (nm) wavelength, is the most effective light for energizing and structuring water. If a breakdown of structured water decreases blood flow, puts stress on the heart, and leads to heart failure, then therapy that exposes the body to infrared light, builds up structured water, and improves blood flow is well worth further investigation.

In fact, a study of 188 heart failure patients who underwent two weeks of infrared sauna therapy showed that all markers of cardiac function significantly improved in the treatment group, with no improvement in the control group.[28] Further research has shown that infrared sauna use in people with heart failure is effective for reducing arrhythmias, improving endothelial function, improving exercise tolerance, improving hemodynamic performance, and improving prognosis by reducing risk of heart attack.[29]

When I was recovering from my heart attack in the hospital, one of the cardiology residents told me they wanted me to take two blood pressure medications to take pressure off my heart to prevent development of heart failure that often develops after a heart attack. I knew that sauna could help me achieve the same result. A 2013 study published in the *International Journal of Cardiology* found that the use of infrared sauna in patients with previous heart disease provided improvements in endothelial function.[30] In a similar 2011 study, researchers induced heart attacks in rats and then exposed them to infrared sauna therapy for thirty-five minutes once a day for eight weeks and tested the effects of it on remodeling of the heart tissue. When it came to the usual decrease in heart function following a heart attack, they found that "decreases were attenuated in ST [sauna therapy] rats compared with non-ST rats" and that "ST attenuates cardiac remodeling after MI [heart attack], at least in part, through improving coronary vascularity in the noninfarcted myocardium."[31] Taken alone, this study is not much, as it is just one study and it was done in rats and not humans. However, if you take it in the context of the information in this chapter it makes complete sense. If the goal is to take pressure and workload off the heart while it is healing, then the best way to do this is to optimize the self-flow mechanisms of the blood in the body. Infrared sauna is proven to do so.

I always like to return to the lens of evolution: Our physiology has evolved to thrive in the context of sunlight, contact with the Earth, and the imbibement of spring water that has been energized by the Earth. Our heart evolved to prefer ketones and fatty acids due to the high-animal-fat diet that was available prior to the advent of agriculture—and certainly prior to the advent of industrial agriculture. Removing ourselves from the way of life that shaped our physiology so profoundly can never be healthy.

CHAPTER 7

Cholesterol and Atherosclerosis

One Christmas, Kinga and I met up with her brother and his wife in Amsterdam for Christmas Eve and Christmas Day. We stayed at a newer, small hotel that had only fourteen rooms, each of them themed after a traditional Dutch craft. Our room, "The Brewer," had once been a beer barrel storage room, and was decorated like a brewery with copper features reminiscent of the large vats that were once used in brewing, including a large copper bathtub.

To celebrate Christmas, the playful hotel staff had put a modest gift in the room safe and hidden candy canes throughout the room with clues to the combination lock. One candy cane under a pillow; a second in the minifridge; a third peeking over the top of the TV; plus one that had been given to us at the front desk. Each was labeled one through four. Candy cane #1 had a note attached, explaining that the first number in the combination lock was equal to the number of candy canes in the room: three. The second number in the combination lock was equal to the number of bar stools in the breakfast area: five. The third number in the combination lock was equal to the first digit in the hotel's address: eight. The final clue told us that the next number in the combination lock was the second digit in the hotel's total number of rooms: fourteen. This gave us a combination of 3584.

Excited to open the safe, we punched in the code. To our surprise, it didn't work. We tried again—nothing. After the third try, we received a message that we had attempted to open the safe too many times and would have to wait thirty minutes before we could try again. Defeated, we realized it was time to get ready for dinner, and the charming little game and the gift in the safe were abandoned. I won't lie, though: It bugged me.

The following morning, I woke up and went to use the bathroom when I saw something in the shower out of the corner of my eye. Tucked under a washcloth was another candy cane! Like a kid on Christmas morning, I grabbed it and found another clue with the number five on it. A fifth clue? That changed everything! I was doing the math in my head with the information from the last clue when my wife asked why I was hogging the bathroom. I walked out of the bathroom and went straight to the safe. "Why did you take a candy cane clue into the bathroom?" my wife asked. "I think you're a little obsessed."

The combination to the safe wasn't 3584. It was 2565. I punched in the numbers, opened the safe, and pulled out a box of Dutch chocolates: Something I don't eat, but I was glad that I had finally solved the mystery.

Later, I thought about how convinced I'd been that I'd found the correct combination to the safe, even though the feedback from the locked safe told me I had not. After three tries, I'd figured there must be something wrong with the safe. I'd even considered calling the front desk to tell them they'd programed it wrong. In reality, I was moving forward without all of the information.

Something similar happened to Ancel Keys in the 1950s and '60s when he used incomplete research to blame cholesterol for atherosclerosis. He was driven to find an answer, and he did, but it wasn't the correct answer. He went forward with his incorrect answer before he had all the information. Unfortunately, Ancel Keys didn't have the immediate feedback of a locked safe to tell him he was wrong. Instead, we have a decades-long epidemic of chronic disease telling us that his "combination" to the heart disease puzzle was wrong. Cholesterol and dietary fat do not cause atherosclerosis.

Cholesterol 101

A book about heart disease would not be complete without a discussion of cholesterol. Unfortunately, the myopic focus on cholesterol and low-density lipoproteins (LDLs) has been a major distraction in the quest to understand and prevent heart disease. It has been the focus of medical teaching and dietary recommendations for far too long. It is time that we set the record straight.

Cholesterol is a fatty, waxy substance synthesized by the body and absorbed from the food we eat; all animals have it and it is essential for many aspects of human physiology. Plants synthesize and use a different type of fat called phytosterol. Plants do not use cholesterol and animals prefer not to use phytosterol, though we can absorb phytosterol through the diet and use it if we need to (and this becomes significant when we discuss diet in chapter 11). First, let's get a basic understanding of how cholesterol is transported and used throughout the human body.

Since cholesterol is a fat, and fat is hydrophobic, it does not blend well into water, and since blood is almost half water, cholesterol needs help traveling though the bloodstream. Enter lipoproteins. Some lipoproteins are famous, such as LDL and HDL, while others are less known, such as chylomicrons, VLDL, and IDL. But all of these proteins can package up cholesterol molecules and transport them to different areas of the body to be used in various ways.

These lipoproteins vary in size. In order from largest to smallest, there are chylomicrons, very-low-density lipoproteins (VLDLs), intermediate-density lipoproteins (IDLs), low-density lipoproteins (LDLs), and high-density lipoproteins (HDLs). The more densely packed with cholesterol the lipoproteins are, the smaller they tend to be.

LDL has, unfortunately, been labeled the "bad cholesterol," taking the rap for clogging our arteries, while HDL has been labeled the "good cholesterol," and is said to help scavenge damaged cholesterol molecules. The terms *good* and *bad* to describe lipoproteins are bizarrely accusatory and should be thrown out, for reasons you will understand by the end of this chapter.

Let's first discuss the many essential roles cholesterol plays in the body. If you ate no cholesterol in your diet, your body would make about 1.5 grams of cholesterol per day. That's how important it is. One thing that cholesterol does is aid in defense against infection. LDL can bind to bacteria and endotoxins and neutralize them before they cause harm.[1] One study looked at the ability of HDL, LDL, apolipoprotein B (apoB), and apolipoprotein A1 (apoA1) to bind and neutralize toxins and concluded that "plasma lipoproteins may represent another line of defense in neutralization of endotoxin when infections progress beyond the initial stage."[2] In fact, there is evidence that using a new drug called a PCSK9 inhibitor to lower cholesterol can leave us vulnerable to endotoxins.[3]

Cholesterol is also helpful in fighting viral infections.[4] The body uses cholesterol to conjugate (meaning "attach") peptides to antibodies that then improve the antibodies' capacity to mount a defense against pathogens. One study found that cholesterol-conjugated peptides can halt the merging of a viral and cellular membrane. The researchers stated that this had "broad implications for antiviral development with application to . . . targets include[ing] influenza A and B viruses as well as arenaviruses (Junin), human metapneumoviruses, filoviruses (Ebola), flavivirus, and coronaviruses (severe acute respiratory syndromes)."[5]

I believe we often see this antiviral effect among people who eat a high-cholesterol diet, especially those on a ketogenic diet. In these cases, LDL on a blood panel will often go way up, as the body starts making ketones from fatty acids, a process that shares much of the same biochemical pathway as cholesterol synthesis in the liver; therefore, cholesterol production goes up as well. Another reason we often see this elevated LDL with a high-cholesterol diet is that plant fats (phytosterol) and animal fats (cholesterol) compete for absorption in the gut. When we eliminate plant fats and eat only animal fats, we get much higher absorption of them and, again, cholesterol levels in the blood go up. Dave Feldman of cholesterolcode.com has labeled people who see a dramatic rise in blood cholesterol levels when they adhere to low-carbohydrate, high-fat diets as "lean mass hyper responders." I would consider myself a lean mass hyper responder as my LDL goes above 300 when I have been on very-low-carbohydrate diets in the past. Among these people there is anecdotal evidence that they rarely get sick. Based on the evidence presented in the previous paragraph I speculate that this is because the higher LDL is protecting them from bacterial and viral infection.

Cholesterol also plays an important role in cell membrane structure, function, and repair. And cholesterol is essential for the communication *between* cells. Without communication, our cells would not be able to come together and form tissues, tissues wouldn't be able to become organs, and organs wouldn't be able to function together. Studies have also shown that the cholesterol packaged in LDL can repair nerve cells that have a damaged—or demyelinated—outer membrane.[6]

Again, the main job of LDL is the delivery of cholesterol, which is the backbone of our hormones. Without LDL transporting cholesterol, we could not make hormones. As cardiologist Nadir Ali has said, "Women would not be as beautiful, and men would not be as handsome without cholesterol." But it is vital to more than just our sex hormones. The body uses cholesterol as the base for the synthesis of all steroid hormones.[7]

You may be surprised to learn that one of these steroid hormones is vitamin D. Vitamin D_2 (ergocalciferol) and vitamin D_3 (cholecalciferol) are both converted to calcitriol, the active form of vitamin D, in the body. Most of us know that our body synthesizes vitamin D when our skin is exposed to sunlight, but you may not know that if we do not have the other essential raw materials, we'll be deficient. Cholesterol is one of them. Having enough cholesterol is essential for the synthesis of adequate amounts of vitamin D. Once vitamin D is made, it is transported around the body in LDL, as are all the fat-soluble vitamins.[8] In fact, long-term use of LDL-lowering PCSK9-inhibitor drugs has been shown to decrease levels of vitamin E, a fat-soluble vitamin that is essential to healthy blood, skin, brain, and eyes.[9]

LDL also delivers *energy* to the body. When we restrict carbohydrates, the body burns more fat and delivers that fat to our cells to be used for energy. This could explain why some people on a ketogenic diet experience high LDL: The body is delivering a lot of energy in the form of fat. LDL also delivers cholesterol to muscles, where it is essential for muscle repair, especially after exercise.[10] Without cholesterol delivered from LDL, we cannot build strong muscles. Given that muscle mass is one determinant of longevity and that we cannot build muscle mass without cholesterol delivered from LDL, a continuous supply is a key to lifelong good health.[11]

The delivery of cholesterol by LDL is also essential for the proper function of insulin receptors on cells.[12] As someone with type 1 diabetes, I have to administer my own insulin. Anecdotally, I noticed my insulin worked better, and I had to use less, when I began eating an animal-based diet. At first, I thought maybe I had eliminated a plant toxin that was interfering with insulin or that I had reduced inflammation, and so I required less. When I learned that cholesterol is essential for the health of insulin receptors and combined that knowledge with the increase in my LDL, I began to realize that delivery of cholesterol by LDL was the most plausible mechanism.

Lastly, let's discuss the ability of LDL to prevent vascular calcification, also known as deposits on our arteries. Yes, you read that right. Cholesterol is blamed for causing atherosclerosis, but it can actually help *prevent* it. Cholesterol does this through another fat-soluble vitamin, K_2. LDL-delivered cholesterol is essential for making vitamin K_2, which aids in depositing minerals where they're needed and keeping them away from where they can cause damage, such as the lining of an artery. K_2 stimulates the matrix Gla protein that inhibits the formation of calcium plaque.[13] In fact, LDL-lowering medications have been shown to stimulate atherosclerosis, and one source of this stimulation is low production and delivery of K_2 due to lack of cholesterol.[14]

Clearly, cholesterol and its transporters (lipoproteins) are incredibly important to human physiology. Unfortunately, because of the belief that high cholesterol causes atherosclerosis, there have been many different types of statin drugs developed to lower cholesterol—they are some of the most prescribed drugs in the United States—as well as the newer cholesterol-lowering drugs, PCSK9 inhibitors.[15] Both are effective at lowering cholesterol in the blood, but that doesn't mean they're good for the heart.

Cholesterol Medications: Helpful or Harmful?

The infamous statin drugs. These are drugs like Zocor, Crestor, and Lipitor. Statins work by directly preventing the production of cholesterol. To understand how, and to understand the consequences, we need to first become familiar with the basic steps through which the body makes cholesterol. The many-stepped process starts with the synthesis of acetyl-CoA from either glucose (glycolysis) or fatty acids (beta-oxidation). From there the basic, though admittedly simplified, steps to making cholesterol go like this:

acetyl-CoA → HMG-CoA → mevalonate → mevalonyl-PP → isopentenyl-PP → geranyl-PP → farnesyl-PP → squalene → cholesterol

You don't have to understand what all these intermediate molecules are to make sense of what I'm about to say: Statins are called HMG-CoA reductase inhibitors because they inhibit HMG-CoA reductase, the enzyme that converts HMG-CoA to mevalonate. Because statins block the production of mevalonate, the next step never happens, nor the next, and we certainly don't make it all the way to cholesterol at the end. Just as importantly, however, we don't make any of the intermediate molecules between mevalonate and cholesterol, some of which are significant and reveal some of the consequences of taking statins.

The first is isopentenyl-PP. When cholesterol synthesis from acetyl-CoA gets to isopentenyl-PP, some of this molecule proceeds toward cholesterol synthesis. But some of it is directed toward other purposes, such as the making of selenoproteins. The most famous selenoprotein is glutathione peroxidase, arguably the body's most important antioxidant. Sufficient levels of this antioxidant are essential for preventing both tissue damage and damage to DNA. If we block HMG-CoA from becoming mevalonate, we never get isopentenyl-PP, and therefore end up with lower levels of protective antioxidants. One study found that as statins rose, antioxidants diminished.[16] This is a recipe for oxidative stress.

Isopentenyl-PP is also important for the conversion of vitamin K_1 to K_2. K_2 helps prevent and reverse calcification in the arteries.[17] It does this through activation of the matrix Gla protein. Again, if the HMG-CoA-to-mevalonate step doesn't happen, the pathway never arrives at isopentenyl-PP, and the body cannot depend on the conversion of K_1 to K_2 to help prevent atherosclerosis. The irony is that statins are touted as drugs that prevent atherosclerosis, but in fact they actually disrupt the protective biochemical pathway.[14]

Farnesyl-PP is an intermediate only two steps away from cholesterol, but also important for other reasons: It is used to synthesize CoQ10, which helps make ATP in our mitochondria. The heart has one of the highest mitochondrial densities of any tissue in the body, which is why CoQ10 is often supplemented for heart health. However, if the intermediate farnesyl-PP isn't made because statins interrupt the cholesterol production chain, we don't get CoQ10, resulting in less-than-optimal ATP production. This could be why statins have been shown to cause fatigue and cardiomyopathy, disease of heart muscle tissue.[18] Since muscles are very metabolically active, this could also explain the muscle pain side effect of statins.[19] A 2003 paper reviewing all the animal and human research on statins and CoQ10 stated that "as the potency of statin drugs increases and as the target LDL cholesterol level decreases, the severity of CoQ10 depletion will increase with an increasing likelihood of impairment in heart muscle function."[20]

Farnesyl-PP is also used to synthesize another molecule, called dolichol, which plays an important role in the function of insulin receptors and, naturally, the prevention of insulin resistance. In fact, a recent study found that insulin resistance in statin users was much higher than in nonstatin users.[21] It comes as no surprise then that statins have been shown to cause diabetes. A study of 3,234 individuals at risk for diabetes placed participants into one of three groups: those taking a drug for diabetes (metformin), those engaging in a prescribed lifestyle change, and a control group. Participants in all groups also started taking a statin. At the end of the study, the researchers found that statin use resulted in a 30 percent increased risk of developing diabetes in each of the study groups.[22] A meta-analysis found that "the weight of clinical evidence suggests a worsening effect of statins on insulin resistance and secretion."[23] In chapter 18, we will discuss how insulin resistance—not high LDL—may be the best indicator of risk for cardiovascular disease. If that's correct, wouldn't it be concerning that the drug most often prescribed for preventing heart disease is actually causing the number one risk factor?

Lastly, the mere fact that statins prevent the synthesis of cholesterol is itself problematic: As you now know, cholesterol helps defend against infection, repair cells, reduce inflammation, synthesize hormones and vitamin D, transport fat-soluble vitamins, deliver energy, support muscle function, support neurotransmitter signaling, and prevent vascular calcification. Given all of these benefits, why would we want to inhibit cholesterol synthesis with statins? Or interfere with the body's ability to use cholesterol, which is the mechanism by which another class of cholesterol-lowering medications called PCSK9 inhibitors work?

PCSK9 is the molecule that blocks or removes LDL receptors on cells so that LDL is not taken out of the bloodstream and into the liver, typically when there's inflammation or infection that the LDL can help mitigate. A PCSK9-inhibitor medication eliminates PCSK9 through an antibody mechanism, leaving all the LDL receptors open to take LDL into the cells and out of the bloodstream. This lowers LDL on a blood lipid panel, but it leaves the individual at risk for all the issues caused by lack of LDL in the blood—including cholesterol transport issues, infection vulnerability, lack of energy delivery, slower muscle repair, less insulin sensitivity, and being more prone to vascular calcification. PCSK9 inhibitors are newer than statins, and while there's a relatively small number of studies on their side effects, those that exist suggest there may be some serious risks associated with the drugs. One study demonstrated that use of a PCSK9 inhibitor resulted in a 16 percent decrease in vitamin E, a fat-soluble vitamin with many essential functions in the body.

Two recent studies cast further doubt on PCSK9-inhibitor drugs. In the first, "Serious Adverse Events and Deaths in PCSK9 Inhibitor Trials Reported on ClinicalTrials.gov: A Systematic Review," the authors concluded that their "meta-analysis of clinical events registered on ClinicalTrials.gov did not show that PCSK9 inhibitors improve cardiovascular health. Evolocumab [the name of the PCSK9 used in the study] increased the risk of all-cause mortality."[24] In the second, not only did the authors find no association between lowering LDL and a reduction in cardiovascular events, they found a "a tendency to harm for all outcomes with PCSK9 antibodies. Therefore, at the moment, the data available from randomized trials does not clearly support the use of these antibodies."[25]

Statins basically interfere in the biochemical steps to synthesize cholesterol. With PCSK9 inhibitors, it is more about sequestering cholesterol, so that it is not in the blood or available to tissues. This is concerning, considering low cholesterol in the blood has been associated with higher risk of stroke, lower cognitive performance, increased risk for Parkinson's disease, increased risk for Alzheimer's disease, higher risk of cancer, and higher general risk of mortality.[26]

The question we haven't considered, however, is this: Do these drugs actually reduce the risk of heart disease? A 2007 study published in The Lancet showed that among healthy women with high cholesterol, there was no benefit from statins in heart attack risk or death. The same study showed that in men and women over age sixty-nine with high cholesterol, there was also no benefit.[27] Research has also shown that treatment with two statins lowers cholesterol more than a single drug alone but does not reduce heart attack risk—and leads to more plaque in the arteries.[28] In people who already have heart disease, statins prevent only 1 in 83 deaths, 1 in 39 nonfatal heart attacks, and 1 in 125 strokes.[29] Finally, a 2016 study of a new cholesterol-lowering drug was halted mid-trial because, despite the drug effectively lowering LDL, "the favorable effects on cholesterol did not translate into any reduction in the study's primary endpoint: the amount of time until cardiovascular death, heart attack, stroke, coronary artery bypass surgery or hospitalization for chest pain due to unstable angina."[30]

Three large studies have concluded statins are beneficial, but the devil is in the details. In a group of 6,605 people, half took the statin drug pravastatin and the other half took a placebo. After five years, 4.9 percent of the statin group had heart attacks versus 6.4 percent in the placebo group, a difference of only 1.5 percent. Sixty-three people would have to take the drug for five years to prevent a single heart attack among them.[31] Further, the deaths from any cause were the same in both groups; this means that while statins slightly decreased the risk of dying from heart disease, the people still died of something else. Another study of 6,595 men with high cholesterol put half on the statin drug pravastatin and the other half on a placebo. After five years the statin group had a 3.2 percent risk of mortality versus 4.1 percent in the placebo group. The "number needed to treat" for this study was 110; 110 people needed to take the drug for five years to prevent one death.[32] Finally, the JUPITER trial examined the effects of a statin on 17,802 men and women with elevated hs-CRP, a marker of inflammation. After two years, the statin group had a 2.2 percent risk of mortality compared to the placebo group's 2.8 percent.[33] Minimal effects yet again. While other studies, like the 4S trial, show a greater benefit—a reduction in cardiac events from 22.6 percent to 15.9 percent—overall the impact is negligible.[34]

Given these meager statistics, I find it curious that the conclusions of the studies, which were funded by the companies that make statin drugs, point to a "significantly" reduced risk of heart attacks, or that the lowering of LDL with statins to reduce the risk of heart attack was "confirmed." These margins do not suggest "significant" or "confirmed." And yet this is the research that supports the use of statin drugs. Further, the marginal benefit of statin drugs may be due to their anti-inflammatory effect, rather than the reduction of LDL.[35] And lifestyle changes are a much more effective way to achieve a decrease in inflammation (see part 3). Add to that: Statins have been shown to cause memory problems, sexual dysfunction, and muscle pain.[36] These drugs just aren't worth it.

Although statins are only mildly effective and cause a whole host of side effects, many cardiologists recommend using them to lower cholesterol. But what happens when cholesterol gets too low? There is a condition called abetalipoproteinemia, in which the body cannot absorb fat and results in very low levels of LDL. Individuals with this condition often have recurrent infections (because LDL cannot help them defend against bacteria), blindness (because fat-soluble vitamin A is not delivered by LDL), ataxia (because of nerve cell demyelination due to lack of cholesterol), and higher rates of liver cancer.[37] They also tend to die earlier, in their forties or fifties.

To play devil's advocate, does LDL become problematic when it gets too high? There is a condition that causes that condition, too: familial hypercholesterolemia (FH). This is a genetic condition, in which patients experience an altered lipid metabolism that creates high LDL cholesterol, and these individuals often do not fare well, but evidence points to the altered lipid metabolism, not the high LDL per se, as the culprit. A study that tracked families with the genetic line of familial hypercholesterolemia for over two centuries found that "the precocious onset of cardiovascular disease and the bad prognosis of familial hypercholesterolemia have been overemphasized." This study also found that the condition "may have conferred a survival advantage when infectious disease was prevalent." The researchers found that 40 percent of the people with familial hypercholesterolemia lived a normal life span, and they concluded that the variation in mortality suggested that "environmental factors" were more important than cholesterol levels in determining life span.[38]

In an article that analyzed extensive research on the topic of cholesterol and heart disease in the context of hypercholesterolemia, the authors disagreed with the idea that people with familial hypercholesterolemia (FH) are more prone to heart disease "based on the absence of support for the diet-heart hypothesis, and the lack of evidence that a low saturated fat, low cholesterol diet reduces coronary events in FH individuals." They concluded that people with familial hypercholesterolemia develop heart disease for the same reasons as anyone else: "The subset of FH individuals that develop CHD exhibit risk factors associated with an insulin-resistant phenotype (elevated triglycerides, blood glucose, haemoglobin A1c (HbA1c), obesity, hyperinsulinaemia, high-sensitivity C reactive protein, hypertension) or increased susceptibility to develop coagulopathy."[39] This suggests that having high LDL does not predispose us to heart disease.

If very high cholesterol doesn't seem to be an issue as far as longevity goes, then why not reap the benefits of it? Now that we have seen the many benefits of cholesterol and reviewed the harm cholesterol-reducing drugs inflict on the body, let's review some research that directly studies the link between cholesterol and heart disease.

Cholesterol and Atherosclerosis

But what about cholesterol and heart disease, specifically? For that, we should start with a definition of *atherosclerosis*. For his 1989 book, *Natural History of Coronary Atherosclerosis*, physician and researcher Constantin Velican surveyed fifty-nine researchers, research teams, and medical and health organizations for their definitions of atherosclerosis, noting great variation and that most were speculative. "To sum up, as there is no unanimity concerning the definition of atherosclerosis, at present each writer should make clear from the onset in his work what this term implies. This absence of an adequate definition is overlooked in many textbooks, monographs, book chapters, and reviews."[40]

Velican's point was that, if there is no consensus among experts on what atherosclerosis actually *is*, researchers should always give their definition of atherosclerosis at the outset of an article, in order for the article to mean anything. But there's another point: If there's no clear definition of atherosclerosis, how do we know atherosclerosis is caused by elevated LDL? We don't. And this becomes a springboard for the revelation that there isn't any high-quality evidence proving that LDL leads to atherosclerosis.

As we discussed in chapter 5, epidemiological studies can show that two things are associated, but it cannot prove that one causes the other. These types of studies have shown a correlation between cholesterol and disease, but they have also shown the opposite. For example, in the Leiden 85-plus Study, researchers in the Netherlands tracked 570 individuals eighty-five years old and over for five years. They found that those who had the highest cholesterol levels had the lowest rates of infection, cancer, and all-cause mortality.[41] The Lothian Birth Cohort Study, which tracked 1,091 people born in 1936 in the Lothian region of Scotland, found that those who had the highest cholesterol levels had the highest cognitive function compared to people with intermediate or low cholesterol levels. This study also found that those who had the highest cholesterol had the lowest rates of high blood pressure, lowest risk of stroke, and lowest incidence of heart disease.[42] Finally, a 2019 study of 347,971 individuals looked at the association of low levels of LDL and mortality. The researchers found that the group with the lowest LDL had the highest rate of all-cause mortality. They concluded that "low levels of LDL-C concentration are strongly and independently associated with increased risk of cancer, CVD, and all-cause mortality."[43]

You may be wondering why I just said that we cannot determine cause from epidemiological studies and then cited three of them. My goal is to emphasize that, while the results sound compelling, we cannot draw conclusions from them. If one of these studies shows that higher cholesterol is associated with higher rates of heart disease and a second shows the opposite, which of the two studies are we supposed to believe? This is the nature of epidemiology. It should be used to create hypotheses and to find associations so that we can design clinical trials to test those associations. Clinical trials didn't happen after Ancel Keys's studies, and his studies became the foundation of public health guidelines to limit intake of saturated fat and cholesterol, without the requisite conclusive data. If LDL were as bad for us as we have been led to believe, you would expect some association between having higher levels of LDL and higher rates of chronic disease. But we don't see that; we see the opposite.

Let's look at some different types of research. One systematic review study—one of the most rigorous and respected types of research because it assesses all available data on a subject and summarizes it in one paper—studied all the published papers on the association of cholesterol and heart disease. The study found a "lack of an association or an inverse association between LDL-C and both all-cause and CV mortality."[44] *Inverse association* means that there was not just no association, but its opposite: The higher the cholesterol, the lower the risk of all-cause mortality and cardiovascular disease.

Another interesting study looked at 136,905 people who were admitted for heart attacks to 541 different hospitals. Medical professionals measured cholesterol levels in these people within 24 hours of admission. They found that 75 percent of the subjects had at least "normal" LDL (under 130 mg/dL) and 50 percent had "optimal" LDL (under 100 mg/dL).[45] These people had "ideal" cholesterol, yet still had a heart attack; this data suggests that what someone's LDL level is when they have a heart attack is not as relevant as many doctors think. Knowing this made it all the more frustrating for me while I was in the hospital after my heart attack listening to the doctors go on and on about my LDL.

In addition to the data from these studies that contradict the idea that high LDL causes atherosclerosis and heart attacks, and the biological science on cholesterol, LDL, and statins, it's simply illogical that high LDL in the blood causes atherosclerosis. Why? Because when LDL is high in the blood, it is not just high in certain areas; it is high everywhere. So why do we only see atherosclerosis in arteries, and not in veins? The only time atherosclerosis occurs in a vein is when a vein is taken from the body and used in bypass surgery. This transplanted vein promptly develops atherosclerosis. Even more interesting is that we only see atherosclerosis pop up in certain areas of the arteries. If LDL is so troublesome to the artery wall and it is everywhere in the blood, why don't we see it develop everywhere? To answer these questions, and to understand the real cause of atherosclerosis, we have to revisit the fourth phase of water.

The Exclusion Zone

In chapter 6, we discussed the formation of structured (fourth phase) water on the lining of the blood vessels. The formation of this fourth phase water creates an energy gradient that drives blood flow without the need of a pump. But the formation of this water in our blood vessels also has another important role: protection of the arteries.

Recall that fourth phase water forms when water molecules cleave off one of the hydrogens and the resultant O–H molecules team up with other cleaved off O–H molecules to create a lattice structure. These lattice structures stack on top of each other to form many layers. But they don't stack up exactly in line. The lattice structure is made up of hexagonal rings, but the rings do not line up; instead, they are slightly offset. One result of this offset

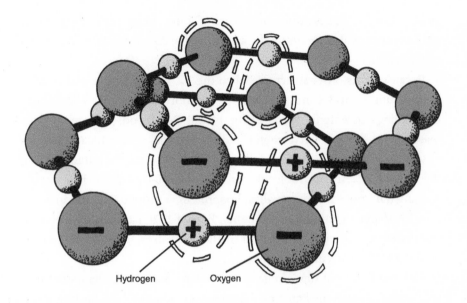

Hydrogen   Oxygen

Figure 7.1. Stacked layers of fourth phase water are offset. This characteristic gives structured water the nickname "exclusion zone" (EZ) water because this offsetting allows for almost nothing to penetrate. Adapted from *The Fourth Phase of Water*.

is that only very tiny molecules can get through the layer of water. This is why the fourth phase of water is also called the "exclusion zone," or EZ. Almost everything is excluded from penetrating it.

This EZ protects blood vessel linings from everything present in the blood. In *The Fourth Phase of Water*, Dr. Pollack stated, "Even red blood cells, several strains of bacteria, and ordinary dirt particles scraped from outside our laboratory were excluded. The protein albumin was excluded." Why mention the protein albumin? Because at approximately 3.8 nm in diameter, it is one of the smallest substances that can be found in the bloodstream.

Conventional wisdom is that excessive LDL will penetrate the lining of the arteries and deposit itself in the endothelium (the cells that make up the lining of the artery), resulting in atherosclerosis. Damaged LDL particles that are smaller in size, the theory goes, can penetrate the endothelial layer more easily, and this is why LDL particle size has become a popular test among doctors. The exclusion properties of fourth phase water suggest that LDL cannot possibly penetrate the arterial wall *if EZ water is there*, regardless of particle size.

Because of its offset structure, when the EZ water is intact and healthy, even albumin—at 3.8 nm in diameter—cannot penetrate it. What about other things commonly found in the blood? Red blood cells are approximately 6,000–8,000 nm in diameter, and bacteria range from 1,000–2,000 nm in width and 10,000–20,000 nm in length. At those sizes, they aren't getting through the EZ. An LDL molecule comes in at around 24–28 nm in diameter, and an HDL molecule, the smallest lipoprotein, is around 7–12 nm in diameter. They aren't getting through either. Even if LDL particles are damaged and therefore smaller, they never get smaller than an HDL molecule, and not even the HDL molecule can penetrate EZ water.

The significance of this is huge. It shows that it is much harder for harmful substances to reach the lining of the artery provided we have healthy, intact EZ water. It also suggests that if we do things to help maintain a healthy EZ layer, *we can prevent atherosclerosis*. I have discussed how radiant energy from various sources can help energize the water in our bodies so we maintain healthy exclusion zones. But what breaks down exclusion zones?

What *Really* Causes Atherosclerosis?

Once again, Dr. Pollack led us in the right direction: "Suppose some electron-hungry process draws off some of the EZ's negative charge, leaving the released lattice unit devoid of its usual negativity. . . . Issues of this nature could upset the default situation."[46] So, what's an "electron-hungry process"? Remember from chapter 1 that free radicals are the body's main electron-demanding molecules. Free radicals play important roles in physiology, but they can cause problems when they accumulate.

These molecules are called free radicals because they have an unpaired electron, which makes them unstable and "electron hungry." They will steal an electron from any source in order to be paired and stable, including from the EZ barrier in our blood vessels. Excessive free radicals will continue to break down the EZ barrier until they reach the inner lining of the artery. When more free radicals are created than the body's antioxidants can handle, this state is known as oxidative stress, which has been shown to cause atherosclerosis due to a chronic state of inflammation.[47]

What, precisely, causes free radicals and oxidative stress? For starters, a glucose-based metabolism. This occurs when people consume carbohydrates as their primary fuel source. Any time we turn the food we eat into energy (ATP), we make free radicals; it's the natural way of things. The human body usually takes care of these free radicals by making endogenous antioxidants. Whether or not this process gets out of balance, leading to oxidative stress, can largely depend on which fuel source we give our bodies to use on a regular basis.

While carbohydrates are not all bad, eating carbohydrates does raise your blood glucose. Insulin is then secreted to bring it back down. This process happens no matter how healthy you are. The only way to get big increases in blood glucose is to eat carbohydrates, especially processed carbohydrates. When we do it multiple times a day, it causes a blood sugar roller coaster—and greater amounts of oxidative stress and endothelial dysfunction (that is, dysfunction in the innermost layer of cells that line the arteries).[48] Researchers have found that this occurs not only among people with diabetes who are expected to have poor blood sugar control, but also among people with good blood sugar control. Regardless, a diet high in processed carbohydrates contributes to the production of free radicals, and development of atherosclerosis.

In fact, simply administering a glucose tolerance test—in which a one-time dose of sugar is eaten to see how well the body can bring the blood sugar back down—has been shown to increase free radicals in the bloodstream and deplete antioxidants.[49] And we know that the smooth muscle cells in the middle layer of the artery lining are very susceptible to the oxidative stress created by high glucose concentrations in the blood.[50]

One way that glucose creates free radicals is through a process called glycation. Glycation happens when too much sugar in the blood damages molecules. These sugar-damaged molecules are called advanced glycation end products (AGEs). AGEs mostly result from spiking blood sugars caused by eating excess processed carbohydrates, but they can also come from eating burnt meat, bread crust, and fats that are excessively heated. The blood test hemoglobin A_1C measures for the red blood cells that have been damaged by glycation. Looking at the percentage of these sugar-damaged red blood cells can give us an idea of blood sugar levels over a time period of about three months, the approximate life span of a red blood cell.

AGEs are dangerous and have been shown to initiate atherosclerosis.[51] A study that examined the interaction between AGEs and the lining of the blood vessels found that "AGEs can initiate and/or propagate atherosclerotic lesions independently of diabetes or dyslipidemia."[52] This is profound. These molecules can *initiate* atherosclerosis all on their own. What's more, AGE molecules did this even in the absence of high cholesterol; this finding provides yet more evidence that high LDL is not the cause of atherosclerosis.

Endotoxemia, which occurs when high amounts of bacteria get into the bloodstream, also causes oxidative stress, possibly as a result of the body's attack on the bacteria, which releases toxins when the cell disintegrates after death. It is no surprise then, that studies have found a connection to endotoxemia and atherosclerosis.[53] Endotoxins have even been found embedded in atherosclerotic plaque.[54] Endothelial progenitor cells travel from the bone marrow to the bloodstream to repair damaged areas in the lining of the blood vessels. When endotoxins are present in the blood, even at relatively low concentrations, it reduces cells' ability to repair the lining of the blood vessels.[55]

How does endotoxemia develop? It usually results from a leaky gut—where the lining of the intestines is damaged and bacteria from the gut leak into the bloodstream—or from poor dental health, including gum disease, root canals, and jaw infections called cavitations that leak bacteria into the bloodstream.[56] (See chapter 15 for more on the connection between dental health and heart disease.) The cause of atherosclerosis is much broader than we've been taught—and it doesn't stop there.

Next up is heavy metals. These are metals such as lead, mercury, aluminum, cadmium, and arsenic. These metals remained safely sequestered in the ground for most of human history; only recently have we started to dig them up and expose ourselves to them. Our physiology has no use for them, and they cause many problems when they get into our bodies, including oxidative stress.[57] Common exposures in our modern world include, but are not limited to, dental fillings, fish/seafood, tap water, cosmetics, antiperspirants, dust, cigarette smoke, aluminum foil and cans, vaccines, lead-based paint, and sunscreens.

Since heavy metals create free radicals, it stands to reason that they might contribute to atherosclerosis as well. Indeed, the amount of mercury in the blood has been directly correlated to the amount of atherosclerosis found in carotid arteries; at 2.81 micrograms per gram of mercury in the blood, the thickness of atherosclerosis has been shown to increase by 35 percent.[58] Mercury is not the only heavy metal that has been linked to heart disease: Lead exposure has been linked to high blood pressure; arsenic exposure has been linked to atherosclerosis and ischemic heart disease; cadmium exposure has been linked to atherosclerosis; and aluminum exposure has been linked to ischemic heart disease.[59]

Lastly, let's take a look at bisphenol-A (BPA). This molecule is known as a plasticizer—it is what makes plastics, well, plastic. BPA has come under a lot of heat for causing all kinds of health issues, which has triggered the BPA-free movement. Unfortunately, rather than searching for nontoxic solutions, product developers have simply replaced it with equally toxic plasticizers in consumer products. BPA is not a free radical per say, but it has been shown to cause oxidative stress.[60] A 2014 study looked at atherosclerosis in the aortic root and brachiocephalic arteries of mice that were fed a diet supplemented with BPA. Compared to the control, these mice had a 104 percent increased atherosclerotic lesion area in the aortic arch and a 120 percent increase in lesion area in the brachiocephalic artery.[61]

In addition to heavy metals and BPA, there are many other toxins that can contribute to oxidative stress and damage to arteries. Air pollution has been linked to cardiac arrhythmias and arterial blood clots.[62] Pesticides have been shown to cause cardiac arrhythmias, electrocardiographic abnormalities including prolonged Q-Tc interval, conduction defects, sinus tachycardia, sinus bradycardia, hypertension, and hypotension, and atherosclerosis.[63] Exposure to perfluorooctanoic acid (PFOA), which is found on many household items, has been linked to increased atherosclerosis of the coronary arteries.[64]

The "electron hungry process" that Dr. Pollack described and that causes oxidative stress may actually be coming from common modern-day products and sources. This oxidative stress may lead to an overabundance of free radicals in our bloodstream, breaking down the EZ that protects our arteries, which are then subjected to the same fate as the EZ itself: damage via free radicals.

Worse, when the body becomes insulin resistant, the endothelial cells that line the artery cannot repair themselves when damaged due to impairment of the insulin-mediated production of nitric oxide, making the cells even more prone to oxidative stress.[65] A damaged artery that cannot repair itself in the usual way is forced to repair itself in another way before it ruptures and clots form. The repair consists of bringing in minerals and cholesterol, kind of like spackle, to patch up the artery wall.

All of this is to say that there are many steps leading up to damage of the inner lining of an artery—before cholesterol is ever involved, or as one research article put it, "The cause(s) of coronary arterial disease are therefore concerned more with these pre-lipid stages than with the lipids themselves, which are complicating rather than causative factors."[66] In fact, when researchers looked at the association of high LDL and incidence of atherosclerosis, they only found an association when high LDL was also found with higher Lp(a), which are lipoproteins that are damaged from inflammation and oxidative stress.[67] This suggests that whatever is causing the damage to the lipoproteins and creating Lp(a) is what is causing the atherosclerosis and that LDL is not involved until damage to the artery occurs by other means first.

Can EZ water form next to an area of atherosclerosis and protect it from further damage? Nobody knows. I suspect that EZ water does not form over atherosclerosis because fatty substances like cholesterol are hydrophobic, and EZ water forms over hydrophilic surfaces. This could be why atherosclerosis continues to grow once it forms; it resists the potential protection of EZ water. It could also be why atherosclerosis contributes to heart failure: If EZ water does not form, blood flow from the energy gradient will diminish, forcing the heart to pump beyond its capacity. This is speculation on my part and I hope researchers someday take up these questions in a laboratory setting.

And why do we only see atherosclerosis in arteries, and only in certain places in the arteries, at that? Because arteries are under more pressure, and some places in arteries experience more pressure than others. In a state of oxidative stress, damaging molecules—endotoxins, heavy metals, BPA, AGEs—float around in the blood. The more pressure, the more those molecules get pushed against the EZ water, increasing the likelihood they will damage the EZ barrier by stealing electrons. This situation is why high blood pressure is associated with the development of atherosclerosis.[68]

Atherosclerosis occurs where pressure is high, such as where an artery splits into two arteries, where it takes a sharp turn, or in the coronary arteries where the contracting heart keeps them under more pressure.

Some Final Considerations

This way of understanding heart disease is predicated on the idea that when endothelia are damaged, the body repairs that damage by creating atherosclerosis from the *inside* of the artery. There is some interesting research, however, suggesting that the reaction of the body to this damaged endothelial lining may come from the *outside* of the artery.

First some background: The artery has many layers. The thin endothelial layer, which belongs to the innermost layer of connective tissue, or intima, where atherosclerosis starts, takes the initial brunt of oxidative stress. The media, or the middle layer, is filled with smooth muscle and elastic fibers that allow for the widening and narrowing of the arteries. Finally, the adventitia is the outermost layer of connective tissue that is supplied with blood by small arteries called the vasa vasorum. That's correct; there are arteries that supply blood to the arteries.

Since atherosclerosis develops in the intima, the layer of the artery closest to the bloodstream, it has long been thought that atherosclerosis develops from molecules *within* the bloodstream. But some curious observations have been made when it comes to atherosclerosis and these layers. The first is that the vasa vasorum—the arteries that supply the arteries with blood—are more numerous and developed in arteries that have developed atherosclerosis.[69] The second observation is that when atherosclerosis develops, the first signs of it appear in the outermost area of the intima layer, with no sign that molecules have traveled from the bloodstream and through the first layers of the intima to arrive to it.[70] This observation suggests the molecules come from the outer layers of the arteries.

In his publications on the topic, Dr. Vladimir Subbotin at the University of Pittsburgh described how atherosclerosis can develop from the outside in.[71] When the inner layer of the artery is damaged due to breakdown of EZ water from oxidative stress, the artery starts growing more cells in the intimal layer. This growth of the intimal layer causes the arteries of the vasa vasorum to grow new arteries from the adventitia into the deeper layers of the artery. Since these new arteries are going through stages of development, they are fenestrated—they have holes in them. The holes cause some molecules to leak into the tissue. Since these arteries are coming from the outer layer to the inner layers, it's no surprise that researchers have observed atherosclerosis starting in the outermost area of the intima layer. This process also explains why the vasa vasorum are more numerous and developed in atherosclerotic arteries; they have to be in order to penetrate deeper into the artery wall.

So, while there may be agreement on the *cause* of atherosclerosis—damage to the inner lining from oxidative stress—the *mechanism* is up for debate. One thing is clear, however: Atherosclerosis is much more complex than we've been led to believe, and much more is required to assess heart health than simply looking at a lipid panel. LDL has been a giant distraction to the real causes of atherosclerosis, and this distraction has been a major disservice to public health. LDL is still relevant, just not in the way we've been told. LDL molecules may actually be protective, since lipoproteins, such as LDL and HDL, neutralize endotoxins.[72] There is evidence that cholesterol has a role as an antioxidant, and could even be directly protective against atherosclerosis.[73]

Dr. Stephanie Seneff, a senior research scientist at MIT, has proposed that the molecule cholesterol sulfate is essential to all cells, especially those in the heart. That's correct: She's proposing that cholesterol is essential for heart health. She argues that when the body is unable to synthesize cholesterol sulfate, the body stores cholesterol in the lining of the arteries so that it can readily become cholesterol sulfate when sulfur-providing molecules such as homocysteine or cysteinylglycine float by in the bloodstream.

Let's dig a little deeper. Normally, cholesterol sulfate is synthesized in skin cells (keratinocytes), red blood cells, and platelets in the skin. This synthesis is dependent on sunlight exposure. Research shows that places with sunnier climates have lower rates of heart disease.[74] It has been thought that this finding was due to higher rates of vitamin D, and yet studies have also shown that supplementing with vitamin D has no effect on rates of heart disease.[75] What explains this discrepancy? Supplementing with vitamin D doesn't give us the sunlight exposure to catalyze the synthesis of cholesterol sulfate—and cholesterol sulfate is the bigger player when it comes to atherosclerosis.

When cholesterol, sulfur, and sunlight are all present in the skin, the enzyme nitric oxide synthase (eNOS) creates cholesterol sulfate.[76] Dr. Seneff hypothesizes that heavy metals, including in sunscreens, and toxins such as the herbicide glyphosate, the active ingredient in the common herbicide Roundup, disrupt this enzyme, interfering with the creation of cholesterol sulfate, resulting in a shortage of cholesterol sulfate in the body.[77]

A few things happen with a shortage of cholesterol sulfate. Since cholesterol sulfate is water soluble, it can travel through the bloodstream without the help of a lipoprotein like LDL. However, if cholesterol sulfate synthesis is impaired, the body's capacity to deliver cholesterol via the bloodstream is also impaired. In this case, the body will increase production of LDL so that fat-soluble cholesterol can be carried to the cells by LDL instead. This process can result in the "dreaded" rise in LDL cholesterol.

Deficiency in cholesterol sulfate can also force the body to obtain it in other ways, including the development of atherosclerosis—because with cholesterol stored in the artery wall it provides quick access to the raw materials to create cholesterol sulfate. As Dr. Seneff explains, "As an alternative means of supplying cholesterol sulfate to the heart, an atheroma is uniquely suited to cholesterol sulfate's manufacture by platelets. The sulfate is supplied by breaking down homocysteine thiolactone, a precursor that is ready to become sulfate under the right circumstances; the lipid stores in the macrophages supply the cholesterol; the red blood cells supply adenosine triphosphate (ATP) to energize the reaction; and the inflammatory response provides superoxide needed to oxidize the sulfur atom in homocysteine."[78]

Dr Seneff's theory suggests that the body will go to great lengths to ensure it has a sufficient supply of cholesterol sulfate. All cells need cholesterol sulfate to maintain health and blood supply, but the heart is such a vitally important organ that this could even explain why the coronary arteries of the heart seem to be so prone to atherosclerosis. Atherosclerosis may be, unfortunately, *necessary* to ensure cholesterol sulfate is provided to the heart in the absence of normal cholesterol sulfate synthesis. There is also evidence that, in the absence of cholesterol sulfate, the body may activate the normally dormant bacteria *Chlamydia pneumoniae* to supply heparin sulfate for the synthesis of cholesterol sulfate. The body may also induce ischemia—reduced blood flow—in the heart to release the amino acid taurine, which can supply sulfur for the formation of cholesterol sulfate.[79] I don't think I need to explain what can happen when the heart doesn't get enough blood.

If Dr. Seneff's theory is correct, our bodies take dramatic steps—such as inducing atherosclerosis, activating dormant bacteria, and inducing ischemia—in order to ensure sufficient production of cholesterol sulfate. When we suppress the synthesis of cholesterol sulfate with statins, inadequate dietary sulfur, having toxic heavy-metal exposure, and inadequate amounts of sunlight, we may be forcing the body into mitigation steps to maintain adequate cholesterol sulfate.

Why does the body go to such lengths to synthesize this molecule? Cholesterol sulfate is an important component of cell membranes, providing stability that protects them from collapsing on themselves. In addition, the cholesterol sulfate molecule has properties that help structure water, which helps keep blood moving and delivering nutrients.[80] Stabilizing cells so they don't die and ensuring the delivery of nutrients are important jobs, and this significance suggests why our bodies might go to such lengths to ensure adequate levels of cholesterol sulfate.

Regardless of why we develop atherosclerosis, the accepted cause for concern about it is that it will build up in coronary arteries, or a piece will break off, and it will restrict blood flow to an area of the heart and cause a heart attack. Atherosclerosis is clearly not a "good" thing, but in chapter 8, we will see just how relevant it is when it comes to assessing the risk of heart attacks.

CHAPTER 8

The Three Imbalances
of a Heart Attack

One summer when I was in middle school, my grandmother took my cousin, Luke, and I to the Outer Banks of North Carolina. Before we left, my grandfather had a surprise for us. Their next-door neighbor, Wayne, was a pilot who owned a small plane and had offered to take us up in it for a ride the day before we left. Luke and I were excited. Wayne even told us we could take turns sitting up front as his copilot. Since he had a stop to make en route, I would sit up front on the first leg of the journey and Luke would sit up front on the way back. My grandfather came along for the ride, while my grandmother busied herself at home packing for the trip.

When Wayne switched control over to me, I gently turned the plane and went up and down. He showed me which dial on the plane indicated if we were flying level to the ground, and he told me to try to fly the plane level by keeping that dial on zero; it was harder than it sounds. When it was Luke's turn, he had a little more fun with it. His turns were a little less gentle, and he liked making the plane go up and down pretty quick. Wayne told him to take it easy. "Okay everyone ready for the barrel roll?," Luke asked through the headset. My grandfather interjected: "Quit it son, you're gonna give me a heart attack!" We made it back to the airport safe and sound, drove back to my grandparents' house, and got ready to leave for the Outer Banks the next morning.

When we arrived at our hotel, Luke and I made a beeline for the indoor pool and hot tub, where my risk-loving cousin said he could breathe the air bubbles coming from the hot tub and stay underwater forever. Of course, you can't really do this, but that didn't stop him. On his third attempt, he stayed down for quite a while. "Where is he?" my grandmother asked, finally. I shrugged my shoulders. She walked over to the hot tub from where she was sitting nearby, looked down into the water, then rolled up her sleeve, reached into the water, and grabbed Luke by the hair, pulling him out of the water. He came up half laughing from the ruse and half screaming from the hair pulling. "You stop doing this or you're going to give me a heart attack!" my grandmother scolded, bitterly.

It's an interesting choice of words if you think about it. We are told that heart attacks are caused by the buildup of plaque in the arteries that restricts blood flow, so does being stressed or suddenly scared induce such sudden buildup? I suppose if an artery was partially blocked by plaque, a sudden stress could restrict blood vessels and blood flow enough to cause a heart attack, but that's uncommon. So why do we talk about "giving someone a heart attack" and what are the origins of that association between a sudden stressor and a heart attack? Because a sudden stress *can* induce a heart attack. There are potential mechanisms that can create this regardless of amount of plaque buildup in the coronary arteries.

Questionable Practices

Most everyone knows "the story" of how a heart attack happens. Something blocks an artery and prevents blood flow (ischemia), resulting in tissue death. That blockage can be an acute blockage (like the one that I had) where a clot forms and gets stuck, preventing blood flow. Or it can be a gradual buildup of atherosclerosis creating stenosis, or narrowing, of the area blood is supposed to move through. But is this the only way we can develop ischemia in heart tissue? Is this the cause of all heart attacks?

Western medicine's approach to heart attack prevention is to decrease the cause of atherosclerotic buildup with low-fat diets and cholesterol-lowering medications. Once a stenosis is present, doctors will use stents, and if it is severe enough, bypass surgeries to give blood a path around stenosis. With stent placement, doctors first perform an angioplasty to open up an area of narrowed artery and then place a wire mesh in the artery to keep it open. These can be lifesaving in acute blockage situations like my heart attack and have been shown to effectively restore blood flow to larger arteries of the heart. However, as a preventative technique in elective, nonacute situations, there's debate as to whether stents can prevent heart attacks or not; they are mostly used to relieve angina and chest pain.

Restoring blood flow to the large arteries, while a good outcome, may not be the most important step to preventing a heart attack. In a study that compared 901 patients with heart disease, 642 of them were treated with only medication and 259 were treated with the same medication plus a stent placement procedure. Researchers found that, regardless of treatment, probability of a cardiac event continued to rise for the next twelve years of follow-up. They also found that "there were no differences in long-term mortality or the composite of all-cause mortality or cardiovascular hospitalization between patients treated with medical therapy alone compared with medical therapy plus PCI [stent]."[1] A similar study of 2,287 patients concluded that stents "did not reduce the risk of death, myocardial infarction, or other major cardiovascular events when added to optimal medical therapy."[2] Summarizing the effectiveness of stent procedures in a research article, Dr. Aseem Malhotra stated, "The elephant in the room is that randomized studies (including patients at low risk and high risk) have not demonstrated outcomes benefit for stenting stable coronary disease in addition to optimal medical therapy despite its widespread use."[3] If narrowing of an artery causes heart attacks, we would expect better outcomes from a procedure that corrects the narrowing.

There is another approach: bypassing, or creating a route around, the area of an artery with stenosis. The first coronary artery bypass surgery was conducted in 1960, and the surgery became common practice shortly after. By the late 1970s, researchers were studying the outcomes after ten years of bypass surgery on 100 thousand patients. They concluded, "The relief of symptoms experienced directly following bypass surgery does not necessarily last. The current data do not indicate that bypass surgery prevents heart attacks, heart rhythm problems (arrhythmias), or the development of heart weakness. The lives of the majority of patients are not prolonged."[4]

But this was 1977—surely over time the results of these procedures would improve, right? In 1984 the Coronary Artery Surgery Study looked at eight hundred patients with coronary artery disease who either underwent bypass surgery or were treated with medication alone. They found that after five years, the number of people who were still alive and had not suffered a heart attack was nearly the same in each group (82 percent and 83 percent). After ten years, there was no difference between the two groups. In other words, the study found that bypass surgery neither prolonged life nor prevented further heart attacks.[5]

What about more recent analyses? A report issued by the Mayo Clinic in 2003 concluded that bypass surgery does not prevent future heart attacks and that only high-risk patients experienced an increased rate of survival. Only one in forty-three operations saved a life long term.[6] Lastly, a study from 2011 that took data from 127 clinical sites in twenty-seven countries and followed patients for five years after bypass plus medication or medication alone found that "there was no significant difference between the two study groups with respect to the primary end point of the rate of death from any cause."[7]

If heart attacks are caused by a narrowing of an artery, then why aren't these procedures that restore blood flow and correct the narrowing, or bypass it altogether, working to prevent heart attacks? More concerning, if analyses of these procedures reveals they don't work, why are they still being performed at such high rates? The bottom line is that lowering cholesterol and opening or bypassing blockages has not improved death rates from heart disease.

According to a 2016 report from the CDC, the number of deaths from heart disease per year since 1950 consistently rose until 1985, when it peaked at nearly 800 thousand. From 1985 until 2011, the number dropped, but since 2011 deaths per year have been rising again.[8] Could it be that the rates continue to rise not only because the dietary advice on preventing heart disease is wrong but also because we are treating the problem once it occurs the wrong way as well?

Baroldi

Around the same time that fat and cholesterol became public enemy number one in the 1950s, the career of an extraordinary Italian coronary artery pathologist named Giorgio Baroldi was just getting started. Dr. Baroldi was fascinated by the heart's arteries and interested in the cause of heart attacks. His research consisted of conducting heart autopsies, including on people who died of heart attacks and those who did not. He also introduced the use of plastic casting of arterial systems to study the arteries after death. At the end of his career, Baroldi was seen as a heretic, however. His work largely contradicted the stenosis or blockage theory of heart attacks, and he was very outspoken about it.

In his most notable study, Baroldi autopsied 305 people: All had neither prior symptoms nor diagnosis of heart disease, but 208 died of sudden heart attacks and 97 died in accidents. He found that of the 208 who died of heart attacks, 28 had minimal to no stenosis (<50 percent narrowing), 23 had moderate stenosis, and 157—about 75 percent—had severe stenosis (>70 percent narrowing). In only 32 cases (15.3 percent) of the people who died of heart attacks did he find evidence of an acute blood clot. Even more interesting is that of the 97 who died in an accident, 28 had minimal to no stenosis, 31 had moderate stenosis, and 38—about 40 percent—had severe stenosis.[9] This data shows that while acute blockages do cause heart attacks, there are times when someone dies of a heart attack despite little to no stenosis or blockage and times when someone has severe stenosis and no heart disease symptoms. Some of Baroldi's earlier work showed us that even severe stenosis may not lead to heart attacks.

I mentioned before that Baroldi was known for using plastic casting to study heart arterial systems. He did this by injecting a latex or neoprene material into the arterial system of the heart after he removed it during autopsy. He filled the entire arterial system and then set it aside and waited for the material to dry in the arteries. Once it had dried, he dissolved away the heart tissue with hydrochloric acid. He was left with a perfect cast of the arterial system. He found that there was a vast network of what he called collateral arteries in addition to the larger arteries and microcirculation that he already knew were there.

What he found in areas of severe atherosclerosis is interesting. The network of collaterals in areas of severe stenosis was dramatically high. Anywhere an artery was 70 percent or more occluded (blocked), he found a dramatic increase in the length and diameter of collateral arteries that would have fully compensated the area with blood. He found that the amount of collaterals varied from five to thirty-three vessels depending on the degree of stenosis.[10]

I have been told by cardiologists that while they know collateral arteries exist, they feel that there is no way that these arteries can form in enough time to adequately compensate the heart tissue in the case of rapidly progressing atherosclerosis. Researchers, however, have tested this. In one study done in dogs, researchers induced a coronary occlusion over seven days and found that the collateral blood vessels grew fast enough to prevent ischemia, or insufficient blood supply.[11] Another study, also in dogs, showed the same result when a total occlusion was artificially produced over four days.[12]

What does all this mean? First, I think it provides a lot of clarity as to why stents and bypass surgeries haven't been more effective at prolonging life and preventing heart attacks. Baroldi showed that the body is capable of compensating for the narrowing of an artery by building collaterals. Opening up a stenotic blood vessel or bypassing the stenotic area is likely to have little to no effect because the body already has it under control.

Second, this tells us that heart attacks can happen without a blockage. Clearly Baroldi showed that an acute clot formation can block an artery, causing ischemia, but he found it only in 15.3 percent of 208 heart attack victims. That number is a small sample, but thanks to Baroldi's work, we know that there are cases where there was no atherosclerosis or acute blockage, yet the person died of a heart attack with evidence of ischemia in the heart tissue. And in cases of severe stenosis but no acute blockage, the body has prevented ischemia by creating a vast network of collateral arteries. This begs the question, what causes a heart attack without a blockage of a blood vessel? We also see obstruction of the blood in other places in the body, such as the kidney and brain, but it is rare in the kidney.[13] There seems to be something unique about the heart and brain that makes ischemia happen more often in them.

The Three Imbalances

In part 1, we went through the history of life on Earth, including human history and how we arrived at the current, but incorrect, medical understanding of heart disease. We discussed multiple species that evolved the ability to survive in low-oxygen environments through various physiologic adaptations that prevent hypoxia (low oxygen). In a way, hypoxia is the same as ischemia (inadequate blood supply); so why do we see ischemia in humans when evolution has protected other species through evolved adaptations?

I believe evolution has protected us from ischemia, to an extent, with our organs' preference for burning fatty acids and ketones for fuel. However, there is no way that evolution could have evolved mechanisms to protect us from the rapidly changing environment that has taken us from nomadic hunter gatherers all the way up to modern-day society in less than fifteen thousand years (an evolutionary blink of the eye). The rapid changes we have experienced have led us to develop many imbalances between our evolved physiology and the modern way of life. The combination of these imbalances has contributed to the development of ischemia in our heart tissue, creating the conditions for a heart attack.

To understand how heart tissues can develop ischemia without a blockage, we first need to understand the imbalances in the body that set us up for this and other chronic diseases. Those imbalances are threefold: (1) the inability to readily burn fat for fuel, (2) an excess of free radicals that leads to oxidative stress, and (3) an imbalance in the stress response of our ANS.

Imbalance 1: Metabolic Inflexibility

When our bodies become metabolically inflexible, they are unable to readily burn fat for fuel. Normally, we have the ability to burn a few different nutrients to make energy, including protein, fat, and carbohydrates. However, just because we *can* burn all three doesn't mean we should. Since carbohydrates are easy to burn, our bodies will burn them first when they are present; this is called oxidative priority. All good, right? Not exactly. Burning primarily carbohydrates can be a fast track to poor health, because it results in excess production of free radicals. Our other options are fat and protein. Protein is only relied upon for energy if we are in starvation, so that leaves fat. Our bodies are more efficient when we burn fat. To do this, we need to limit our carbohydrates, especially processed ones, so that our bodies can relearn to burn fat and the ketones made by fat.

Compared to the rest of the body, the heart seems to have a special preference for fatty acids and ketones. The heart is always utilizing some glucose, some fatty acids, and some ketones, but changing the levels of ketones in the heart seems to regulate which fuel the heart will preferentially burn. In one experiment, if ketone levels were dropped below 34 mg per 100 ml, the heart had to burn more glucose, but if they got the levels up to between 34 and 80 mg per 100 ml, the heart switched over to burning primarily ketones.[14] Supplying the heart tissue with more ketones has been shown to result in a

30–60 percent reduction in use of other fuel sources.[15] This suggests that the heart prefers ketones as a fuel source.

The body even has mechanisms to ensure this happens. One mechanism is that the fat we eat is packaged into chylomicrons and then delivered more or less directly to the heart by way of the lymphatic system; this delivery system gives the heart first dibs on the fat before it can be used by other tissues. Another mechanism is that the heart has a signaling pathway that allows it to communicate directly to fat cells.[16] Even though our hearts are special in this way, if we don't ensure our bodies can burn fat and therefore make adequate ketones for heart tissue, we are predisposing ourselves to the possibility of a heart attack. This is especially true when the other imbalances I discuss below develop as well.

The thing to remember from this first imbalance is that the heart prefers to burn ketones. To provide it with this preferred fuel source, we have to restrict carbohydrates enough to avoid metabolic inflexibility so the body will learn to burn fat and make ketones. If this doesn't happen the heart is likely to burn more glucose. I believe heart attacks without a blockage happen when a series of events take place that force the heart to burn predominantly glucose for fuel; metabolic inflexibility makes this more likely to happen.

Imbalance 2: Oxidative Stress

Every time the human body makes energy from a protein, fat, or carbohydrate, it makes a waste product called a free radical. Burning primarily carbohydrates (glucose) for fuel produces more of these free radicals than if we were to burn fats for fuel. Having too many free radicals can damage our bodies, including the lining of our arteries. Other things that can contribute to excess free radicals include elevated blood sugar (from developing insulin resistance), endotoxemia, and excess exposure to toxins in our environment. This overload can lead us to a state of oxidative stress, in which there are more free radicals than our bodies can handle.

When it comes to how this imbalance can lead to ischemia and a heart attack without a blockage, it's important to remember that oxidative stress can deplete nitric oxide (NO) when excessive free radicals damage the arterial linings where NO is made. Also, because NO can act as an antioxidant, it gets depleted in the battle against too many free radicals (oxidative stress).

This has been shown to be true when processed carbohydrates in the diet burden the body with excessive free radicals.[17]

Imbalance 3: Imbalanced Stress Response

The third imbalance is a dysfunctional stress response in our ANS. This is the system that allows the human body to sense if our current environment is safe or threatening. Our evolved acute stress response is supposed to work by being activated only when it needs to be, such as when our life is in danger (see chapter 2). However, because of the mismatch between the evolution of our stress response and our modern environment, our stress response can become imbalanced. Instead of going back and forth between a stress response and a nonstress state, we can get stuck in a stress response that causes our bodies to be on constant high alert.

Dr. Robert Sapolsky, who has spent his life studying the difference between the stress response of mammals in their natural environment compared to the stress response of humans in the modern world, stated in his book *Behave*: "Mobilizing energy while sprinting for your life helps save you. Do the same thing chronically because of a stressful thirty-year mortgage, and you're at risk for various metabolic problems, including adult-onset diabetes."[18] This perpetual state of high alert can alter the signaling of our ANS. Our ANS is always supposed to send a balanced signal to our heart cells. If this balance is interrupted, it can trigger a series of events that can lead to a heart attack.

Our ANS consists of two parts. There is the "rest and digest," or parasympathetic nervous system (PNS), which is more active in a nonstress situation. And there is the "fight or flight," or sympathetic nervous system (SNS), reserved for those times when a stress response is necessary to get us away from a threat. These two states should be in balance, and a surge in one normally includes a lesser surge in the other.[19] The signal for this system is conducted through the vagus nerve. Many believe this nerve only communicates to the right atrium, where the heart's pacing signal is received from the nervous system. However, research has shown that this nerve reaches all areas of the heart and can therefore affect the whole heart.[20] While there is a combination of factors that have to happen for a heart attack without a blockage to occur, when this system gets out of balance it is one important aspect that can trigger the event.

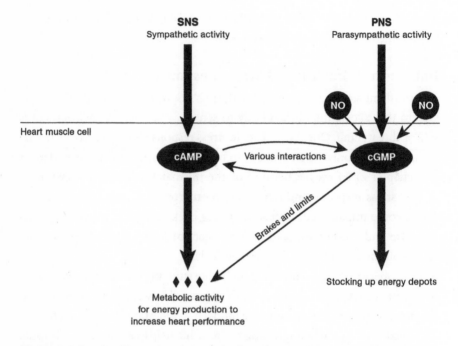

Figure 8.1. In a healthy autonomic nervous system, cAMP and cGMP keep each other in check. NO (nitric oxide) is needed to signal cGMP.

This next part gets a bit technical, so bear with me. Balance of the ANS in cardiac cells, and many other cells, relies on two messenger molecules called cAMP and cGMP. cAMP levels rise in the heart cells when we have a stressful response, and cGMP levels rise when we are in a relaxation state. The only difference is that when it comes to cGMP, the relaxation molecule, something else is also needed: nitric oxide.[21] NO is produced in the cells of the walls of arteries called endothelia. These two molecules—cAMP and cGMP—keep each other in check within heart cells. When we experience a stressful response and the nervous system causes spikes in cAMP, then cGMP, provided there is enough NO, also has an increase to keep the system in balance.[22] This is depicted in figure 8.1.

But the system can become unbalanced. When we have increased levels of cAMP due to prolonged periods of stress and, at the same time, not enough stimulation of the relaxation response, we can lose the ability to move between these two states; in other words, we get stuck in our stress state. This is called decreased vagal tone, because the vagus nerve carries this specific signal.

The best measure of balance in our stress response is heart rate variability (HRV). The higher your HRV the more balanced you are. To show you the significance of HRV—and therefore of the ANS balance in heart attacks— one study of HRV in people who later had heart attacks found that "the vast majority (95%) of transient myocardial ischemic events in our study is preceded by an almost complete suppression of HRV."[23] Another study that measured HRV before and after myocardial ischemic events in 110 adults concluded that "the gradual shift in balance before the onset of the ischemic event, suggests the hypothesis that this is probably a causal factor and not a consequence of myocardial ischemia."[24] This means that through HRV, changes in our stress response are detected prior to a heart attack and play a role in the cause of it.

Imbalances in stress response have been shown to have negative effects on the heart and cardiovascular system.[25] When this happens, the failsafe within the cardiac cells is that the consistently high levels of cAMP are balanced by also rising levels of cGMP. But remember that cGMP can only rise if nitric oxide is present. If NO gets depleted, it is really bad news. Having elevated free radicals, or oxidative stress, can deplete our NO.[26] Remember, free radicals are molecules with an unpaired electron, and they do not like to be unpaired. One place they can find another electron is NO.[27] This decreases the NO available for cGMP stimulation.

How do these imbalances come together to directly cause a heart attack? Let's say that someone is living life with a high-stress job and is so consumed by that job that there is just no time to care about eating for optimal health and avoiding toxins. This is unfortunately the case for many people in our fast-paced world. Combined with aging, it is the scenario that predisposes us to many diseases, but especially a heart attack.

The Main Event

Now that we have set the stage, it is time for the main event. When humans experience long-term, decreased vagal tone from a stress state on overdrive paired with decreases in NO due to free-radical overload, a sudden surge in stress response can create an elevation in cAMP in our heart cells without the balanced rise in cGMP.[28] This situation is shown in figure 8.2.

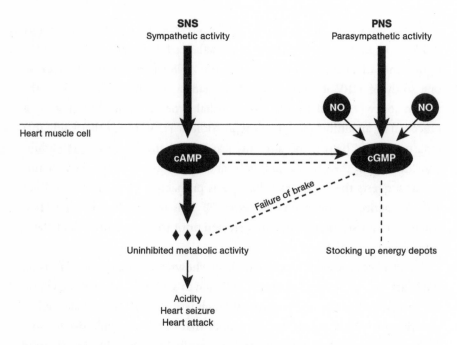

Figure 8.2. A surge in stress response elevates cAMP in our heart cells without the balanced rise of cGMP, leading to heart attack.

When this happens, the cascade of events known as a heart attack plays out. A sudden unchecked rise in cAMP has been shown to cause an increase in lactic acid production within cardiac cells.[29] This increase happens because the heart usually prefers to burn fatty acids and ketones. But in a stress-response situation, the body thinks it needs to burn energy more quickly, and goes to the faster-burning option: glucose.[30] Burning glucose causes the buildup of lactic acid and hydrogen ions within the heart cells, creating a state of acidity. Studies have shown that the production of lactic acid increases by a factor of eight in this situation, and that no change in oxygen levels is seen during these events.[31] No change in oxygen means blood flow has not been restricted; rather, the body has shifted its metabolic mechanisms, resulting in this acidity. The response is similar when you do a sprint or a hard, fast workout: Your muscles get a stress signal and start burning more glycogen (stored glucose) and lactic acid builds up in the muscles and produces a burning feeling, but oxygen levels are not affected. During intense exercise, if the burn in our arms or legs gets severe, we simply stop moving the affected muscles; the lactic acid will move along, and we'll feel relief from that burning. The heart muscle, of course, cannot simply stop contracting.

When we have this increased metabolism to an area, we will also have increased waste products. These waste products (carbon dioxide, hydrogen ions, and lactate) need to be evacuated in a timely manner. However, when too many are present it can result in the dilation of blood vessels, which slows blood flow and can cause a swelling of "dirty" blood in the area. This blood is low in oxygen, which forces the area into anaerobic glycolysis. Since anaerobic glycolysis is less efficient and produces more waste products than oxidative phosphorylation, the tissue is unable to maintain proper physiologic function.[32] It makes sense that the most metabolically active organs—the kidney, brain, and heart—are also the most common locations of infarction: renal infarction, stroke, and heart attack.[33]

In an imbalanced stress response, the presence of lactic acid in heart tissue prevents calcium from being able to bind to muscle fibers to create contraction of heart muscle.[34] Low calcium in heart cells results in slower conduction velocity (the speed of the electrochemical impulse that contracts the heart muscle) and elevated arrhythmia risk.[35] This situation eventually leads to decreased muscle tension and contractility, which then causes a stretching of the wall of the heart that leads to increased pressure. This increased pressure prevents blood from getting to the tissue, creating ischemia, and the blood instead stagnates, becoming oxygen and nutrient depleted.[36] The lack of new blood quickly results in tissue death—a.k.a. a heart attack—before any drop in oxygen is seen in heart tissue.

Other Observations Explained

This "metabolic theory of heart attacks" also explains related trends and statistics on heart attacks, including the fact that heart attacks are more prevalent on stressful days of the year, including Mondays.[37] When someone is already imbalanced, a stressful experience can be enough to trigger the events described above. A study that followed heart disease patients for six months after they were released from the hospital found that psychological stress was the number one predictor of future events, including cardiac death, cardiac arrest, and heart attack.[38] Heart disease patients also tend to have a more difficult time—and in fact are more likely to die—in winter, which makes it no surprise that we see lower HRV during the winter, most likely due to decreased exposure to sun and the outdoors in the winter months.[39]

And while heart attacks are seen across many age groups, they are most prevalent among the elderly, as heart cells become less efficient at burning fat and ketones for fuel; because older people have had more time to be exposed to toxins that contribute to oxidative stress; and even due to the social isolation many elderly people experience.[40] Heart rate variability also declines naturally as we age.[41] It is also known that men suffer from heart attacks more than women. It's possible this is partly because women tend to have a healthier vagus nerve, which is stimulated by menstrual cycles, creating healthy HRV.[42] Perhaps men suffer from heart attacks earlier in life than women do because women experience the "protective" effect of a monthly parasympathetic stimulation, balancing their HRV until after menopause.[43]

Certain heart disease drugs have been shown to prevent a heart attack, even though they are not specifically designed for that purpose. Beta-blockers, for example, are probably useful because they have a desirable effect on HRV.[44] The same goes for ACE inhibitors.[45] And nitroglycerin tablets are sometimes used to treat angina because they are thought to dilate the blood vessels, restore blood flow, and provide relief. Since blocked arteries are compensated by collateral arteries and blood flow is not actually compromised, however, perhaps the relief provided by nitroglycerin is due to its restoration of NO levels. Decreased NO will lead to dysfunctional signaling of the ANS in heart cells via cGMP. Nitroglycerin increases the expression of cGMP in tissues, which allows for balanced ANS signaling to the heart.[46]

Finally, we also know that nearly 100 percent of heart attacks happen in the left ventricle, which is supplied mainly by one artery, the left anterior descending artery. This is curious because severe stenosis and clots occur evenly among the vessels supplying all areas of the heart.[47] The left ventricle is under the most pressure, making it more susceptible to fluctuations in pressure caused by the stretching and decreased contractility that happens once lactic acid builds up and interferes with calcium. This metabolic theory of heart attacks also explains why oxygen usage of the heart muscle remains largely unchanged during some heart attacks. With a blockage, you would think that oxygen levels would drop, instead of remaining unchanged, but studies have shown that a shift in metabolism after the stimulation of a stress response in heart cells can lead to the events described above without any effect on oxygen consumption in heart cells.[48]

While this metabolic theory of heart attacks, in which there is no blockage, can help explain some of the common observations seen in heart attacks, events like mine where a clot forms, blocking blood flow, do happen often. However, chronic stress, like I was experiencing prior to my event, can lead to an imbalanced stress response and can be just as much of a contributor in these cases. One review paper looked at all the evidence on stress and clot formation. The researchers concluded that "catecholamine surge [acute stress] may trigger a hypercoagulable state and enhance the odds of overt thrombosis in patients with atherosclerotic disease."[49]

Another research article discussed the many triggers of transient myocardial ischemia and plaque rupture. It drew particular attention to the patterns seen in transient myocardial ischemia that seem to follow circadian rhythm. An imbalanced circadian rhythm can be caused by an imbalance in the signaling of our ANS. The author concluded that "these concordant temporal patterns of transient ischemia, myocardial infarction and sudden cardiac death probably represent independent manifestations stemming from the consequences of increased sympathetic activity."[50]

One final study, though done in mice, showed more direct evidence of what could have possibly caused my event, and it seems more relevant to what I was going through as well. In this study, researchers put mice through twenty hours of "restraint stress" and then assessed the potential of arterial thrombus formation. They found that the mice exposed to the stress "displayed an increased arterial prothrombotic potential" compared to mice not put through the stress, and that this was due to an increase in blood-borne tissue factor. Further, when they chemically inhibited the SNS, the observed increased prothrombic potential disappeared.[51]

Atrial Fibrillation

Atrial fibrillation, or Afib, is an irregular and often rapid heartbeat, causing the atria of the heart to contract in a chaotic fashion. It can cause palpitations, weakness, inability to exercise, fatigue, lightheadedness, dizziness, shortness of breath, and chest pain. It can be occasional, which is called paroxysmal atrial fibrillation, or it can be more frequent and persistent; it can even occur in someone constantly. It has been estimated that by the year 2030, 12.1 million people in the United States will have Afib.[52] In 2018, Afib was mentioned on 175,326 death certificates and was the underlying cause of death in 25,845 of those deaths.[53] It is a growing concern.

When looking for a cause of this condition, it makes sense to start with the nervous system because the conduction of the heartbeat is controlled by two signals from the nervous system to the right atria of the heart. The sinoatrial (SA) node is known as the pacemaker of the heart and the atrioventricular (AV) node is known as the pacesetter of the heart. One can imagine that if the signal to the heart from the ANS is imbalanced, the heart could be getting confused, mixed, or wrong signals on how to contract. The research backs this up nicely. In studies done on patients with paroxysmal Afib, one study found that stimulation of the vagus nerve through the skin "suppresses AF [Afib] and decreases inflammatory cytokines."[54] A similar study found 85 percent less Afib burden in the treatment group than the control.[55] There are various medical interventions that can stimulate the vagus nerve with a therapeutic effect on Afib, although too much artificial stimulation can be causative in Afib.[56] For this reason, my favorite ways to balance the ANS are not the medical interventions but a more natural approach (see chapter 13).

However, there is more to the story of Afib than the ANS signaling to the heart. Alterations in metabolism that change fuel sources result in greater production of oxidative stress in cardiac tissue.[57] In fact, I believe that many of the imbalances we see in heart attacks without a blockage are also in play in Afib, to a lesser degree. These imbalances can also be complicated by nutrient deficiencies, including magnesium.[58] In fact, I believe that being metabolically inflexible, having high oxidative stress, and having imbalances in our stress response, especially when complicated by nutrient deficiencies, are the underlying causes of most all chronic disease. Becoming familiar with these imbalances allows us to understand how best to prevent heart disease and create a thriving, healthy heart.

CHAPTER 9

How the Heart Evades Cancer

One Saturday when I was a kid, my cousin, Luke, and I were hanging out at my house. Usually we were outside throwing a ball around, but this day it was raining, so we were inside and restless. We came across one of my mom's cookbooks in the kitchen and started looking through it when we stumbled upon a recipe for peppermint taffy. We scoured the cupboards for the ingredients.

We had everything we needed . . . sort of. The recipe called for white sugar, cornstarch, corn syrup, water, butter, salt, and peppermint. We had everything except for the corn syrup and peppermint, and not quite enough sugar. So naturally we found some replacements. We did have regular syrup, so we used that instead of corn syrup, and we used a candy cane left over from Christmas instead of the peppermint. To make up for the shortage of granulated sugar, we added some powdered sugar. This still wasn't enough sugar, until we found a package of Jell-O mix with sugar in it. We were all set.

We carefully followed the directions by mixing the ingredients into a pot and bringing it to a slow boil. At this point, we decided we wanted the taffy to be green, so we added in some food coloring. The mixture turned bright green, and we were pleased, until it continued to boil and turned a light shade of brown. We decided brown taffy would be fine.

We poured the liquid out into a pan to cool, but impatience got the better of us and we put our creation in the refrigerator. By then the rain had stopped so our next move was obvious: go out and play basketball. After about two hours, we went inside and once again got so excited to bite into the chewy sweetness. Instead, we were greeted by wiggly brown Jell-O. To our dismay, it tasted burnt, and after a few bites, we threw it out.

To this day, I look back on that memory and laugh at how far our results were from peppermint taffy. Of all the things we did wrong, it was probably the Jell-O packet that had the most impact. This is because the Jell-O contains gelatin and when it's combined with water and heated, gelatin forms a gel. A gel is very different from the chewy taffy we were attempting to make! But as it turns out, the body makes gel in a similar way, with the fourth phase water in the lining of our arteries. This process also happens in cells, which is significant because it explains why cancer of the heart is so rare.

A Rare Disease

When trying to fully understand an organ, it is important to understand all the pathologies it develops. It is equally important to understand the pathologies the organ resists, and when it comes to the heart, it seems to enjoy protection against a disease that decimates so many other organs: cancer. Heart cancer does occur, but it is among the rarest forms of cancer.

According to Dr. Timothy Moynihan of the Mayo Clinic, the majority of heart tumors are benign. Even then they are rare. In fact, the Mayo Clinic sees, on average, only one case of heart cancer each year, and among more than twelve thousand autopsies only seven cases of primary cardiac tumor were found.[1] Dr. Robert Cusimano, a cardiac surgeon at the Peter Munk Cardiac Centre in Toronto, also confirms that the majority of heart tumors are benign. When a malignant tumor does occur in the heart, it is often due to metastasis of primary tumors from other nearby organs such as the kidneys or lungs. Even Dr. Cusimano, who often gets referred heart cancer patients, only sees around twelve heart tumors a year.[2] Primary cardiac tumors are 0.3–0.7 percent of all cardiac tumors, meaning it is very rare for a tumor to originate in the heart; metastasis from other primary cancers are thirty times more common. While heart cancer is rare, it does have a very poor prognosis when it is malignant. Without surgical resection, the survival rate at nine to twelve months is only 10 percent.[3]

Cancer is a disease that affects more and more people every year. Yet as cancer rates grow, the heart continues to be the least affected. To understand why, we first have to understand cancer, and how wrong the approach to cancer has been for the last fifty years.

Cancer as a Metabolic Disease

The prevailing theory about cancer is that mutations in our DNA trigger a healthy cell to become a rapidly dividing cancer cell. There is a belief that with enough research, scientists will discover so-called cancer genes and we can prevent cancer. However, epigenetics—when genes alter their expression based on their environment—has put a wrench in the genetic theory of cancer. While you may have genetic predisposition to a certain disease, whether or not your genes express in a disease-creating way is dependent on the environment, including food, toxins, and stress, that your body is exposed to.

In one set of experiments, researchers took cancer cells and healthy cells and switched their DNA through transplantation. That is, they took DNA from the nucleus of cancer cells and put it into the nucleus of healthy cells and vice versa. You would expect that transplanting DNA from cancer cells into healthy ones would cause those healthy cells to become cancerous, but that's not what happened. Instead, when the cells with transplanted cancer DNA divided, they were healthy. This fascinating research also demonstrated that when cancer cells received noncancerous DNA into their nucleus, the cells remained cancerous when they divided.[4] What does this suggest? Cancer is driven by events in the cytoplasm (the environment), not by events in the DNA.

The explanation for this is known as the metabolic theory of cancer and was first proposed by Nobel Laureate Dr. Otto Warburg in 1924, and more recently researched by Dr. Thomas Seyfried, a professor of biology at Boston College. The metabolic theory of cancer posits that the metabolic health of the *mitochondria* determines whether a cell will become cancerous. I mentioned in chapter 1 how cells become cancerous once they lose mitochondrial health and stop using oxygen, but numerous research studies have also shown that the mitochondria in cancer cells are reduced in number, size, and shape.[5] Changes of this nature have been highly correlated with mitochondrial dysfunction.[6]

What causes that mitochondrial dysfunction? As it turns out, dysfunction is directly correlated with how our mitochondria produce the ATP (energy) our cells need. If the cell is healthy, about 89 percent of our ATP is produced through oxidative phosphorylation, with either glucose or fatty acids for the fuel.[7] But the cell can use another process to make ATP without using oxygen, even if oxygen is present. That process is aerobic fermentation, also called glycolysis. In this case, oxygen is still around but for some reason the cell can't—or chooses not to—use oxygen and instead makes energy through fermentation. This way of making energy is characterized by a large uptake in glucose by the cell for fuel. Nearly all cancers have been shown to function through elevated aerobic fermentation.[8] This is why tumor detection imaging is based on putting labeled glucose into the body and seeing which cells use more of it.

The most significant issue with aerobic fermentation compared to oxidative phosphorylation is the amount of energy that can be made through each process. In oxidative phosphorylation a human cell can produce thirty-six ATP molecules from one molecule of glucose; in aerobic fermentation it can only make two. Clearly, oxidative phosphorylation is more efficient, which helps explain why cancer cells uptake glucose so rapidly: They have to keep burning it to keep up with the energy demands of the cell. Not only does aerobic fermentation lead to less ATP production, it also creates by-products like alcohol and lactic acid, which are toxic to our cells. So why would our cells ever "choose" to use fermentation? When mitochondria—the structures that allow our cells to use oxygen—become damaged, the cell cannot use oxygen as well and must get energy in another way.

Our cells need to make energy. If they are provided with oxygen and fuel to burn in the form of glucose or fatty acids, they will make energy through oxidative phosphorylation. If oxygen is absent but mitochondria are still healthy, the cell will survive through fermentation without oxygen, or anaerobic fermentation. And if oxygen is present but cannot be used because mitochondria are damaged, the cell will survive through fermentation even in the presence of oxygen, or aerobic fermentation. Fermentation that occurs when oxygen is available tells us that mitochondria are damaged to the point that oxygen cannot be utilized by the cell. In this state, the cell will not live much longer. To ensure the furthering of its cell line it starts to rapidly divide into many undifferentiated cells that do not use oxygen: This is the start of cancer. It is a survival mechanism that the cell uses to stay alive in the hopes that mitochondrial health and oxidative phosphorylation will soon be restored. If they are not restored, then the cancer will continue to progress.

The things that damage mitochondria are the same things that lead to oxidative stress. When damage happens, in most cells it can lead to cancer. The heart, however, seems to be different.

Heart Cells Are Unique

In chapter 8, I discussed how a certain set of circumstances could cause a heart attack without stenosis or blockage of a coronary artery. That process involves a shift in metabolism from the heart burning primarily fatty acids and ketones to the heart burning more glucose than it wants to. This shift is forced by an imbalanced stress signal to the heart.

In a way, this shift in metabolism is similar to what I just discussed regarding cancer. In cancer, the mitochondrial respiration of oxygen is compromised, and the cell has no choice but to use a large amount of glucose through aerobic fermentation to produce ATP. In the heart, not being fat-adapted, experiencing oxidative stress, and having an imbalanced stress response can give a signal to burn too much glucose. Both of these situations are characterized by an increase in lactic acid production. Yet we get two different outcomes. In cancer, the cells turn into rapidly dividing, undifferentiated, acidic, and anaerobic cells. In heart attacks, the buildup of lactic acid causes biochemical and biomechanical changes that cause tissue death.

The difference between the two is one reason why cancer in the heart tissue happens so rarely: Heart cells cannot divide. These cells are what researchers call terminally differentiated because very early in their development they leave the cell cycle indefinitely and stop dividing. The only growth of heart tissue that can occur after that point is through expansion in cell size and not through cell division. Some have speculated that the heart evolved this way as a kind of trade-off because of the high metabolic activity, and therefore energy demand, of a constantly contracting heart tissue. Cell division uses a large portion of the ATP the cell produces. If you eliminate cell division, a lot of ATP is freed up for metabolically demanding tissue.

When the criteria are met for the development of cancer in normal tissue, it results in tissues that rapidly divide—because they cannot stay alive for long under fermentation circumstances—but what if this happens in a tissue that cannot rapidly divide? If increased glucose utilization leads to buildup of lactic acid in the heart where cells cannot divide, the cells die quickly and result in necrosis. In his early work on cancer, Otto Warburg stated that cells that die can never become cancerous.[9]

Remember that the heart, which prefers burning ketones for fuel, has mechanisms for ensuring it can burn fatty acids and ketones, such as having "first dibs" on fatty acids delivered through chylomicrons and direct communication with fat cells for mobilization of fats as needed. The only way cells can use ketones is through oxidative phosphorylation. In fact, it has been shown that in human tissues higher amounts of ketones have increased mitochondrial respiration, or oxidative phosphorylation, by 128 percent.[10] The heart cells' priority access to ketones guarantees the heart can always use oxidative phosphorylation. I believe these mechanisms were a trade-off when evolution selected out the ability of heart cells to divide—if that ability ever existed in mammals. Preventing too much glucose utilization in heart cells protects against the altered metabolism that is cancer (which results in cell death in the case of heart tissue), making it a rare occurrence. Unfortunately, due to the metabolic inflexibility, oxidative stress, and imbalance in the ANS that often occur within the context of our modern way of life, the events that result in metabolic heart attacks that we discussed in chapter 8 can still occur.

The fact that the heart has mechanisms to prevent it both from using too much glucose and from the downstream effects that the use of too much glucose would have, explains some of the reasons why heart cancer is rare. And even if those mechanisms fail, heart cells usually die rather than become cancerous. This is a metabolic reason why the heart rarely gets cancer, but there is another reason, too. To understand, I'll have to revisit fourth phase water.

Cells and Gels

I have heard my whole life that the human body is around 70 percent water. But when I think about it, I don't really feel like I am mostly water. If all my cells were little sacs filled with liquid water, I feel like my body would have the consistency of a waterbed. I would be sloshing around. However, if I find a group of soft tissues, like the musculature of my forearm for example, and I push into it, the tissue gently gives way and then returns to form once I remove the pressure. This is similar to if I poked Jell-O. Body tissues behave much more like gels than they do like liquids.

We are mostly H_2O, but most of that water is in the fourth phase gel state. We have already discussed how this fourth phase water can form an exclusion zone next to the lining of our arteries and how this EZ protects the arteries and drives blood flow. But fourth phase water is also *in* our cells. Recall the ingredients needed to build fourth phase water in the arteries: water, the hydrophilic surface of the artery, and radiant energy. The same is needed in the cell, with one addition.

The cell already has water, and exposure to radiant energy comes from various external sources, including the Sun, but what's the hydrophilic surface? In the cell, it is intracellular proteins suspended within the cytoplasm, including protein strands called the microtrabecular lattice, which can be seen with standard electron microscopy.[11] More than half the water in the cell lies within 5 nm of a surface of this cellular protein network.[12] It is because this microtrabecular lattice provides a surface for gel to form that when you damage a cell membrane, the fluid and contents don't leak out; they are all held in place by the gel.[13]

Being made up of fourth phase water gives our cells unique properties. The one most significant to this discussion is the distribution of ions. A cell holds a charge due to a concentration of potassium ions in the cell and a concentration of sodium ions outside the cell. It is thought that this distribution is maintained by pumps within the cell membrane that work to keep these ions in place. However, there is evidence to the contrary. For starters, these pumps would require a large amount of energy to handle this distribution. It's also been shown that when the cell's energy source is removed, the distribution of ions remains, even after eight hours with no cellular energy.[14] The ability of fourth phase water to exclude some things and include others may play the bigger role in this distribution.

To see how this ion distribution is maintained, we need to look at something called the Hofmeister series of ion sizes. This series arranges ionic forms of common solutes in order from biggest to smallest according to their hydrated diameters. The order is $Mg_2+ \rightarrow Ca_2+ \rightarrow Na+ \rightarrow K+ \rightarrow Cl- \rightarrow NO_3-$. Because of how fourth phase water is structured in the cell, the dividing line of what is and what is not allowed to pass through the membrane falls precisely at the middle of the Hofmeister series. Anything the size of sodium (Na) or larger is excluded, and anything the size of potassium (K) or smaller is allowed in. Sodium and potassium are the most abundant solutes in and around cells, and so, with the help of fourth phase water, we see the following distribution of these ions in our cells: Potassium is more concentrated inside the cell and sodium is more concentrated outside the cell.

This distribution of ions, which has been proven experimentally, gives the cell a low net negative charge.[15] Both sodium and potassium have positive charges (Na+ and K+), so if the cell is concentrated with potassium, how can it have negative charge? There are other things in the cell, too. The protein structures of the cell hold a high negative charge and there is also chloride (Cl-) in the cell. If not for the concentration of potassium, there would be a highly negative charge instead of a low net negative one.

This charge allows cells to maintain spatial "awareness" and separation from other cells near them (see figure 9.1). The negatively charged cells are attracted to the positive area outside them but are repelled by other negatively charged cells if they get too close. This keeps the cells evenly spaced. Up to this point I have discussed that cells are filled with fourth phase water, fourth phase water distributes ions in an orderly way, and this distribution gives the cells their charge. Next, I'll discuss what happens if this situation fails.

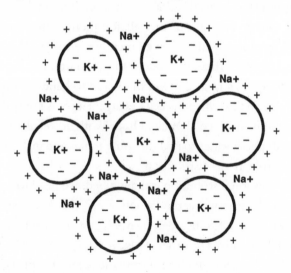

Figure 9.1. Depiction of properly charged and therefore evenly spaced cells.

If the cell loses the structure in its cytoplasm, the ion distribution will become chaotic, and the cell will lose both its charge and its proper spatial orientation. If this happens to many cells in the same area, the cells will clump together, and the spatial orientation and integrity of the tissue will fail (see figure 9.2). When this clumping happens, the tissue feels very different from soft, healthy tissue filled with gel. It feels

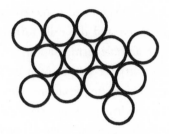

Figure 9.2. "Clumping" that occurs when cells lose their charge and therefore proper spacing.

more like a hard nodule within the tissue: kind of like what a tumor feels like.

To be clear, I am saying that a breakdown in fourth phase water in cells is what initiates the beginnings of tumor formation. So what leads to the cell failing to maintain the fourth phase water in its cytoplasm? To answer this question, let's look at how other gels—like Jell-O or bone broth stored in the fridge—form.

The basic ingredients needed to form a gel are water, collagen or gelatin, and an energy source. A packet of Jell-O mix contains these ingredients along with sugar and food coloring. When you boil down bone joints to make bone broth you get similar ingredients, though the broth usually has fat and salt, too. Remember that in order for gel to form, water needs hydrophilic surfaces. Proteins, like the gelatin found in Jell-O mix and bone broth, provide this surface. However, they are usually folded up and don't provide enough of a surface for gel to form. This is where an energy source comes in. When you first stir the Jell-O mix, it is still liquid because the proteins are still folded tightly together. Heat is the energy that unfolds the proteins, giving the water more surface area to form gel. As the solution cools in the refrigerator, the gel forms on the proteins, creating the wobbly consistency of Jell-O.

A cell has water in the form of cytoplasm and, throughout the cytoplasm, proteins in the form of the microtrabecular lattice—though the proteins are usually folded tightly together. Since we obviously cannot boil our cells to the point where the proteins unfold, we need a different energy source. The energy source that unfolds proteins in our cytoplasm is ATP.[16] This unfolding creates more surface area and allows our cells to maintain enough gel in the cell for it to function properly. Remember that in cancer the ability of the mitochondria to use oxygen and make energy through oxidative phosphorylation is compromised and the cells turn to aerobic fermentation. Also remember that with aerobic fermentation, we get around two ATP molecules compared to the thirty-six we get with oxidative phosphorylation. This decrease in ATP sets the cell up for failure: There is limited ATP to unfold proteins, cytoplasm starts to lose protein surface area for fourth phase water, and gel cannot form. (As an interesting aside, an early twentieth-century bone surgeon and cancer researcher named William Coley once induced fever for thirty days in cancer patients and saw a 40 percent cure rate among them.[17] Since the cells did not have enough ATP to denature cellular proteins, could the *fevers* have heated them enough to denature them and give him the results he saw?)

It is no surprise, then, that another characteristic of cancer cells is that they lose their structure. Dr. Warburg himself summarized, "The irreversible injuring of respiration is followed, as the second phase of cancer formation, by a long struggle for existence by the injured cells to maintain their structure, in which a part of the cells perish from lack of energy, while another part succeeds in replacing the irretrievably lost respiratory energy by fermentation energy. Because of the morphological inferiority of fermentation energy, the highly differentiated body cells are converted by this into undifferentiated cells that grow wildly—the cancer cells."[18]

This loss of structure happens first, then cells lose their charge and therefore their spatial orientation. On a tissue level, the clumping is what causes the hard mass we call a tumor. At a cellular level, loss of proper cellular charge can cause all kinds of things to go wrong.

One characteristic of cancer cells is all the gene mutations we find in them. These are not the cause of the cancer; they are a result of the loss of structure. Mutations cannot be the cause because there are a large number of mutations and chromosomal abnormalities found in tumor cells and the number and type of mutations are different when cancer cells of the same tissue are tested.[19] If mutations in individual cancer cells from the same cancer are different, searching for a cause for cancer through single gene mutations makes little sense.

The breakdown of structure within cells offers some clarity, and arises during the process of cell division. Cell division requires a substantial amount of the ATP that the cell produces, about 40 percent. If cells rely on fermentation for production of that ATP, they probably won't have enough. When this happens, we will get mistakes in the process of cell division and since cell division involves the dividing of chromosomes, this results in mutations and chromosomal abnormalities we see in cancer cells. The cell structure, gel, is also important in cell division; it gives the cell a framework within which to properly perform the division. Without a framework, mistakes are likely to occur. This division can be so dysfunctional that some cancer cells don't even end up with the right number of chromosomes. Since this chromosomal number is what makes us human, you might consider that cancer cells are not human.

Getting back to the heart, remember that the heart has a unique metabolism that keeps it preferentially burning fatty acids and ketones instead of glucose for fuel. This preference makes it less likely to revert to aerobic fermentation, which means it is less likely for the heart cells to end up in a low-ATP situation, causing a breakdown of fourth phase water and cancer formation. The heart's metabolism is protective not only from a metabolic standpoint, like I discussed with heart attacks, but also in maintaining the structure of our cells.

The Electromagnetic Heart

When I first described fourth phase water, I said that in order for it to form, it needs a hydrophilic surface and an energy source. In the case of our cells, ATP is the energy source. That energy source creates the hydrophilic surface by unfolding proteins. We still need radiant energy sources to energize the water in our cells so that they can form fourth phase water on the hydrophilic surfaces. I have discussed how radiant energy can come from the Earth, the Sun, vortexing water in the presence of oxygen, and other living things. But the heart is special in this department as well.

The body can actually serve as its own source of radiant energy because it gives off an electromagnetic field. These are different frequencies from the electromagnetic fields we are exposed to from modern-day electronics and wireless signals. While I do not think the body can provide enough radiant energy to sustain health on its own, it does contribute to the overall amount of radiant energy. Every organ in the body gives off an electromagnetic field, some bigger than others, the heart biggest of all.

One would think that the organ with the most electrical activity, the brain, would be the one producing the strongest electromagnetic field, but research has shown that the heart emits an electromagnetic field five thousand times stronger than the one emitted by the brain.[20] The electromagnetic field of the heart can be detected by a device called a magnetometer from about eight to ten feet away.[21] If radiant energy is needed to form fourth phase water, and this is key for preventing cancer, it seems the heart has yet another advantage.

Understanding why cancer of the heart is so rare has shown us some unique characteristics of the heart. Heart cells cannot divide, and so they die in the face of metabolic derangement instead of rapidly dividing, as we see in cancer cells. Heart cells also have mechanisms to keep the heart burning ketones and fatty acids so that it is less likely to revert to fermentation; this keeps ATP available for the denaturation of proteins to maintain proper cell structure. The heart also has the electromagnetic energy needed to constantly provide the water in its cells with at least some radiant energy to form fourth phase water. All of these protective mechanisms make sense from an evolutionary perspective, but less so in the context of our modern world.

When our hearts evolved to trade off heart cell division for high metabolic activity, it was long before modern life created an imbalance in our stress response strong enough to derail the heart's fatty acid and ketone metabolism. There have been very few times during our evolution when excessive carbohydrate consumption was an option; therefore, for most of our history, nothing prevented our bodies from making ketones and using oxidative phosphorylation to make enough ATP to keep our cells in a healthy structured state. The heart used to receive more than enough radiant energy from our environment, in the form of contact with the Earth and sunlight. This and the addition of the intense electromagnetic signal of the heart meant we could easily maintain fourth phase water in all of our cells.

These characteristics of the human heart largely protect it from cancer. As a whole, though, our hearts and our entire bodies still falter in the face of the drastic shifts in our environment. On the bright side, these underlying causes point to clear preventative solutions. But we still have one more crucial piece to discuss to fully understand the connection between our modern lifestyles and heart disease.

CHAPTER 10

The Ceaseless Signals of High Blood Pressure

Remember that long trip I took in the back of that pickup truck from Guatemala City to the hostel in the middle of the jungle in Semuc Champey? The very next day I had another adventure. Across the river and upstream from the hostel, there was a cave coming out of the side of a mountain. Coming out of the cave was a small river that flowed into a bigger river, Río Cahabón. The hostel gave guided tours of the cave for its guests, and I decided to go for it.

Once I got to the mouth of the cave, I was met by three other travelers. Our guide handed each of us a small candle, lit them, and we headed into the cave. We started out walking along the banks of the river within the cave, but soon we were wading through ankle-deep water, as the banks disappeared beneath the water's edge. The river got deeper and deeper, until I was swimming with one hand and holding my candle above water with the other. A moment later, I heard what sounded like a waterfall, and sure enough, we came up on the source of the sound, falling into the pool we were swimming in. We climbed out of the water and up onto a little ridge with a rope dangling over a rock face. We then used the rope to scale the rock face next to the waterfall, candles gripped longways between our teeth.

We walked for quite some time next to and through the river, sometimes taking turns holding each other's candles so we each could climb up a rock wall and jump back into the river. We eventually started our return trek out of the cave, but then veered off where the river split into another cave opening. This route was much narrower than the other, and many times we had to crouch to get through and repel down small waterfalls. When my candle went out, I lit it again with the help of someone else's candle, or watched in amazement as our guide pulled a hidden lighter out of the cave wall. Twice I needed a new candle because mine had gotten too wet. Candles seemed hidden everywhere in the cave walls, too.

The cave became rounded, still large enough for us to stand and walk through, but cylindrical in shape. As it grew narrower, we had to crouch in order to press on, and the speed of the flowing water picked up. Eventually we came to a little opening where the water was flowing into a small room. The guide jumped through the opening, and we all followed, finding ourselves in a space where we all fit comfortably. Because this area of the cave had been getting narrower and narrower, the water flowed through quickly to the other side where it flowed even faster and through a chute carved out of the rock, like an enclosed waterslide at a water park. I jumped into the chute, and three seconds later I plunged into a pool of water. Once I got my bearings, I realized we were very close to the mouth of the cave. When everyone had come down the slide, we headed out.

Exploring a cave in a foreign country with nothing but candlelight was an exciting and, at times, nerve-wracking excursion. There were many moments when my blood pressure jumped. One of the ways our bodies regulate blood pressure is not dissimilar to something I saw in the cave: At the end, when we were about to head down the chute, the cave became much narrower, causing the water to flow faster. It got so narrow that it was moving intimidatingly fast through the chute I was about to go down. The body does the same sort of thing by constricting blood vessels. In the cave, the water flowed quickly and was under more pressure because of the narrowing of the cave. Our blood pressure responds in a similar way when we get signals from the environment to crank up the pressure.

———————

Most people know that high blood pressure means an increase in pressure in the blood vessels. If we think about a tube with fluid flowing through it, we can imagine what would increase pressure in this system. More fluid would do it, such as when the kidney gets a signal to retain fluid. An increase in the speed at which blood needs to pass through would also do it, such as when the body is signaled to increase blood in tissues. A decrease in the amount of space in the tube would also do it, such as when the body is signaled to constrict the blood vessels or when there is a buildup of atherosclerosis. All of these things can happen at the same time, which is often the case.

To measure blood pressure, we most commonly take systolic and diastolic pressure measurements from the brachial artery in the arm. Systolic pressure (the top number) measures pressure when the heart is contracting, and diastolic pressure (the bottom number) is taken when the heart is not contracting. You now know the heart is not the main mover of the blood, and that a contracting heart cannot create enough force to move the blood through the whole body. However, the contraction of the heart and the opening and closing of valves does create momentary pressure changes. This gives us blood pressure measurements and the sensation of a pulse in our arteries.

I think of the pulse not as feeling the force of a pumping heart on the arteries, but as the feeling of changing pressure in arteries as the heart valves open and close. It is similar to a room with a door on both ends. In college, I used to study in a room in the library that had two doors, one on either end of the room. Because of the heating and cooling system and the ventilation in the rooms, the pressures would differ in adjacent study rooms. Oftentimes in my study room, one door would be closed and the other one slightly ajar. Then someone would come in the closed door and the pressure in the room would change, travel across the room, shift the blinds in the windows, and slam the open door. There was no pump in the library to force air through the room; it was just high pressure flowing into a lower pressure area. This is what happens in the arteries when the heart valves open and close; it can be felt all throughout the arterial system.

The body regulates blood pressure in an automatic way, meaning it is not under conscious control. Like breathing and the heart beating, the body just does it. Blood pressure regulation starts in the kidney, which is always sensing fluctuations and responding accordingly. If blood pressure drops too low, the kidney will secrete renin into the bloodstream from its juxtaglomerular cells. Meanwhile, the liver is continuously making and releasing angiotensinogen into the bloodstream. When the renin encounters angiotensinogen, it converts it to a substance called angiotensin I. Once angiotensin I is present in the blood, an enzyme called angiotensin converting enzyme (ACE), which is always present

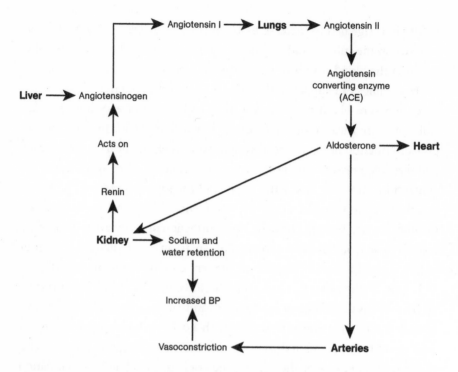

Figure 10.1. Flow chart of blood pressure regulation of the body. The body is constantly monitoring multiple metabolites for the regulation of blood pressure. This is a classic negative feedback loop used in many other places in the body as well.

in the blood, starts converting angiotensin I to angiotensin II. The presence of angiotensin II then triggers mechanisms in the body that raise blood pressure. It stimulates the production of aldosterone in the adrenal glands, which triggers sodium and fluid retention that increases the volume of blood, raising blood pressure. It also stimulates vasoconstriction of blood vessels, also increasing the pressure, and stimulates the SNS, which constricts blood vessels and quickens the delivery of blood to tissues. Once the pressure in the blood has been increased sufficiently, the kidney lowers production of renin, allowing the whole system to downregulate. This is depicted in figure 10.1.

The system is a classic negative feedback loop seen in many of the body's regulatory systems. But when the system gets improperly stimulated, it creates chronic high blood pressure, which is associated with atherosclerosis, heart attacks, heart failure, and strokes, as well as dementia, kidney disease, and eye damage. But I want to make something clear: I do not think that high blood pressure *causes* all of these things. I think the imbalances that lead to high blood pressure are also the driving forces behind these diseases. High blood pressure is coincidental with many of these conditions and can worsen them, but there is no direct evidence that it causes them. Chronic high blood pressure usually does not happen unless other imbalances, the same ones that cause those other chronic diseases, are present first.

The elevation of blood pressure is a normal and essential process. It is one of the ways the body adapts to ever-changing environments. This is why when they measure your blood pressure at the doctor's office and see that it's high, they cannot diagnose you with high blood pressure right away. They have to test it at the end of the visit and during a few subsequent visits to make sure that your body isn't just adapting to the stress of the doctor's office. This reaction is called "white coat syndrome."

One of the best indicators of health is the ability to adapt to different environments. For example, if someone were to go from standing still to a dead sprint, this is a large and quick change that the body must adapt to. The average teenager would much more likely successfully adapt to that change than, say, an eighty-year-old person would. As a matter of fact, being forced to do this just might kill an eighty-year-old. Elderly individuals lose the robustness of their adaptive mechanisms over time. This is why I think things like heart rate variability (which measures your ability to transition between a stress and nonstress state) and metabolic flexibility (the ability to readily adapt to burning different fuel sources) are extremely good indicators of health, especially as we age.

This reshaping of our understanding of high blood pressure alters our understanding of disease in important ways. Primarily, if blood pressure stays chronically elevated, it is not because the body is doing something it is not supposed to; it is because the body is getting the signal to keep the blood pressure elevated. The body is being told to adapt to a situation. It is doing exactly what it is supposed to. If the body didn't create high blood pressure when signaled, this would indicate a failure to adapt, a much bigger issue than unnecessarily high blood pressure. When the body gets constantly oversignaled to adapt to conditions with an increase in blood pressure, the increase becomes chronic. The causes of improper signaling are the true culprits that create the diseases associated with high blood pressure. High blood pressure itself is not the cause.

The Three Signals of High Blood Pressure

There are three main culprits when it comes to imbalances that create chronic signaling for high blood pressure. The first is insufficient radiant energy. Remember that the ability to maintain blood flow is dependent on enough radiant energy to maintain adequate fourth phase water on the lining of arteries. Without enough radiant energy, primarily in the form of infrared light from the Sun and contact with the Earth, water won't structure as efficiently. If the body cannot create adequate blood flow via fourth phase water, it will adapt by signaling for the constriction of blood vessels. Less space creates higher pressure and quicker flow, similar to the increase we see when we put our thumb partially over the spout of a water hose. The amount of fluid does not change, but decreasing the flow area creates more pressure and quicker flow, just like I saw in the cave in Guatemala.

A 2012 study in rats found that exposure to artificial infrared light resulted in "significant decreases in heart rates and systolic and mean blood pressure."[1] In humans, the use of an infrared sauna for only twenty minutes three times a week over three months has been shown to decrease blood pressure.[2] Sunlight, the original source of infrared, has also been shown to decrease blood pressure.[3] One study examined whether vitamin D from sunlight exposure could explain the decreases in blood pressure, and concluded it couldn't.[4] Vitamin D is not what causes the drop in blood pressure; the drop is caused by radiant energy boosting the self-propel mechanism of the blood. By applying infrared light, we improve blood flow through fourth phase water production, so the body can relax the constriction of the blood vessels and decrease arterial pressure.

The second cause of improper signaling to increase blood pressure is an imbalance in our ANS, which interprets our environment as safe or threatening. When our body perceives we are in a stressful situation, it does things that will help us fight or flee. One of those things is increasing blood flow in order to deliver oxygen and energy to tissues. To increase blood flow the body has to raise blood pressure by constricting blood vessels and increasing blood volume. A stressful situation—or a perceived stressful situation—activates this system.

One issue in the current epidemic of chronic disease is that modern humans unnecessarily stimulate the stress state of our ANS, mostly because our higher-level cognition gives us the ability to think about the future and worry about things. Recall Dr. Robert Sapolsky in chapter 8: "Mobilizing energy while sprinting for your life helps save you. Do the same thing chronically because of a stressful thirty-year mortgage, and you're at risk for metabolic problems like diabetes and high blood pressure." An imbalance in our ANS, where the stress state is chronically but unnecessarily turned on, is a recipe for chronic signaling to increase blood pressure.

Remember that the best measure of balance and health of the ANS is heart rate variability (HRV). Studies have established the relationship between psychological stress and decreases in HRV, as well as increases in blood pressure.[5] A study of medical students looked at the effects of a stress-relieving relaxation therapy on HRV and blood pressure, and concluded that "short-term practice of relaxation therapy can improve autonomic balance and promote cardiovascular health of medical students."[6] Our stressful society exacerbates the imbalance of our ANS, a huge contributor to the oversignaling that creates chronic high blood pressure.

The third cause of improper signaling of our blood pressure regulating system is poor metabolic health. I saved the biggest and most important for last. What I mean by *poor metabolic health* is when the body becomes insulin resistant. When we eat, it raises our blood sugar and insulin is secreted to (among other things) take that sugar and put it into cells to be utilized or stored as fat. When we are insulin resistant, the body does not respond as well to that insulin. High blood pressure is highly correlated with ailments like diabetes because the defining characteristic of diabetes is high blood sugar due to insulin resistance, which has been shown to directly upregulate the renin-angiotensin system that raises blood pressure.[7] This is due to the elevation of insulin in the bloodstream.

In a 2014 study that looked at the mean fasting insulin levels of fifty people newly diagnosed with high blood pressure compared with fifty healthy individuals, the experimental group had more than twice the level of fasting insulin as the control group had.[8] The experimental group was so resistant to insulin that their bodies had to secrete twice as much to get their blood sugar down. Another study looked at biomarkers in people with type 2 diabetes as they initiated insulin therapy, and the research turned up some unexpected results: "The study was not primarily designed to examine blood pressure. The preliminary conclusion from the present study, however, is that the initiation of insulin treatment in poorly controlled type 2 diabetes causes a temporary and possibly clinically significant elevation of blood pressure."[9]

Insulin increases blood pressure and creates a state of insulin resistance that leaves high amounts of insulin in the blood. Insulin resistance is created when we constantly eat excess calories, especially in the form of polyunsaturated fat and processed carbohydrates at the same time. This would rarely, if ever, have happened during the course of human evolution, until very, very recently. If we do it consistently, as people do in society today, we can wear out the systems that signal and receive insulin, creating insulin resistance.

On a personal note, and to illustrate the sometimes backward ways of modern medicine, a common treatment for high blood pressure, the beta-blocker metoprolol, has actually been shown to cause insulin resistance.[10] This is the drug I was prescribed long term when I was in the hospital. It is well established in the research that insulin resistance is detrimental to the endothelial lining of the blood vessels,[11] and one study even found that these insulin resistance effects of metoprolol can alter the insulin sensitivity of the endothelial cells on the arteries, decreasing their function.[12] The endothelial cells of arteries were the very part of the body that I needed to be functioning optimally while recovering from a heart attack! Another study of people who already had decreased insulin sensitivity found that "after metoprolol treatment, insulin sensitivity further decreased significantly by about 14%, whereas it increased after carvedilol [a different type of beta-blocker]."[13]

I want to reemphasize that high blood pressure does not cause all the conditions and ailments it is associated with. The things that cause high blood pressure—lack of radiant energy, ANS imbalance, and insulin resistance—are also highly causative of the conditions associated with chronic high blood pressure. High blood pressure is just another *consequence* of these three imbalances; it is not *causative* of those conditions, though it can certainly exacerbate them. For example, increased pressure in the arteries can worsen atherosclerosis because the pressure pushes the molecules that damage the artery wall up against the wall even harder. But this would not happen if the insulin resistance wasn't already there.

Sodium and High Blood Pressure

I also want to address the misconception that salt causes high blood pressure. The fact that the body starts to hold on to fluid and sodium when angiotensin II is produced, and that this results in increased blood pressure, has led doctors and scientists to believe that eating a lot of salt results in high blood pressure. This is not true. It is also observed that people with kidney failure have trouble holding on to sodium and regulating its levels, but that does not mean that high sodium intake will *cause* kidney disease. It means that when someone has kidney disease (from metabolic dysregulation), they often have trouble managing sodium.

Researchers have found that increasing salt up to eight times the normal amount for three days in people without diagnosed high blood pressure created only minimal increases in blood pressure, and that "moderate dietary salt restriction may have adverse effects on both vascular and systemic sensitivity to insulin."[14] That's right: *restricting* salt leads to insulin resistance, something that we know causes high blood pressure. One study of an increase of salt intake in those with high blood pressure found that the mechanisms that increase blood pressure were downregulated with salt intake. The researchers in this study felt that their results gave them "reasons to search for other mechanisms in the genesis of increases in total peripheral resistance and arterial pressure."[15]

People with heart disease, especially heart failure, are often told to restrict salt because, it's thought, eating salt causes high blood pressure and fluid retention. However, there is not much evidence for this recommendation.[16] A 2014 study published in the *International Journal of Cardiology* compared the use of a diuretic alone to a diuretic with a hypertonic saline solution and found that those that received the saline solution had "improved weight loss, preserved renal function, and decreased length of hospitalization, mortality and heart failure rehospitalization."[17] So eating a lot of salt does not cause high blood pressure, restricting it can lead to insulin resistance, and more salt might actually bring blood pressure *down* in those with high blood pressure, benefiting those with heart disease. For the record: I am not an advocate of table salt; I believe that unprocessed mineral salts are the salts we should be consuming.

ACE Inhibitors

ACE inhibitors are one common type of blood pressure–lowering medication and they work by preventing the conversion of angiotensin I to angiotensin II by inhibiting ACE, which is what triggers the body to increase blood pressure. When this is prevented the body doesn't get the signal to hold on to fluid and sodium or constrict blood vessels to increase pressure. Therefore blood pressure comes down. However, this is another example of chasing a symptom instead of correcting the problem. When taking a blood pressure medication, we are artificially lowering the increased pressure in arteries. That increased pressure is not caused by an ACE-inhibitor deficiency; high blood pressure is a symptom of the imbalances we just discussed.

By cheating and lowering the blood pressure with a medication rather than attempting to rebalance the system, the imbalances are allowed to get worse and the individual's health continues to decline. What's more is that, because the drug blocks ACE activity, the ACE II receptor never gets to give the signal to hold on to fluid, sodium, and other minerals, which does need to happen sometimes. This can cause mineral deficiency symptoms in people on those drugs.[18] Remember the study that showed how restricting sodium can actually *cause* high blood pressure and insulin resistance? This makes it clear that attempting to correct high blood pressure with medication is a backward approach.

High blood pressure is not a state that causes damage but instead is a normal response to our environment. If the environment inside or outside the body signals the body to increase blood pressure, it will. To correct this, we need to change our environments. This requires focusing on the same changes that will help us combat all the chronic conditions or ailments of the cardiovascular system. We need to maintain metabolic flexibility by restricting excess consumption of carbohydrates and vegetable oils and eating more animal fat, provide energy to our bodies in the form of radiant light, reduce oxidative stress, and strive for balance in our ANS.

PART III

A Heart Healthy Lifestyle

CHAPTER II

The Real Heart Healthy Diet

While I was living in Portland, Oregon, for chiropractic school I was invited by a cousin who lived in the area on a three-day backpacking trip on the Oregon Coast Trail. I wasn't new to backpacking, but I had recently switched to a vegan diet and this was my first backpacking trip on a plant-based diet. Since it was the Pacific Northwest, we went prepared for rain, and the weather didn't disappoint. Three of us—me, my cousin, and his friend Philip—spent most of the trek in our rain gear, but the trail was exciting, as it took us through many different types of terrain. We hiked right next to the ocean and past Haystack Rock on Cannon Beach; through coastal forest among huge evergreen pines in Ecola State Park; and along cliffs that dropped off to the ocean at Cape Falcon.

We were walking on the beach when we arrived at a huge rock formation that jutted into the ocean and blocked our path. This was Hug Point, and the trail took us on a path on the perimeter of the rock next to the ocean. We had read in the guidebooks that this part of the trail was only passable at low tide; at high tide the path along the rocks was under water. It was getting dark and the waves were crashing up against the rock as the tide was coming in, but the path was still above water. We decided to run for it.

We ran as fast as we could around the rock formation, fearing that the next wave would be the one to crash over the rocks and onto our path. As we reached the last straightaway and headed for the beach on the other side, our path was suddenly overflowed with the ocean. We turned and ran back the way we came, with the waves crashing up onto the rocks, threatening to overtake our path.

We made it back to the beach we'd come from but there was nowhere to go. Looking inland, we saw steep embankments and rock faces. We didn't dare camp on the beach with the rising tide. We knew that the Oregon Coast Highway ran along the top of the embankments and we decided to go for it. The climb was tough, but after thirty minutes we reached the top and found the road. We found a little road that led down to the beach on the other side of the Hug Point Rock formation we'd tried to pass and decided to set up camp there for the night.

By then, I was starving. My usual fare on backpacking trips was packaged tuna or chicken, some type of beef jerky and cheese, and lots of nuts and dried fruit. Since I was now vegan, I had brought the nuts and dried fruit, as well as some avocados, an instant vegan rice and vegetable meal, and crackers. The avocados were bruised and squished, but I salvaged what I could and cooked up the instant meal.

My two companions asked why I'd chosen to become vegan. I told them the usual reasons: Humans aren't set up to digest meat, animal farming was destroying the planet, and plants were more nutrient dense. Philip politely told me he disagreed with everything that I said. He said he respected the way anyone chose to eat, but that he thought there were flaws in the "facts" on which I had based my decision. He argued that there was no society in the world that had ever been completely vegan, and that it was clear animal foods had been important for human survival throughout history and prehistory—there is no way those people could have gotten all the nutrients they needed from plants throughout the year—and was still important among present-day Indigenous tribes in the Pacific Northwest. Some of those tribes revered salmon, one of their primary food sources, and while he had no idea if my food was nutritionally complete, he did know that it wasn't natively in the area, so there wasn't much of an environmental case to be made.

I was resistant to what he said. Our conversation was polite, but in my head I kept thinking how wrong he was. Over time I realized he was correct and, as a matter of fact, there was way more information about diet that he didn't mention that night that made him even *more* correct. People have relied on animal foods since the dawn of humanity. Oh, and I was hungry throughout that entire trip—no matter how much plant food I ate.

I now believe that the best diet to prevent heart disease is a diet based largely, but not completely, on animal foods. When I say "animal-based diet" I mean eating in a way that the majority of your energy and nutrients come from whole animal foods. This means prioritizing animal protein and getting the majority of your energy in the form of animal fat by mainly eating foods such as beef, pork, fish, poultry, eggs, raw dairy, and bone broth. When it comes to plants, we should focus on plants that are lower in (but not necessarily free of) carbohydrates, and diligently avoid foods like vegetable oils, grains, legumes, and processed sugar. We should also eat fruits and vegetables with an awareness of how plant toxins may affect us, and use strategies like fermenting, soaking, sprouting, and cooking to make nutrients bioavailable and neutralize toxins. As military surgeon Dr. Thomas L. Cleave said about the notion that animal foods lead to poor health, "For a modern disease to be related to an old-fashioned food is one of the most ludicrous things I have ever heard." And yet, we've been told that meat should only be eaten in moderation and that too much causes heart disease and cancer.

The goal of this chapter is to clear the name of animal foods, which have been unjustly and inaccurately maligned, and focus on their benefits for heart health. But first I want to explain something about diet in general. Some people claim that animal foods are better for heart health and some say that plant foods are, but I think the real issue with diet in society today is not necessarily a matter of plant foods versus animal foods. Rather, it is an issue of excess energy, poor metabolic health, and nutrient deficiency. To me, metabolic health is the ability of our bodies to metabolize what we eat in a way that doesn't harm us. We metabolize foods in a way that harms us when we take in too much energy, especially in the form of processed food, requiring "storage" of this extra energy, leading to poor metabolic health.

Our bodies mainly use fat and carbohydrates for energy, and while I think fat is healthier, it is possible to eat primarily one or the other and achieve metabolic health. A 2018 study published in the *Journal of the American Medical Association* tracked participants who ate either a "healthy low-carbohydrate" diet (which included more animal foods) or a "healthy low-fat" diet (which included more plant foods). Both groups saw improvements in metabolic markers and weight loss.[1] The key was that in both groups, participants reduced energy intake and ate whole-food diets. Eating too much of either carbohydrates or fats leads to poor metabolic health, and this is especially true if we eat polyunsaturated fats or processed carbohydrates, especially at the same time. Unfortunately, this is exactly what many peoples' diets consist of.

Which should we choose as our primary energy source, fats or carbohydrates? Most people agree that it's easy to overeat foods with lots of sugar, like cakes and candy, but it is hard to overeat steak and eggs. With simple processed carbohydrates we always seem able to have a little bit more; with foods high in animal protein and fat, there comes a point when you just can't eat anymore. And two hours after a higher-carbohydrate meal, we are often hungry again, whereas animal fat and protein leave us satiated longer. This makes eating animal foods a better route to prevent us from overconsuming energy as well as to help us focus on getting nutrients.

While it's possible to achieve metabolic health with a carbohydrate-based diet, especially in the form of whole foods, such as root vegetables, whole grains, and many fruits, it's more difficult. A 2007 study, also published in the *Journal of the American Medical Association* and using similar methods, compared four different whole-food diets with various amounts of carbohydrates and fats. The researchers found that a whole-food, high-fat diet was better for weight loss and markers of metabolic health, like triglycerides and fasting insulin, than any whole-food, higher-carbohydrate diet.[2]

A 2020 study compared an animal-based, low-carb (ABLC) diet to a plant-based, low-fat (PBLF) diet, putting participants into two groups for two weeks and then switching each group to the opposite diet for the next two weeks. All participants were allowed to eat as much as they wanted of the food provided to them. Participants in both groups experienced weight loss, and both had improved metabolic health markers like fasting insulin, fasting glucose, and inflammation. The PBLF diet showed decreases in cholesterol, increased fasting triglycerides, higher blood sugars after meals, and higher lactic acid concentrations. The ABLC diet showed unchanged cholesterol, decreased fasting triglycerides, lower blood sugars after meals, and lower lactate concentrations.[3]

These findings support the idea that metabolic health is not entirely about plant versus animal foods, but they're also a little misleading. Participants only spent two weeks on each diet, and adapting to fat as a fuel source on a low-carbohydrate diet can take longer. As the body becomes more efficient at using fatty acids and ketones for fuel, energy intake is likely to drop in the ABLC group. The researchers acknowledged that, given the limited time frame, "whether long-term adaptations to the ABLC diet would result in reduced appetite and energy intake compared to the PBLF diet is unknown."

While there's a legitimate argument that either animal-based or plant-based diets can support metabolic health, I still have concerns with the plant-based approach. Aside from higher blood sugar spikes after meals, higher triglycerides, and higher lactic acid concentrations, it's less effective in delivering nutrients such as fat-soluble vitamins and bioavailable amino acids (also known as protein). I do not believe that carbohydrates are inherently bad, and eating small amounts of whole-food carbohydrates (honey, low-sugar fruit, squash) is fine, so long as the quantities preserve metabolic flexibility.

And while dietary carbohydrates are not needed—because the human body can run off of fat and ketones and synthesize the glucose it needs—they do not cause diabetes, like many low-carb advocates may think. Heart failure is a condition that makes one intolerant to exercise, but that does not mean exercise causes heart failure. Kidney failure makes one intolerant to a high-protein diet, but that does not mean that a high-protein diet causes kidney failure. Likewise, diabetes makes one become metabolically intolerant to carbohydrates, but that does not mean that whole-food carbohydrates cause diabetes; only excess energy consumption in the form of processed grains, sugar, and vegetable oils do that. All that being said, animal foods are the way to go due to higher nutrient availability. And since animal foods get such a bad rap when it comes to heart disease, I'm going to dedicate the rest of this chapter to discussing why they're superior to plant foods for heart health.

While I am arguing that a diet centered around animal foods is better, I want to be clear that from an evolutionary perspective, I do not think that there is one perfect diet for humans, or for any living thing. In his 2017 book *Evolution's Bite* Peter Ungar stated, "When I think about food choice in nature, I envision the biosphere, that part of our planet that harbors life, as an enormous buffet. Animals belly up to the sneeze guard with plate in hand. What do they take? That depends in part on the utensils they've got to eat with, but also on what's left when they get to the front of the line. In other words, food choice is a matter of matching needs with items that teeth make accessible and nature makes available in a given place at a given time."[4] Throughout history, humans ate what was available in order to survive and pass on our genes. Humans became proficient at attaining meat from the environment and our digestive system evolved along with that, which is why meat is so healthy for the heart. It is clear that humans can also eat plants. As such, plants can play a role in our diets, even though early modern humans likely only ate them when necessary.

Although humans have retained the ability to eat and digest plant foods, that does not mean they are optimal. Let's say that the ideal diet of a particular species is one consisting entirely of pudding. Yet, for a few months out of the year, pudding is not available, and this species must instead rely on hard nuts as a food source; it is not an ideal food, but it keeps them alive during these few months of the year. While their ideal food source of pudding would not require teeth, the hard nuts would. Since they rely on those nuts for survival during one part of the year, they need to maintain the evolved characteristics to ingest and digest that food, even though it is not ideal for them. A species may retain the ability and evolved biological tools to use a certain food for survival, like humans did for plants, but those evolved characteristics do not necessarily mean it is the ideal food source.

In the 1980s, T. Colin Campbell of Cornell University undertook a major epidemiological study looking at the health outcomes of people who ate meat-based diets compared to those who ate plant-based diets. The China Study, as it's known, concluded that people in China who ate more meat had higher rates of heart disease, and this study is frequently summoned as evidence that a plant-based diet is superior for health.[5] But, again, the devil's in the details. The people who ate more meat lived overwhelmingly in cities, meaning they had more access to processed foods, more exposure to toxins, and a fast-paced, more stressful life compared to those who ate less meat and lived in rural areas. The China Study failed to account for this. Given heart disease is caused by processed fats and carbohydrates, oxidative stress from toxin exposure, and ANS imbalances from unnatural stresses, it's hardly surprising the people living in cities would be at higher risk.

The study authors also left out some data. One of the counties included in the data collection had very high levels of meat consumption. The residents of Tuoli ate 134.55 grams of animal protein per day on average, and were essentially carnivores. This is an incredible 110.63 grams higher than the residents of the county with the next-highest average animal protein consumption per day, but the Tuoli data was omitted for some reason. The three counties whose residents ate the *lowest* amount of animal protein on average (0, 0.15, and 0.19 grams) had a much higher incidence of heart attack and atherosclerosis than the residents of Tuoli.[6] This is epidemiology, so it can't *prove* that animal foods prevent heart disease. But the point is that the researchers of The China Study didn't report their findings accurately, and that matters.

Dietary recommendations that go out to the public are often based on studies like these, often with the help of companies and interest groups that stand to gain. Assessing whether an animal-based diet is best for the human heart requires far more depth and rigor. While I can't point to one particular research study, I can present a more complete picture of what the research shows. We will start by showing how an animal-based diet can balance the three imbalances that contribute to heart disease, specifically heart attacks without a blockage (see chapter 8): metabolic inflexibility, excess free radicals, and an overwhelmed stress response.

The Diet to Prevent Heart Attacks

First up is ketones. As you know, the heart prefers to burn fatty acids and ketones over glucose as a fuel source. And because it has mechanisms to ensure access to at least some fatty acids and ketones, it takes a lot to force it to burn primarily glucose—and for good reason. Supplying the heart with ketones "acutely lowers cardiac workload during exercise for the same amount of work performed," according to a 2012 study published in *Molecular Genetics and Metabolism*.[7] A 2016 study published in the *New England Journal of Medicine* described ketones as a "superfuel" for the heart after researchers noticed that the diabetes drug they were studying led to an increase in ketone use in heart tissue—and a decrease in cardiovascular death and all-cause mortality.[8] Luckily we don't have to take a diabetes drug to get the same effect.

The thing is, we have to *teach* the body to make and use ketones. The human body has what's called an oxidative priority that dictates which fuel sources it will burn if multiple ones are available. The body first burns what it can't store: alcohol and exogenous ketones (these are ketone supplements, for example, not what your body synthesizes from fat). Next, it goes for carbohydrates, then protein, and finally fat. While protein is usable for energy, it is an extremely energy-depleting process, and therefore is used only in times of starvation. To get our bodies to make ketones, we must be using fat as a fuel source. So, if we continuously supply the body with carbohydrates and fats, carbohydrates will have priority; we have to restrict carbohydrate intake to get the body to start burning fat for fuel and making ketones.

A diet of this nature is termed *ketogenic* because in the absence of carbohydrates, the body upregulates the production of ketones from fatty acids. This puts the body into what is called ketosis. In ketosis, the body has ketones in the blood, which is very different than ketoacidosis, a serious condition that can occur in uncontrolled diabetes.

Our bodies cannot store ketones, so from a weight-loss perspective, the body converting fatty acids to ketones is a good thing. Those ketones will either be used for energy or, if there are too many, excreted through sweat, urine, or breath. Extra energy in the form of ketones is not stored as body fat. As far as the heart is concerned, there will be plenty of ketones available to burn.

While I do not think it is inherently dangerous to be in ketosis all the time, I also do not think that we evolved in perpetual ketosis. The only diet that would put us in that state would provide 70 percent or more of our calories from fat. Health boils down to the body's ability to adapt to its environment. For optimal health, we should be readily able to adapt to different stressors, different temperatures, and different fuel sources. Indeed, this adaptability is a big part of what has enabled humans to be such a successful species; we have even taken it as far as adapting our environment to suit us. Unfortunately, we're now inundated with a constant source of calories in the form of processed carbohydrates—so much so that most of our bodies have lost metabolic flexibility and have forgotten how to burn fats. This is why the ketogenic diet has an adaptation phase. It has to relearn how to burn fats.

Again, the key to a heart healthy diet is metabolic flexibility. The heart is more efficient when burning ketones, making it less likely to have to burn glucose. Remember, if the heart is forced to burn more glucose than it prefers, it will begin using fermentation to make energy, which can predispose us to the events that lead to the "metabolic heart attacks" (see chapter 8). When researchers inhibited oxidative phosphorylation in the heart cells of rats, but supplemented the rats with ketones, the ketones prevented the transition to fermentation as a fuel source.[9] Ketones can have a powerful effect on the heart, and an animal-based diet takes us in and out of ketosis while never fully depriving the body of ketones. This allows the heart to thrive and maintain its preferred metabolism.

The second imbalance is oxidative stress, resulting from an excess of free radicals. An animal-based diet reduces oxidative stress in a few ways. The first is that it is blood sugar stabilizing. When we eat high amounts of carbohydrates, our blood sugar rises substantially, and a lot of insulin is required in order to bring it back down. Eating protein causes a much smaller spike in blood sugar, and fat does not spike blood sugar at all. An animal-based diet, which consists of primarily fats and protein, will create a much more stable blood sugar situation. Among people with type 2 diabetes, blood sugar that frequently goes up and down causes more oxidative stress and damage to our blood vessels than having blood sugar that is a little higher than normal but stays stable.[10] Since carbohydrates cause the most blood sugar oscillation, limiting them is a good strategy for preventing oxidative stress.

The second way an animal-based diet reduces oxidative stress is that the presence of ketones reduces the production of free radicals. Multiple studies have shown this. One study published in the journal *Science* found that when ketone levels increased through supplementation or through fasting in mice, they experienced "substantial protection against oxidative stress."[11] Another research article published in *Epilepsy Research* discussed how research has shown that a ketone-increasing diet produced lower levels of the molecules 4-HNE and H_2O_2, which are markers of oxidative stress, because the diet increased production of the antioxidant glutathione.[12]

While those studies were in animal models, one study in humans showed these effects as well. When twenty female subjects followed a ketogenic diet for fourteen days, researchers found that "14 days of a ketogenic diet elevates blood antioxidative capacity and does not induce oxidative stress in healthy subjects."[13] There is even evidence that ketones can act as antioxidants directly.[14]

There is one more aspect of an animal-based diet that helps prevent oxidative stress. No matter what we do, our bodies will have a free-radical burden simply as the by-product of normal, even healthy, metabolism. Our bodies even synthesize endogenous antioxidants to "mop up" these free radicals. The problem comes when there are too many. Conventional wisdom holds that eating foods high in antioxidants, such as fruits and vegetables, will assist our *endogenous* antioxidants and prevent oxidative stress, but actually this may not be true. A 2018 study published in *Oxidative Medicine and Cellular Longevity* gave nineteen research participants at risk for cardiovascular disease a diet high in vegetables, and a control—also at risk for cardiovascular disease—a diet low in vegetables. After four weeks, researchers found that "no significant changes were detected in clinical, immunological, and antioxidant markers in biological samples."[15] Though the sample size was small and the study duration short, the results were surprising considering how important the antioxidants in these foods are supposed to be.

Another 2011 study of forty-nine postmenopausal women found that when they ate more vegetables for three weeks, the women experienced an increase in carotenoids (a polyphenol thought to act as an antioxidant), but when tested for metabolites in the urine that are markers of oxidative stress and inflammation, the women were "not affected by any administered vegetable dose."[16] Finally, a study of forty-three individuals published in *Cancer Epidemiology, Biomarkers, and Prevention* tested this for a longer duration. Researchers divided participants into three groups: one group ate no fruits and vegetables, one group ate 600 grams of fruits and vegetables daily, and a control group. Among all three groups, "the level of oxidative DNA damage was unchanged. . . . this suggests that the inherent antioxidant defense mechanisms are sufficient to protect circulating mononuclear blood cells from reactive oxygen species."[17] Translation? There's some good evidence that the "antioxidants" in fruits and vegetables don't do much to help our body reduce oxidative stress.

There is one takeaway, here, however. We can focus on eating foods that help our body synthesize endogenous antioxidants, and this is where animal food comes in. An animal-based diet is likely to include more than just muscle meat, especially if we include things like bone broth and organ meat, and don't shy away from the connective tissue parts of a steak. These tissues have a different protein content and contain higher amounts of certain amino acids. For example, connective tissues are higher in glycine and proline, which is important because glycine combines with cysteine to produce the endogenous antioxidant glutathione peroxidase.

Remember that elevated blood sugar can damage tissues, causing oxidative stress. When researchers examined glutathione production in people with uncontrolled type 2 diabetes, they found it was "severely deficient," although levels could be restored through supplementation with glutathione precursor amino acids, decreasing damage from oxidative stress.[18] Researchers have also found that when rats were fed a sugar-based diet, inducing damage to the lining of their blood vessels, glycine supplementation increased available glutathione and superoxide dismutase (another endogenous antioxidant). This decreased damage and increased nitric oxide, which produced a relaxation response and decreased pressure in the arteries.[19]

Remember, the reason we want to decrease oxidative stress is because it breaks down fourth phase water in the arteries and then damages the arteries, leading to the development of atherosclerosis. This damage will also deplete nitric oxide, which is vital for the proper signaling of the ANS to the heart to prevent some forms of heart attacks. An animal-based diet—low in carbohydrates and higher in connective tissue proteins—is effective at preventing oxidative stress.

Lastly, an animal-based diet helps balance our ANS. Usually when we talk about balancing our ANS people don't think about diet. However, many aspects of an animal-based diet have been shown to contribute to ANS balance. The first is the fact that this diet provides us with higher ketone levels. A 2011 study published in the *Proceedings of the National Academy of Sciences* examined the effects of ketones on our stress response and found that the ketone beta-hydroxybutyrate was able to help balance the ANS by inhibiting sympathetic activity.[20] Another study found an association between metabolizing a high-carbohydrate beverage and a relatively higher sympathetic modulation of heart rate, resting energy expenditure, and respiratory quotient. Conversely, metabolizing stored and ingested fat was associated with relatively lower sympathetic modulation, energy expenditure, and respiratory quotient.[21] An animal-based diet will increase ketones and result in increased fat burning, both of which will contribute to ANS balance.

There is another aspect to an animal-based diet that will help with ANS balance that has less to do with metabolism. Remember that the ANS is what enables us to "read" our environment, using our senses, to interpret safety or danger. This is essential for survival, of course. What you may not know is that the digestive tract is one of the ways our ANS gets a feel for the type of environment we're in. Just like there is a reason we say "I love you with all my heart," we also have "gut feelings" about things. These two organs are innervated by the vagus nerve, the main line of the ANS. The heart is sensing our emotional environment and the gut is, in a way, sensing our external environment.

Our gut is basically an external environment: It is sealed off all the way through. In an intact state, the gut allows some things into the body and prevents or excretes others. This makes the gut an important source of environmental information for the ANS. Sometimes described as a sensory organ, the gut has also been called a "second brain." The gut actually sends more signals to the brain than the brain sends to it.[22]

So how is the ANS affected when the gut is damaged? Poor digestive health has been linked to abnormal function of the vagus nerve, which can trigger acid reflux and the poor intestinal motility associated with irritable bowel syndrome (IBS).[23] Healing the gut can also help balance the ANS. The question then becomes what causes damage to the digestive tract. One way we get damage to the digestive tract is through the ingestion of plant toxins.

All living things on Earth defend themselves from being killed and eaten. Animals have claws, teeth, and legs to fight humans or other animals or to run away, while plants make toxins to discourage animals from eating them. Yes, our plant foods are sprayed with pesticides and this makes them toxic, but you may be surprised to learn that pesticides are actually negligible compared to toxins that plants themselves make. Researchers at UC Berkeley found that 99.99 percent (by weight) of the pesticides in the US diet are actually chemicals that plants produce to defend themselves.[24] What kinds of toxins do I mean? The most infamous is gluten, a lectin found in wheat. One of the proteins in gluten (gliadin) is extremely damaging to the gut and causes intestinal permeability, or leaky gut. You do not have to have celiac disease or be gluten sensitive to experience intestinal damage from gluten.[25]

Glycoalkaloids are another plant toxin that can damage the gut. These are found in nightshades, including potatoes, tomatoes, eggplants, and peppers, and can damage the intestinal lining by "embedding themselves and disrupting [the] epithelial barrier."[26] Oxalate is found in many leafy greens, including spinach, chard, mustard greens, and beet greens, as well as almonds, sweet potatoes, chocolate, beans, and grains. Under a microscope oxalates look like sharp pointy crystals; imagine that going through your digestive system. A description in a food toxicology textbook reads, "oxalic acid ingestion results in corrosion of the mouth and gastrointestinal tract, gastrointestinal hemorrhage, renal failure, and hematuria."[27]

Remember that when our gut is in poor health it sends out distress signals, which contribute to an imbalance in our ANS, and we become stuck in a stress response. Nervous system signals are not the only thing that can travel through our nerves, however. Plant toxins have been shown to travel through the vagus nerve. In fact, a groundbreaking 2016 study looked at whether this might contribute to the etiology of Parkinson's disease. The study showed that lectins can travel via the vagus nerve to the brain.[28] Studies have also shown that during their travel via the vagus nerve lectins can also destroy the nerve in a process called transport suicide.[29] There is a significant body of research that investigates this relationship between brain health and plant toxins. And what better way to signal that you are in a stressful environment than plant toxins traveling through your vagus nerve to your brain?

It's clear that plant toxins are harmful to our digestive systems. This damage can contribute to an imbalance in our ANS, as part of the recipe that predisposes us to heart attacks. A review of the scientific literature concerning heart rate variability (the best measure of ANS balance) and IBS found that people with IBS have decreased tone in their vagus nerve.[30] Reducing plant toxins by eating an animal-based diet can allow the gut to heal. This can happen fairly quickly, as the cells lining the gut have one of the fastest turnover rates in the body. By simply hitting the pause (or stop) button, healthy cells replace damaged ones relatively quickly. By lifting stress off the digestive system, we help relieve our stress response and help create ANS balance. I am not saying that we have to eliminate all plants from our diet, but becoming familiar with which plants have high amounts of plant toxins and learning how they affect us can give us great insight into how to markedly improve digestive health with diet.

Gut damage from plant toxins is a huge contributor to inflammation, not only in the digestive tract but throughout the entire body. Inflammation damages many tissues in the body and can lead to plaque rupture or clot formation that can block an artery. The amazing thing is that the elimination of plant toxins not only helps heal the gut and restore ANS balance, it is also extremely anti-inflammatory. Inflammatory markers (hs-CRP, homosysteine, Lp(a), lipid peroxides, etc.) in people on an animal-based diet tend be extremely low. So an animal-based diet can provide the heart with ketones, reduce oxidative stress, and help balance our ANS. All this will help prevent heart attacks regardless of mechanism of cause.

I have focused thus far on how an animal-based diet helps balance the imbalances that drive heart attacks that happen without a blockage. There are other aspects of an animal-based diet that make it better for the heart as well.

Cholesterol Versus Phytosterol: Which Is the Healthier Sterol from Fat?

All living things have sterols that fulfill vital functions in their bodies, especially providing structure and integrity to cell membranes. Since animals have cholesterol and plants have phytosterol, does that mean, de facto, that cholesterol is better for humans than phytosterol? The answer is yes.

Most humans eat both forms of these sterols because most humans eat an omnivorous diet. Cholesterol in our diets obviously comes from the animal foods we eat. The overwhelming majority of phytosterol in people's diets come from what are known as vegetable oils (seed oils) such as corn oil, soy oil, canola oil, sunflower oil, and safflower oil, because these oils have more phytosterols than other plants that have fat and because they are abundant in modern diets. We also get phytosterols in smaller amounts from foods such as olive oil, coconut oil, and avocados. When we eat these two sterols together, they actually compete for absorption in the intestines. Humans are well designed to absorb fat because of our developed gallbladder; this is a characteristic we share with carnivores. Since the human body is a mostly watery environment, and fat does not dissolve in water, we need the bile salts secreted from the gallbladder to absorb the fats we eat. They do this by surrounding the fats in what are called micelles that shuttle them to where they need to go.

Sometimes when people supplement vitamin D, they don't see the rise in blood levels that they expect. I see this frequently on blood work of people taking high doses of vitamin D. This is probably because they're not taking the vitamin D with a high-fat meal; while D supplements come packaged in fat, it is not enough fat to stimulate enough bile. Without enough bile, not much fat is absorbed, and since vitamin D is fat soluble (transported in fats), the vitamin D is not absorbed either.

By eating both phytosterols and cholesterols, the body attempts to absorb both types of fat, often resulting in less absorption of cholesterol and decreased blood levels of cholesterol. This is why, since it is thought that lowering cholesterol will prevent heart disease, many doctors recommend foods with lots of plant sterols such as margarine and vegetable oils. Interestingly, in the case of phytosterols, the gut has a mechanism, an ATP-binding cassette transporter protein in the gut lumen, that places as much of the phytosterols it absorbs back into the intestines to eliminate it with other waste. In other words: The body doesn't want too much of it.

Sitosterolemia is a genetic condition in which this mechanism to return absorbed phytosterols into the intestines is not present. The condition is characterized by phytosterol deposits in the skin (xanthomas) or eyes (xanthelesma and arcus senilis). People with this condition also have increased risk of stroke and heart disease because the phytosterols build up in arteries, as well as in red blood cells, which causes the red blood cells to clump up. People with this condition can have platelet dysfunction causing abnormal bleeding, and they are at higher risk for diabetes because the phytosterols interfere with cholesterol, impairing insulin receptor function.

Some of these symptoms are from the body's inability to get rid of the phytosterols efficiently, but the more problematic symptoms are due to the effects of phytosterols on red blood cells. A red blood cell is shaped like a disc with a slight depression in the middle, sort of like a doughnut. The cell can maintain this shape because it has cholesterol in its membrane. When there are too many phytosterols and not enough cholesterol in the body, the red blood cells use phytosterols for the cell membranes instead. When this happens the red blood cells lose their pliability, become more rigid, and often clump together or get more easily stuck in tight spaces. This increases the risk of stroke and heart disease, interferes with delivery of nutrients, and causes microcirculation issues.

Hopefully, you are starting to see what can happen from eating too many plant sterols. There's an interesting body of research to back this up. For example, in one study published in the *Journal of the American College of Cardiology*, researchers fed two groups of rats an animal-fat-based diet, but supplemented one of the groups with phytosterols. In the unsupplemented group, the rats' arteries stayed dilated, and in the supplemented group their arteries became restricted. The researchers also induced strokes, noting that the supplemented group experienced bigger, more dramatic strokes because the phytosterols in the red blood cells led to more bleeding. In a second part of the same study, the researchers looked at people who needed replacement heart valves and found a correlation between diets high in plant sterol and plant sterols deposited on the heart valves.[31]

In another study, researchers used rats that had been genetically altered to make them more prone to stroke. They fed one group of these rats a diet high in animal fat, one group a diet high in corn oil, and a third group a diet high in olive oil (corn and olive oil both have phytosterols). They then waited to see which group had strokes first and which had strokes last. The group of rats that ate the high-animal-fat diet lived much longer than the other groups. The last rat to die from stroke in the olive oil and corn oil groups died at around the 100-day mark while the last rat to have a stroke in the animal-fat-diet group died at the 250-day mark.[32] The researchers concluded that with high amounts of phytosterols present, the phytosterols were used in the cell membranes of red blood cells instead of cholesterol. This made the red blood cells more rigid and less able to squeeze through small arteries, leading to blood vessel damage and stroke. It's possible to criticize the study's conclusions because it was done in genetically altered rats, but when you combine it with the following epidemiological study in humans, it becomes quite more compelling.

Researchers surveyed 48,188 people about their diet, placing them in one of three groups—those who ate any kind of meat, those who ate no meat except fish, and vegetarians—and then looked at health outcomes among the groups. They found that the meat eaters had a slightly higher risk of ischemic heart disease—but remember, this is epidemiology; they only looked at meat eating, not whether the participants *also* ate processed grains, sugars, and vegetable oils. They found that the vegetarians had 20 percent higher risk of hemorrhagic and total stroke.[33] In order for the researchers to put them into the vegetarian group, the participants had to have claimed to eat no meat, fish, or eggs, so it is reasonable to assume that they would have had much less animal fats in their diet and therefore much higher amounts of plant fats, which possibly led to an increase in stroke. It seems likely that the phytosterols are problematic, especially in high amounts. All this said, it's important to acknowledge that people with a genetic predisposition to high levels of plant sterols in their blood develop atherosclerosis prematurely, so this genetic predisposition is a factor in outcome.

In 2015, researchers reviewed all the associational literature on high levels of plant sterols in the blood and development of cardiovascular disease and found four studies that showed no association, four that showed an association between higher presence of plant sterols and less cardiovascular disease, and nineteen studies showing presence of higher plant sterols in the blood linked with higher risk of cardiovascular disease. These are associational studies, but the association is heavy in one direction. The authors of the review are hesitant in their conclusion yet clear about what their work signals: "These discordant findings make it impossible to draw any firm conclusions, even though the largest prospective trials have suggested that high plasma levels of plant sterols increase CV risk. The available data are still not sufficient to confirm whether plant sterol consumption increases CV risk, although they do suggest the presence of such a risk and so cannot be ignored."[34]

Basically, large amounts of plant sterols in your diet seems to be a bad idea. But before we discuss the main sources of these phytosterols in food, it's important to note that diet is not the only source. As you know, the body tries to rid itself of as many of these plant fats as it can when too many are ingested, by depositing absorbed sterols back in the intestines. However, if the intestines are overloaded, we end up with *more* absorption. What can overload the system besides food? Cholesterol-lowering drugs. Interfering with the production of cholesterol with a statin drug prevents the reabsorption of cholesterol in the liver and therefore more plant sterols are absorbed instead.[35] Another reason not to take statin drugs.

Some sources of plant sterols contribute to insulin resistance. Plant fats are much higher in unsaturated fats, and when we burn these fats rather than saturated fats for fuel, they change the way our cellular metabolism works. This changes the resulting ratio of $FADH_2$ and NADH, which determines if our fat cells are sensitive to insulin or resistant to it.[36] The tricky thing is that we don't want an insulin-resistant body, but we do want insulin-resistant fat cells. The reason for this is that insulin is the number one fat-storing hormone, and if our fat cells are insulin resistant, we will not store excess fat. Eating unsaturated fat creates a ratio of $FADH_2$ to NADH that makes fat cells insulin sensitive and eating saturated fat creates a ratio that makes our fat cells insulin resistant.[37] This phenomenon has led to the misconception that saturated fat leads to insulin resistance.

But it gets worse. If we eat lots of unsaturated plant fats, we create insulin-sensitive fat cells that take up glucose and fats and store them, creating weight gain. This happens because the mitochondria of those fat cells become dysfunctional when burning plant fats.[38] As those fat cells expand, they send out insulin-resistant signals called lipokines to the rest of the body.[39] This leads to the metabolic derangement that underlies the chronic diseases that plague our society, including cardiovascular disease.

So where are these plant sterols found? In fats derived from plants. That includes avocados and avocado oil, olives and olive oil, coconut oil, nuts, seeds, and all the vegetable/seed oils (soybean, corn, canola, sunflower, etc.). The seed oils have higher levels of plant sterols than any of the other plant oils and so it is no wonder that we have seen a steady increase in heart disease since seed oils entered mass production and became widely available in the early 1900s. While olive oil, avocado oil, and coconut oil do have plant sterols, they contain much smaller amounts than the seed oils do, and I believe they are a safer option if you are going to eat plant fats. Be cautious though: Many olive oil and avocado oil companies are not honest about what is in their oils. One study found that 82 percent of the avocado oil brands they tested had soybean oil in them, and some of the brands tested to be near 100 percent soybean oil![40] We also should be careful about how we source our animal foods. If the animals we eat are fed a diet high in soy and corn, then in some animals (namely chickens and pigs), the fat in their bodies contains plant sterols that are passed on to us when we eat them.[41] Because of differences in their digestive systems, this is not the case for ruminant animals like cows.

All this is to say that humans are designed to eat and use animal fats, but we can use plant fats to survive when animal fats are not available. Plant fats are not ideal and long-term high use of them can lead to many health problems. When we can, we should stick to fats that come naturally from animals. This makes intuitive sense: We don't have to overprocess lard, beef tallow, butter, bone marrow, or suet to get a fat from them. Long-term use of the industrially derived seed oils and plant fats will lead to disease. Natural animal fats are the route to health.

The Misconceptions About Animal Foods

There has been a lot of misinformation about the effects of consuming meat and animal foods and the impact it has on our health. As discussed in part 2, we've been fed inaccurate, broad generalizations that eating meat causes an increased risk of heart disease and cancer; there are also misleading misconceptions that meat will cause insulin resistance and that metabolites such as TMAO, mTOR, and homocysteine lead to disease. Let's start with insulin resistance. I have already discussed some studies that show that a low-carb, high-fat diet will improve markers of metabolic health. However, one thing we do observe in people on very-low-carbohydrate diets is that they test positive for insulin resistance on an oral glucose tolerance test or a glucose clamp test. This test result has led some people to conclude that a low-carb, high-fat diet causes insulin resistance and can therefore lead to all the issues that come with insulin resistance, like metabolic syndrome and diabetes. This conclusion is not true.

There are two kinds of insulin resistance in the body: pathologic and physiologic. I have to get a bit technical so bear with me; this is a very important part of understanding the prevention of heart disease through metabolic health. When there is minimal glucose available to the tissues—such as when someone is on a low-carb, high-fat diet—the body distributes available energy (in the form of carbohydrates, fats, and ketones) differently than when there is ample glucose around.[42] Certain tissues, like the brain and red blood cells, need some glucose. However, through a process called gluconeogenesis, the body can make all the glucose these tissues need from fats and proteins, meaning we do not have to ingest any carbohydrates.

In a state where the only available glucose is the glucose the body makes, the tissues that can easily run off fat and ketones, like the muscles and liver, will stop taking in glucose to leave it for the tissues that do actually need it.[43] This "glucose sparing" effect is the key mechanism of physiologic insulin resistance. In order for this effect to happen, the muscle cells have to become insulin resistant so that they stop receiving the signal of insulin to uptake glucose. In this situation the mild insulin resistance in the muscle tissues is healthy; these tissues have plenty of other fuels to run on.

The misconception occurs when someone in a glucose-sparing state gets tested for insulin sensitivity. Because some of their tissues have become insulin resistant to spare the glucose for other tissues, when you challenge the body with a large exogenous load of glucose, the cells that are insulin resistant don't react to the insulin that is secreted to bring that blood sugar down.[44] This can make it look like they are pathologically insulin resistant. In reality, they are metabolically healthy and if they were to eat more carbohydrates over a few days the insulin-resistant cells would easily turn back on their insulin receptors and the insulin/glucose balance would be normal again.

This misconception is based on a limited understanding of what insulin does in the body. Because of the discovery of being able to use injected insulin to control the blood sugars of type 1 diabetics, it was thought that the main role of insulin is to push glucose into cells. However, insulin has many functions, and aside from various ones like activation of the immune system, it has multiple roles within the regulation of our metabolism.[45] When blood sugar is in the normal range, the body is always mobilizing fat from cells and, to an extent, breaking down protein in the body so that the liver can convert it to glucose for our cells to use up. This is a catabolic, or breakdown, activity. If we eat carbohydrates and raise the level of glucose in our blood, the body secretes insulin to bring it down. Many people know that insulin decreases blood sugar by turning on insulin receptors on cells and pushing glucose into the cells. While insulin does do that, it is not its first action.

If we increase blood sugar by eating carbohydrates, insulin will first signal the body to stop the breakdown of tissue that provides the liver with metabolites to turn into glucose because we have enough glucose and don't need to make more. Glucagon is the hormone that signals the body to break down tissues. Both glucagon and insulin are secreted from the pancreas. When the pancreas senses that insulin has been secreted, it shuts off production of glucagon in order to stop production of glucose.[46] Second, once the insulin gets to the liver, it further halts production of glucose by signaling the liver to stop using any breakdown products that may already be in circulation.[47] And third, it further halts production of glucose once it arrives to the peripheral tissues by also signaling those tissues to stop breaking down those products.[48]

It is thought that insulin is largely anabolic, meaning it initiates building and repair. But when we look at these first three functions of insulin, in reality it is sort of anticatabolic. By turning off the breakdown of tissue, it allows the continually happening anabolic activities to get ahead, creating a net anabolic effect.

The fourth role insulin plays in metabolism is to open the doors of the cells to allow excess glucose in the blood to get in, which is why it lowers blood sugar. Whether insulin performs this role depends on how much glucose rises. If we eat a small amount of carbohydrates and our cells are metabolically flexible, then the anticatabolic effects of insulin could be enough to level out the small rise in glucose. Larger rises in insulin would require more insulin so that there is enough to shuttle the excess glucose into the cells. The more carbohydrates—especially processed carbohydrates—we eat, the more glucose will rise, and the more insulin will be needed to perform its role of pushing glucose into cells. We should note here again that when we look at the priority of the body to burn certain fuel sources, glucose comes first. Because of this, if we eat carbohydrates and fats, especially polyunsaturated fats, at the same time, the body uses the glucose first and stores the fat as body fat. As discussed in the Cholesterol Versus Phytosterol section, these polyunsaturated fats largely come from plant fats and directly contribute to insulin resistance and poor metabolic health.

The high-carb, high-polyunsaturated-fat dietary path to insulin resistance is called pathologic insulin resistance; over time it forces the body to stop responding to insulin because our fat cells become overburdened by the abundance of energy. Conversely, the low-carb, high-fat dietary approach can lead to physiologic insulin resistance, in which the body makes some tissues stop responding to insulin and taking up glucose to spare it for the tissues that need it. These are two different metabolic states: physiologic insulin resistance is heart healthy and pathologic insulin resistance contributes to the development of heart disease.

Now let's move on to those individual metabolites: TMAO, mTOR, and homocysteine. Philosophically speaking, the idea that a single biochemical molecule can, by itself, create serious disease is not logical. The human body is a complex biological ecosystem that is impossible to fully understand or predict. One of the major flaws in modern medical science is the belief that we can study one chemical reaction, pathway, or molecule in the body in order to understand the complexities of what creates health and causes disease.

Take trimethylamine N-oxide (TMAO) for example. TMAO is a metabolite made by gut bacteria when we eat certain foods. For example, it has been shown that eating red meat results in higher levels of TMAO, and some epidemiological studies (which, again, have their drawbacks) have shown an association between higher TMAO levels and heart disease.[49] The curious thing is that fish is touted as being heart healthy, but it creates higher levels of TMAO than either meat or eggs.[50] This illustrates the flaw of narrowly focusing on one metabolite and concluding that it alone creates a higher risk of disease, as well as some of the limitations of certain types of research. For example, in isolated lab experiments, the metabolite N-glycolylneuraminic acid (Neu5Gc) is shown to be harmful, but other research shows that eating animal foods stimulates changes in gut bacteria that easily minimize the effects of Neu5Gc.[51] The same has been found for TMAO.[52]

Even if we entertain the idea that single metabolites could cause disease on their own, looking further into the research suggests there is little to worry about. An associational study that tracked TMAO levels in 817 people over ten years to see if higher TMAO levels correlated with higher coronary artery calcium scores or carotid intima media thickness found that higher TMAO levels did not associate with higher amounts of atherosclerosis based on these measures.[53] While another study found that high TMAO was associated with increased cardiovascular disease, it also found that those with cardiovascular disease also had higher previous incidence of hypertension, diabetes, and prior heart attack.[54] So was it the TMAO that was causing this association or the metabolic dysfunction?

Let's move on to mTOR, or "mammalian target of rapamycin." mTOR is a metabolite that triggers growth and repair, but some research suggests that too much will lead to excess growth, and a predisposition to cancer. In fact, we need mTOR signaling; it is important to our health. There are a few things that stimulate mTOR. One is the amino acid leucine, found in high amounts in animal foods, and the other is insulin, secreted by the body in higher amounts when we eat carbohydrates. But the stimulation of mTOR by these two things is not equal. One study compared the stimulation of mTOR by insulin and leucine and found striking differences. The stimulation of mTOR by a meal high in leucine (animal foods) did so in a transient fashion; it was stimulated for about thirty minutes after eating a meal that contained leucine. With a carbohydrate meal that causes higher levels of insulin, mTOR was stimulated for two to three hours after the meal.[55]

This study showed that the stimulation of mTOR can be quite distinct for different eating patterns. When people eat a high-fat and animal-protein diet, many tend to eat only a few times a day because they are satiated, fat burning, and less hungry. Therefore, they are only activating mTOR a few times a day and for a shorter, thirty-minute to one-hour duration. If someone is eating the standard American diet, or even a paleo diet with lots of whole-food carbs, then they are triggering mTOR with a spike in insulin. This will stimulate mTOR for that longer two-hour to three-hour duration. Further, since excess carbohydrate meals are less satiating and tend to trigger people to eat three or more times a day, then we could potentially be getting mTOR stimulation for two to three hours, three or more times a day—pretty much all day long. So yes, animal foods trigger mTOR, which is important for growth and repair, but they are not going to stimulate it for very long, or lead to undue harm from overstimulation.

Finally, the metabolite homocysteine is a product of metabolizing the amino acid methionine (which is high in animal foods) to the amino acid cysteine, and is associated with damage to the arteries and atherosclerosis.[56] It is thought that since high levels of homocysteine are an indicator of inflammation, that animal foods that are high in methionine will result in higher levels of homo-cysteine production and predispose us to atherosclerotic heart disease.

But this is not fully understood, and research results are inconsistent. One study looked at 139 male subjects: eighteen were vegan; forty-three were vegetarians; sixty were moderate meat eaters; and eighteen were heavy meat eaters. Researchers found that "an inverse trend was observed with plasma homocysteine concentration, with vegans showing the high-est levels and high meat eaters the lowest."[57] In other words, these results suggest the opposite of what we're told (we're told that animal foods will elevate homocysteine levels). The cause of elevated homocysteine is more likely a lack of B vitamins, which are important for proper metabolism in the liver. This is especially true for people with different polymorphisms, or variants, in their genes that regulate metabolism in the liver. The best source for bioavailable B vitamins is animal foods like beef liver and egg yolks.

What about inflammation? We've discussed how inflammation caused by oxidative stress plays a role in atherosclerosis, heart failure, and heart attacks. Given that meat is often blamed for creating loads of inflammation, it seems natural to conclude that meat would cause heart disease. However, research shows that this is not the case, including two important interventional trials. (Interventional trials are experimental studies that establish cause-and-effect relationships.) In the first, a six-week interventional trial, thirty-seven people with type 2 diabetes were assigned to two groups; one group was fed a high-plant-protein diet and the other was fed a high-animal-protein diet. After six weeks, researchers measured many markers of inflammation. Although many people claim that plant protein is less inflammatory, these researchers found that the diets of both groups were effective at lowering various mark-ers of inflammation.[58]

In another interventional study, six participants change their diet by increasing the amount of red meat they ate over an eight-week period. When researchers compared the inflammatory marker levels with their baseline lev-els, they found that the participants had lower F2-isoprostanes, a marker of fatty acid damage from inflammation; lower leukocytes, markers of inflam-mation in the body; and lower serum C-reactive protein, a marker of general body inflammation. The researchers concluded that "partial replacement of dietary carbohydrate with protein from lean red meat does not elevate oxidative stress or inflammation."[59]

Not only are the claims that animal foods cause heart disease incorrect, animal protein is actually best for warding *off* heart disease. In 2013, researchers published the results of a study in the *American Journal of Clinical Nutrition* comparing diets in certain Asian countries. Researchers expected to find higher rates of disease in countries where people ate more meat, but instead found an inverse association with red meat, poultry, and fish / seafood —meaning those who ate the most of these things had the lowest risk of mortality. "Red meat intake was inversely associated with CVD mortality in men and with cancer mortality in women in Asian countries," the study reported.[60] A 2019 systematic review of all the randomized controlled trials on red meat and cardiometabolic and cancer outcomes stated that their findings "do not support the recommendations in the United Kingdom, United States, or World Cancer Research Fund guidelines on red meat intake" and that they "highlight the uncertainty regarding causal relationships between red meat consumption and major cardiometabolic and cancer outcomes."[61]

Heart Healthy Animal Food Nutrients

Before we jump into the nutrients in animal foods that support heart health, I want to discuss a "nutrient" that is absent in animal foods that is touted as being very heart healthy: fiber. By definition, fiber is undigestible by humans. It passes right through and does very little for us.

However, according to the Harvard T.H. Chan School of Public Health, "High intake of dietary fiber has been linked to a lower risk of heart disease in a number of large studies that followed people for many years."[62] This is true, if you are looking at the epidemiological studies the statement is based on. The Harvard T.H. Chan School of Public Health is considered a standard bearer of nutritional epidemiology studies—and also accepts substantial funding from food industry companies that produce and sell many foods loaded with fiber.[63]

Looking at other research on the relationship between fiber and cardiovascular health, however, paints a different picture. The only long-term interventional trial, to my knowledge, on fiber and cardiovascular risk looked at the effects of changes in fat, fish, and fiber intakes over two years among 2,033 men who had already experienced a heart attack. In the group that increased fiber intake, the researchers recorded 109 deaths from heart disease (among 123 deaths from any cause) compared to only 85 deaths from heart disease (among 101 deaths total) in the control group. Though the researchers concluded that these findings were not statistically significant, they also stated that "subjects given fibre advice had a slightly higher mortality than other subjects."[64]

A meta-analysis on fiber and heart health assessed the results of twenty-three randomized controlled trials (RCTs), which are the most conclusive form of interventional studies. However, none of the studies lasted longer than twelve weeks and "none of the studies reported on mortality (total or cardiovascular) or cardiovascular events." The meta-analysis concluded that "there is a need for longer term, well-conducted RCTs to determine the effects of fibre type (soluble versus insoluble) and administration (supplements versus foods) on CVD [cardiovascular disease] events and risk factors for the primary prevention of CVD."[65] A similar study that used whole grains for the fiber source in the search criteria came to similar conclusions.[66]

The bottom line? There is really no evidence that fiber prevents heart disease. The idea that fiber is helpful in preventing heart disease arose because it has been shown to lower cholesterol, but we have seen how cholesterol does not cause heart disease and can even be beneficial. People cling to the idea that fiber is necessary for a good balance of gut bacteria, for proper digestion and elimination, and to prevent colon cancer. However, it has been shown in carnivorous animals that fiber is not needed for a healthy gut because the gut flora can digest protein in place of fiber.[67] One RCT showed that removal of fiber actually relieved constipation in the study subjects.[68] Lastly, multiple studies show that fiber has no effect on preventing either colon cancer or diverticulosis.[69]

While I don't think that eating some fiber is inherently harmful, the need for lots of fiber is a myth. The benefits of plant fiber for heart disease have been overstated and overmarketed. In contrast, some important nutrients are found in high amounts, and sometimes exclusively, in animal foods. I have discussed vitamin K_2, CoQ10, and cholesterol itself. I have discussed the importance of fatty acids as a fuel source for the heart, as well as the

importance of collagen protein from animals for cellular health and the production of antioxidants to combat oxidative stress.

Collagen, which makes up our connective tissue and is the most abundant
protein in the body, has other benefits. For starters, it holds us together and
gives us structure. Our body can recycle collagen relatively well, but when
it comes to building new tissue, having plenty of new collagen around is
important. If you remember the discussion of atherosclerosis (see chapter 7),
there is a theory that it can develop from the outside layers of the artery in
response to injury of the lining of the blood vessel on the inside layers. It was
the formation of new blood vessels from the outside in—blood vessels in the
middle of developing—that were more prone to leak molecules from the
bloodstream into tissue, leading to the deposition of cholesterol molecules
and minerals in the intima layer of the arteries.

It turns out that collagen protein is important for limiting leakage in the
blood vessels, especially when new blood vessels are forming. For example,
researchers have bred mice to be deficient in certain collagen-forming metabolites and found that they had enhanced permeability of large and small
blood vessels and greater formation of atherosclerosis.[70] Scientists bred these
mice to have a deficiency in development of collagen tissue in newly formed
arteries, so the study doesn't quite show that eating collagen protein will
prevent arteries from being leaky; however, given all the other good things
that collagen does for us, it's clear that having plenty of collagen is important
to good health (see chapter 12 for additional discussion of collagen).

There is also a group of nutrients found almost exclusively in animal foods
that seem to play important roles in heart health: carnosine, carnitine, creatine, and taurine. Carnosine is key for regulating calcium concentrations in
cardiac cells, which is important because calcium is required for proper muscle contraction. Remember that in the end stages of heart attacks that occur
without blockages, the swelling from the buildup of lactic acid and hydrogen
ions interferes with calcium in the heart cells by preventing calcium from
getting into cells.[71] Carnosine is important to prevent interference in calcium
absorption in cardiac cells. Without enough carnosine, interference with the
uptake of calcium in cardiac cells is more likely to occur.

I learned about carnitine in my medical training because my biochemistry
teacher was certain that carnitine's role in the uptake of fatty acids into the

mitochondria to be used as fuel would be a question on our biochemistry national board exam—and it was. The fact that our mitochondria require carnitine in order to use fatty acids as fuel suggests that carnitine is crucial for tissue, like the heart, that prefers fatty acids for fuel. In fact, the shuttling of fatty acids into the mitochondria of heart cells has been shown to be cardio-protective against oxidative stress, inflammation, and heart cell death. There is even a genetic mutation that results in depletion of carnitine and is associ-ated with increased cardiovascular disease. A 2018 research article published in the journal *Life Sciences* discussed all the available research on carnitine and stated, "Hence, exogenous carnitine administration through dietary and intravenous routes serves as a suitable protective strategy against ventricular dysfunction, ischemia-reperfusion injury, cardiac arrhythmia and toxic myo-cardial injury that prominently mark CVD. Additionally, carnitine reduces hypertension, hyperlipidemia, diabetic ketoacidosis, hyperglycemia, insulin-dependent diabetes mellitus, insulin resistance, obesity, etc. that enhance cardiovascular pathology. These favorable effects of l-carnitine have been evident in infants, juvenile, young, adult and aged patients of sudden and chronic heart failure as well."[72] While some plants do have small amounts of carnitine, they cannot compete with animal foods when it comes to quantity and bioavailability of this heart healthy nutrient.

Next, creatine. Again, creatine is a nutrient found almost exclusively in animal foods, and it is higher in meats like beef, pork, chicken, and fish rather than in animal products like eggs, dairy, or shellfish. Due to the role of creatine in muscle contraction, weightlifters sometimes use it as a supplement. Of course, the heart is also a muscle. In one study, conducted with rats, research-ers artificially inhibited the activity of creatine in heart tissue. They found that under nonstress conditions, the end-diastolic pressure, left-ventricular-developed pressure, and heart rate of the rats was unchanged. However, under stress conditions they saw huge changes. Major decreases in the ability of the heart to maintain proper contractility under stress were observed with a depletion of creatine.[73] Since a stress response can trigger a heart attack without a blockage by affecting normal heart metabolism, having nutrients around that help us maintain normal heart physiology is clearly important.

Lastly, taurine. Taurine is a sulfur-containing amino acid important for the metabolism of fats. There are a few plant foods, including seaweed and brewer's yeast, that contain some taurine, but animal foods are by far the main source. Taurine has been shown to decrease cell damage during reperfusion (return of blood to tissue) after ischemia in heart tissue, possibly due to its ability to act as an antioxidant.[74] Taurine is also essential to the production of cholesterol sulfate. Research has also suggested that taurine can help prevent atherosclerosis formation by interfering with its early stages. When high blood levels of an enzyme called myeloperoxidase (MPO) are caused by ischemia in heart tissue, it is considered a risk factor for cardiovascular disease.[75] The risk is because in response to MPO, the body produces hypochlorite, which oxidizes many proteins, leading to activation of platelets causing white blood cells to attach to the walls of blood vessels. Research has suggested that taurine can prevent this activation from happening by neutralizing hypochlorite.[76] Taurine has also been shown to prevent the hardening of arteries by reducing the activity of the cells that calcify plaque, and protect against loss of mechanical function in heart failure (in rats).[77] A 2008 paper dedicated to the protective effects of taurine in preventing cardiovascular disease stated, "Taurine was found to exhibit diverse biological actions, including protection against ischemia-reperfusion injury, modulation of intracellular calcium concentration, and antioxidant, antiatherogenic and blood pressure-lowering effects."[78]

Carnosine, carnitine, creatine, and taurine are micronutrients, but there's also an important discussion to be had about a macronutrient found in animal foods: protein. This is not as much about heart disease specifically, but more about how important animal foods are for reduction of all-cause mortality and increased longevity. Many studies have shown that maintaining of muscle mass as we age is a huge predictor of reduced mortality and increased longevity.[79] The more we lose muscle mass and strength, the greater the risk of chronic disease and death. One study looked at the skeletal muscle mass index (SMMI) in relation to total mortality and cardiovascular disease specifically. The researchers found that "those with a low (1st quartile) SMMI had a 2-fold increase in total mortality and cardiovascular mortality risk compared to those with a normal [2nd, 3rd, or 4th quartile] SMMI."[80]

Getting adequate protein is essential for maintaining our muscle mass. Unfortunately, because so many people eat the standard American diet of processed food, they're not getting nearly enough protein. And not all protein is created equal. For example, beans are considered a good plant source of protein. However, just because a food has a high amount of protein does not mean that humans can use that protein effectively. There is a big difference between crude protein (the amount of protein in a food) and true utilizable protein (the amount of protein that can actually be used by the body). Beans come in at about 58 percent, compared to beef at 92 percent.[81] Further, plant proteins do not have the full complement of amino acids we need. To get enough true utilizable protein from plants to maintain muscle mass, someone would have to eat way more calories' worth of plant food than they would of animal food. Even then, they would not get all the necessary amino acids.

Studies looking specifically at frailty of individuals show some pretty striking results; these are epidemiology studies so they cannot show causation, but they still show some important associations. For example, a 2019 study published in the *European Journal of Nutrition* determined that "protein intake ≥ 1.1 g/kg BW and higher intake of animal protein may be beneficial to prevent the onset of frailty in older women."[82] I consider 1.1 grams per kilogram of body weight per day a *minimum* target. Other research shows that for every 15 grams per day increase in animal protein intake, bone mineral density [BMD] increased by 0.016 g/cm$_2$ at the hip, 0.012 g/cm$_2$ at the femoral neck, 0.015 g/cm$_2$ at the spine, and 0.010 g/cm$_2$ for the total body. Conversely, a negative association between vegetable protein and BMD was observed in both sexes. In conclusion, "this study supports a protective role for dietary animal protein in the skeletal health of elderly women."[83]

Fasting and Heart Health

If we think back to what life would have been like between 6 million years ago (when the last common ancestor between humans and apes lived) and today, there are many massive differences in our eating habits. One of those massive differences is that there were probably times where our ancestors were forced to fast. It wasn't an intentional act; it was just the way of life because food wasn't as readily available, and our ancestors had to work hard to get it.

This was especially true for Neanderthals and the first modern humans that evolved around 250 thousand years ago. These particular ancestors were high-level carnivores, who ate a diet almost entirely made up of animals. At that time, humans and prehumans were prolific hunters, but finding, hunting, and killing the next meal took a lot of time. There would have been times when food was scarce. This would have been especially true in winter.

In summer, if hunting was unsuccessful, some plant foods probably were eaten to prevent starvation. However, in winter, those seasonal foods would not have been available and fasting for extended periods would have been a reality. On a weekly basis, there were likely ebbs and flows of feasts and famine. This likely occurred for a very long time (from about 2.5 million years ago until about ten thousand years ago), so these evolutionary adaptations to fasting would have become deep-seated into our physiology. From this perspective, it's hardly surprising that humans began experiencing a decline in health, including metabolic syndrome, when people began eating more frequently throughout the day.

The Agricultural Revolution, about ten to twelve thousand years ago, was probably the first time humans began eating multiple times a day. This was also the first time humans stayed in one place and farmed crops. Farming provided an abundance of calories, though they were nutritionally poor and lower-quality calories. Yet these abundant, nutrient-poor calories did the job of allowing us to reproduce and grow in numbers very quickly. While the population grew, there is evidence that health suffered.[84]

I believe the poor health that those first farmers experienced was in part due to eating a lesser quality food (crops) but also due to overconsumption of the energy in these foods in an attempt to get enough nutrients. Since these foods were less nutrient dense, and less bioavailable to our bodies, they had to eat more calories throughout the day in order to get the necessary nutrients. This was the beginning of the "constantly eating" society we have today.

That said, throughout history, various civilizations have found value in not consuming food constantly. Historians say that the Romans were known not to eat breakfast because it was thought to be healthier. Eating more than one meal a day was sometimes said to be a form of gluttony. Even in the Middle Ages, fasting was common, especially among monks. If we fast forward to today, we have a society in which huge quantities of food are available to us all day, every day, especially in westernized countries. In the early 1900s, John Harvey Kellogg invented the first breakfast cereal, and the beginning of marketing breakfast was underway. By the 1920s and '30s, the government was promoting a breakfast of processed grains and sugars as the most important meal of the day.

This was around the time of major changes in human health, including the rise in obesity and heart disease. Of course, there were many other changes during this time, including the introduction of seed oils and increased toxin exposure, but breakfast was a big part of it: Our consumption of nutrient-poor calories first thing in the morning likely played a major role in this increase of chronic disease.

So, our physiology was shaped over millions of years in a time when calories were not always available, and fasting was a part of life. Then, in a relatively short amount of time, we began eating constantly and overtaxing our metabolism with the introduction of plentiful, nutrient-poor calories, leading to an increase in metabolic chronic disease. Returning to a more restrictive eating regimen guides us toward health by effectively putting our physiology back in an environment for which it is more evolved.

There is compelling research to support this: Restricting calories through intermittent fasting or a low-carb/ketogenic diet is good for life span and health span. One study conducted in mice found that "energy-controlled high-fat LCD's [low-carb diets] are not detrimental to health, but rather a KD [ketogenic diet] extends lifespan and slows age-related decline in physiologic function in mice."[85] That is an enticing finding for anyone who wants to live a long and fulfilled life. Cut the carbs and empty calories and go with the more satiating nutrient-dense fats.

This longevity effect may be related to autophagy—the cleaning up of old cells to make room for new ones—that is induced by fasting. For the heart specifically, fasting-induced autophagy benefits the heart in many ways, including that a "preponderance of evidence suggests that autophagy and mitophagy are important protective mechanisms across the spectrum of ischemic injury."[86] But the effects of fasting could be due to other longevity effects as well; for example, periodic fasting is associated with maintaining muscle mass, one of the best indicators of health as we age.[87] Other research has uncovered changes in physiology associated with fasting. For example, when researchers instructed people to fast for one week, total cholesterol, LDL, and apo-B levels all went up substantially. In fact, LDL increased from an average of 114 mg/dL to 190 mg/dL—a 40 percent increase.[88] This is likely because the process of making ketones, which the body has to make for a fuel source during fasting, is the same pathway for making cholesterol. So, cholesterol goes up as well.

In another study, researchers fed one group of rats on an intermittent fasting schedule and another group more frequently. They then induced heart attacks in all the rats. The intermittent fasting group had smaller heart attacks, lower amounts of apoptosis (programmed cell death of the heart tissue), and lower inflammation overall.[89] The practice of intermittent fasting seemed to lessen the damage done by a heart attack. Other studies have shown and given explanations for the cardioprotective effects of fasting. Intermittent fasting has been shown to raise levels of what is called adiponectin, a protein hormone in the human body that helps protect heart tissue from ischemic injury.[90]

Fasting also seems to help prevent atherosclerosis. People who had been fasting intermittently for from three to fifteen years, showed lower levels of "markers of atherosclerosis," like triglycerides, trig/HDL ratio, blood pressure, insulin sensitivity, and high sensitivity c-reactive protein. Those individuals who practiced intermittent fasting also had about 40 percent less atherosclerosis in their carotid arteries than the control group. This is even more dramatic than it seems: Because the research defined atherosclerosis as "more than 1 mm [millimeter]" of increase thickness of the carotid artery, a 40 percent decrease means that they didn't have just less atherosclerosis; none of the intermittent fasting group had *any* atherosclerosis.[91]

If fasting increases cholesterol yet also reduces the size of induced heart attacks, reduces cell death during heart attacks, decreases levels of inflammation, and significantly reduces development of atherosclerosis, how could cholesterol cause heart disease?

I recommend fasting. You can do this in various ways. I like to eat two meals a day within a six- to eight-hour window. Implementing these strategies brings us closer to living in a way more compatible to our evolved physiology and can give us huge health benefits, especially for the heart.

A Sustainable Heart Healthy Diet

In my first book, *The Health Evolution: Why Understanding Evolution Is the Key to Vibrant Health*, I argued that creating a personal environment where your body can thrive is also a strategy for having the least environmental impact and, therefore, for ensuring a positive future for humans and other life on Earth. You now also know that I advocate for an animal-based, metabolically flexible diet for heart health, and for health in general. And yet, we're always hearing that animal agriculture is bad for the environment. So, can these things coexist? Can I have a healthy heart by eating an animal-based diet, without having a heavy heart from harming the Earth and the well-being of animals?

Since the environmental impact of raising meat goes beyond the scope of this book, I recommend *Defending Beef* by Nicolette Hahn Niman, *The Vegetarian Myth* by Lierre Keith, *Sacred Cow* by Diana Rodgers and Robb Wolf, and the work of Dr. Peter Ballerstedt for in-depth analysis of this issue. But looking at it from a health perspective is well within the scope of this book: To do that, let's revisit the imbalances that cause a heart attack without a blockage and discuss how correcting those imbalances in our body is also better for the environment. The first two imbalances I will discuss together: ensuring our bodies are fat-adapted because the heart prefers to burn fat, and reducing oxidative stress so that we don't get atherosclerosis or deplete the nitric oxide in our bodies. Both of these can be accomplished by restricting carbohydrates. Restricting carbohydrates will make us efficient at fat burning by encouraging our body to make ketones. Since burning fat produces fewer free radicals, there is also less oxidative stress.

But how is burning fat rather than carbohydrates kinder to the environment? Most of the carbohydrates humans consume come from processed forms of four crops: corn, wheat, soy, and sugar. The vast majority of these crops are produced via industrialized plant agriculture, which is incredibly damaging to the Earth. In *Primal Fat Burner*, Nora Gedgaudas told us that 70 percent of the world's grasslands have been degraded and soil is being degraded 13 percent faster than it can be rebuilt through industrial farming. Large-scale monocropping is at odds with a natural ecological system, which thrives on diversity.

When left alone, nature creates diversity. If you walk into a natural land-scape, you will never see a single dominating species; there is always a range that makes up a natural space. Industrial farming and monocropping clears diversity from a plot of land, and often degrades it to the point of infertility. The once Fertile Crescent is now desert because of relentless farming. But this way of producing food is still happening today, at far greater scale, and the only reason it has not resulted in failure of the food system is because we have chemical fertilizers made from oil, which we will one day run out of. By eating an animal-based diet, I significantly reduce the amount of processed carbohydrates consumed and opt out of supporting the unsustainable prac-tices of industrial plant farming.

Unfortunately, there is a lot of incorrect information about plant-based versus animal-based diets and their respective effects on the environment. The details of how that came about are, again, beyond the scope of this book, but I recommend the work of Dr. Gary Fettke and Belinda Fettke as an introduction to how ideologies have influenced our dietary guidelines.

What about the idea that animal agriculture is bad for the environment? First, let's discuss ruminants, the grazing grass eaters. The main grazer in animal agriculture in the United States is cattle. Cows are amazing animals in that they can take something like grass, a plant we can't eat, and turn it into meat, something we can eat. Cows do this with a specialized digestive system that can take the grass, break it down, and ferment it into short-chain fatty acids. Yes, the end product of a cow eating grass is fat, so in a way a cow eats a high-fat diet.

Humans do not have a digestive system that can turn plants into fat, and therefore, we must eat fat directly. This is the digestive system that evolved during the millions of years of human evolution when our prehuman and human ancestors were eating large ruminant animals. Ruminants turned grass into meat and fat and then we ate the ruminants. Not only that, but the large ruminants that roamed the Earth played a large part in creating the healthy topsoil that we now use to farm crops. Unfortunately, our farming practices have destroyed this topsoil.[92] If ruminant agriculture is so import-ant for ecosystem health, why does it get such a bad rap?

One argument is that animal agriculture produces a large amount of green-house gases that contribute to global warming. However, the US Environmental

Protection Agency estimates that the total percentage of US greenhouse gases produced from all agriculture (plant and animal) is around 10 percent.[93] Of that 10 percent, only 4 percent is attributed to animal agriculture, with the beef industry contributing around 2 percent.[94] By contrast, transportation, industry, and energy production account for 77 percent of the greenhouse gas emissions in the United States. More importantly, studies have shown that properly raised cattle, appropriately rotated on land, sequesters carbon in the soil and contributes to overall ecosystem health.[95] When soil is carbon-rich, it can hold water. When soil is depleted—which happens when we practice large-scale industrial monocropping—rainwater runs off into our rivers, lakes, and oceans, carrying soil with it along with herbicides and pesticides.

There are many farms practicing regenerative animal agriculture that sequesters carbon in the soil. Farms like Polyface Farms in Virginia, White Oak Pastures in Georgia, and Brown's Ranch in North Dakota are leading the way. Organizations like the Savory Institute are showing how ruminant agriculture can be effective in reversing desertification and restoring soil and ecosystems to good health. Remember that it was millions of ruminants in the form of bison, buffalo, and elk (at least in the United States) that built up the topsoil in the first place.

Currently, 11 percent of the Earth's land is being used for plant-based agriculture and 26 percent is being used as rangeland. Sixty-three percent cannot be used for agriculture of any kind.[96] Some argue that if we farm plants on the land being used for rangeland for animals, we could produce enough plant food for everyone to eat only plants, but not all that rangeland is suitable for farming; some rangeland is too rocky to grow crops. Plus, without animals, obtaining enough protein from plants (58 percent utilizable protein) versus animals (92 percent utilizable protein) would require us to produce substantially more plant protein. Trying to produce enough plants to feed humans without eating animals is not only unsustainable—it's impossible.

Reducing processed carbohydrates produced by industrial agriculture in our diet is not only better for our bodies, it is also better for the planet— if done properly. Eating an animal-based diet that does not support the processed-food industry will accomplish this—especially if we only eat animals that are raised in a regenerative way—and is the best approach to accomplishing health and sustainability at the same time.

There is another aspect to eating animals that leads us right to the third imbalance that drives heart attacks: a dysfunctional stress response in our ANS. This dysfunction can result from the mismatch between our evolved stress response and a lifestyle that creates constant unnatural stressors that our bodies are not evolved to handle.

For some people, the killing and eating of animals weighs heavy on their hearts, and I'm sympathetic to this. However, through destroying ecosystems and displacing animals for industrial plant monocropping, the killing of animals to protect crops, and even the accidental death of animals during harvest, a large number of animals are in fact killed to produce vegetarian and vegan diets. Dr. Steven Davis, an emeritus professor of animal and rangeland sciences at Oregon State University argues that in each hectare of all 120 million hectares of cropland harvested each year in the United States, fifteen animals that live in those fields are killed on average per year during harvest. Based on those numbers, this means that an estimated 1.8 billion animals would be killed to produce a vegan diet in the United States.

He goes on to discuss how of the 8.4 billion farm animals killed each year for food in the United States, approximately 8 billion of those are poultry and only 37 million are ruminants (cows, calves). The remainder are pigs and other species. He argues that if the number of cows and calves killed for food each year was doubled to 74 million to replace the 8 billion poultry, the total number of animals that would need to be killed under this alternative method would be only 1.424 billion, which is less than the number of animals he estimates would die in harvest each year if the United States were to try and grow an entirely vegan diet for the population.[97]

I understand that these numbers are just estimates and that getting the actual numbers may be impossible. Regardless of what the actual numbers are, the point is that growing plants the way we do does not avoid killing animals. Living things have been killing other living things in order to survive since life has existed on this Earth. To think that we can somehow avoid killing animals and still sustain ourselves will, I fear, take us down a path of even more self-destruction and environmental degradation. Instead of being so uncomfortable with death that we go to extremes to avoid it and sacrifice our health and the health of the planet along the way, we should embrace and accept the natural way of the world. There are ways to ethically and sustainably feed ourselves through small-scale pasture-based (local) animal husbandry. This practice gives the animals the best quality of life, creates the healthiest food, and has a positive impact on the environment. Confronting an animal's death forces us to acknowledge that we have a responsibility to other life on the planet and that we must protect the ecosystems for all of us. When it comes to ensuring humanity is provided with high-quality nutrition and to restoring health to our planet, eating animals is not the problem; it is a vital part of the solution.

CHAPTER 12

Reducing Oxidative Stress

One summer, my wife and I took a trip to Italy that included a stay on the Amalfi Coast, where the mountains seem to rise straight out of ocean, and the roads, homes, and villages seem to be carved right out of the sides of the mountains overlooking the dark blue Tyrrhenian Sea. The day after our arrival, Kinga and I decided to hike the Sentiero degli Dei, or the Path of the Gods. The receptionist at our hotel lived nearby and offered to show us to the trailhead, so the three of us took a bus to the mountaintop town of Agerola, where she gave us directions and then continued home. On the trail, we walked in fields, along cliffs, and through forest. Many small, man-made monuments were scattered along the path. There even seemed to be some homes. The hike was full of many ascents and descents, and there were spectacular views up and down the mountainous coast and out into the sea.

Our plan was to walk 4.8 miles to Nocelle, another small town nestled into the side of the mountains before descending into the town of Positano and catching a ferry back to Amalfi by dinner. We figured it was no problem: We were high up in Nocelle and Positano was down on the coast—the hike from Nocelle would be all downhill. In fact there were stairs, and we moved quickly, sometimes two steps at a time, through little mountainside neighborhoods following signs for Positano. But the stairs just kept going. We would turn a corner only to find another long stretch of stairs. Eventually our muscles started to burn, and our knees started to ache. The constant compression of taking step after step was taking a toll. Over time we found ourselves in pain and going quite slow down the stairs, all the while worrying if we would catch the ferry. Later, I learned that we had descended between 1,600 and 1,700 steps.

To the relief of our legs, we finally reached the bottom of the stairs and had to walk along the road, through the crowds in Positano, and find out how to buy a ticket for the ferry. Although we didn't have time for sightseeing, we caught the ferry with five minutes to spare. The ferry ride offered a view back up at the coast from the sea and we arrived in Amalfi, enjoyed our dinner, and returned to our hotel for the evening.

The stairs in this story are an analogy for oxidative stress, because the sources of oxidative stress are often things that make life easier or more convenient. Kinga and I assumed that the trek down to Positano would be easy because it was all downhill, but once we started, it caused us pain. My quads, calves, and back were sore the next day. There are many things in our lives today that have made some aspect of our lives easier, but in the end, they damage our bodies. When it comes to oxidative stress, these can be anything from the abundant energy sources we have access to in the form of processed carbohydrates and fats to the many toxic chemicals that help us make things smell better or allow us to clean more easily. While these things may make our lives easier in the short run, they make it harder in the long run.

I have discussed the different sources of excess free radicals or oxidative stress in the body. These things—like a carbohydrate-based metabolism, endotoxemia, and various toxins—can all lead to oxidative stress and therefore contribute to atherosclerosis and heart attacks. So how do we limit the things that cause oxidative stress to begin with?

Seed Oils

I've detailed how a fat-burning metabolism will reduce free-radical formation, but there is a form of fat I briefly discussed but did not fully review, and it is a fat we want to avoid because it is a major cause of oxidative stress. These are the infamous seed oils in the form of margarine, vegetable shortening, canola oil, safflower oil, soy oil, and corn oil, among others. They worsen cardiovascular outcomes and harm our metabolism; they also provoke oxidative stress.

People have only started to eat these processed forms of plant fats, or seed oils, in the last one hundred years or so, which is no time at all when we're talking about the evolution of the human body and the food we need to thrive, and indeed the research on seed oils and oxidative stress is a little scary. One marker of oxidative stress in the body is called lipid peroxidation, which measures damage to fats. When rats on a high-cholesterol diet were supplemented with a seed oil (sunflower oil) or with olive oil and then tested for markers of fats damaged by oxidative stress, those that were supplemented with the sunflower oil had much higher levels of two different markers of damaged fats (malondialdehyde and diene conjugate) compared to the olive oil group and the control group. The sunflower oil group also had decreased levels of the master antioxidant glutathione, which is one of the main antioxidants our bodies use to combat oxidative stress.[1]

We can also assess oxidative stress by looking at the damage to cellular DNA from free radicals. Another study, also done with rats, did just that. The researchers fed a base diet to one group of rats and then in four other groups they fed the base diet plus various types of processed seed oils (sunflower oil, rapeseed oil, olive oil, and coconut oil). While each of the four intervention groups saw a rise in the DNA damage marker 8-oxo-deoxyguanosine compared to the control group, the rapeseed and sunflower oil groups had significantly higher levels than the coconut and olive oil groups. The sunflower oil group was the highest by far.[2]

Higher oxidative stress from consuming high amounts of polyunsaturated plant fats has been shown in humans as well. One study took thirty-eight subjects and fed them a diet of saturated fat for four weeks and then switched some of them to eating a high amount of two different kinds of polyunsaturated fats (linoleic acid and oleic acid) while leaving thirteen subjects on the higher-saturated-fat diet. Four weeks after the switch researchers found that when compared to the control group, the high-polyunsaturated-fat diet "increased oxidative stress and affected endothelial function [through depletion of nitric oxide] in a way which may in the long-term predispose to endothelial dysfunction."[3] Remember that depletion of nitric oxide by oxidative stress is one imbalance that contributes to some heart attacks; this study showed that consuming high amounts of polyunsaturated fat (like we find in seed oils) does just that.

The obvious way to avoid damage from these oils is to eliminate them from our diets. This means being diligent about looking for them in foods. These oils are found in most baked goods and fried foods and are used abundantly in the restaurant industry. They are often labeled as hydrogenated or partially hydrogenated oils. The only thing worse than eating these damaging oils is damaging the oils before they even get into our bodies, which is what heating them does. Consuming these oils that have been heated over and over again—like what happens when frying foods—has been directly linked to the development of heart disease.[4]

Reducing Toxicants from the Major Five Sources

I can't do a comprehensive assessment of all the toxins that can contribute to oxidative stress in the space of this book, but I do hope to create awareness of how you can most substantially decrease the toxin burden on your body. I often guide clients and patients through the five areas of our modern-day lives that expose us to the most toxins, so that they can alter things in each area to the best of their ability and reduce their toxin exposure.

The first area is food (of course). This is the most important change when it comes to lessening your toxic burden, because if we don't pay attention to toxins in our food, we put them directly into our body. I have already discussed how plants make toxins to defend themselves from being eaten. By now you know that I think complete avoidance of these toxins by excluding all plants in the diet, while not always necessary, is perfectly safe and healthy. However, if you do want to include plants in your diet, it is important to make sure they have had as few toxins added to them in the form of herbicides, pesticides, and fertilizers as possible. The best method of doing this is to choose organic plants. Research has shown that organic produce consistently has less toxins and more nutrients than conventional produce.[5] If you cannot afford to buy all organic food, then at least get the organic versions of the Dirty Dozen, the fruits and vegetables that are known to have the highest amount of known toxins sprayed on them. You can find the list of the twelve most highly sprayed foods on the Environmental Working Group website (www.ewg.org/foodnews/dirty-dozen.php).

The other aspect of food to pay attention to is packaging. There are many toxins that come in contact with our food through the process of packaging it. You can reduce this by eating as little prepackaged food as possible and sticking to whole foods. Being this selective is hard to do even for me, because much of the meat I buy comes vacuum sealed in plastic. When I get it from a butcher, I ask for them just to wrap it in paper, but when I buy in bulk, the plastic is hard to avoid. I make sure that I sweat often by working out and using saunas to help my body eliminate these toxins. I also make sure I get plenty of connective tissue proteins so that I boost my body's own antioxidant production to help me mitigate oxidative stress they may cause.

Tap water is also a big source of toxin exposure, including heavy metals, chloride, fluoride, herbicides and pesticides, medications, and plastics.[6] A good water filtration system will reduce this exposure. AquaTru and Berkey filters are two good countertop options. You can also go to www.friendsofwater.com and look into getting filters installed in your sink or for your entire home. It is worth noting that a good enough filter is going to get everything out, including the minerals that you *want* in your water. Drinking mineral-depleted water has been associated with many symptoms in humans, including various forms of cardiovascular disease.[7] An easy fix is to remineralize the water with a mineral solution. All of this may sound like a hassle, but it is the reality if we want to avoid toxins in water. Another option is to drink mineral water from a natural spring (www.findaspring.com) or that comes in glass bottles at the store. A few of my favorites are Topo Chico, San Pellegrino, Mountain Valley, and Gerolsteiner.

Another area of toxin exposure is the air we breathe. Studies in mice and rabbits have shown that when they are exposed to samples of the air pollution we are exposed to, they have accelerated rates of atherosclerosis, as well as more instability of the atherosclerosis that is created.[8] Obviously, we have limited control over the air we breathe, but one solution is to live in places with less pollution. This obviously means living farther away from big cities. If that is not possible, the next best thing is to control the air you can control, which is the air inside your home. Avoid air fresheners with artificial scents (use essential oil diffusers instead), fabric softeners, or colognes and perfumes. These are all very toxic and get trapped in our homes, where we breathe them over and over again. You can also have your home tested for mold and make sure your air filtration system is up to par. It will filter many particles out of circulation. To take it a step further, you can get an air filter like the AirDoctor, Air Oasis, or Molekule that will help clean and sanitize the air in your home. A good strategy is to get one of these for your bedroom so that you can be sure you are at least breathing the best-quality air while you are sleeping.

The fourth area to clean up is your cleaning products themselves. It's ironic that we have to be careful to choose clean versions of the products we use to clean. There are so many toxins in cleaning products that add to our toxic load—everything from the powerful disinfectants to the artificial fragrances in these products. Luckily, there are many brands that make an effort to limit or eliminate the amount of toxins they have in them, and a good move is to support those companies for making that effort. However, in reality, all we really need to clean is a water and vinegar solution. You could also add some essential oils for a nontoxic fragrance.

Finally, toxins are in many cosmetics and self-care products: These are also important because we put them directly on our bodies. If we put something on our skin, it is going to get into our bodies. I won't provide an exhaustive list, but we need to be very conscious of the products we use, including makeup, soap, shampoo, deodorants, moisturizers, sunscreens, and tooth-paste. Do your research on these products. When we think about all the little toxin exposures we experience each day, it may not seem like that big of a deal, but when they all come together it can drastically increase the amount of oxidative stress in our bodies. Most of the toxins we come in contact with are water soluble and easily eliminated, but if we constantly expose ourselves, our bodies never have time to catch up, so the toxins begin to get stored in our bodies. This is how we get oxidative stress that can contribute to atherosclerosis and depletion of nitric oxide, making us more vulnerable to heart disease.

Vaccines, Childhood Illness, and Long-Term Health

I want to briefly touch on another source of toxins: vaccines. I am not going to argue for or against vaccines here, but the choice of whether to get a vaccine or vaccinate your children should not be taken lightly. For more complete information on vaccines, I recommend *Vaccines, Autoimmunity, and the Changing Nature of Childhood Illness* by Thomas Cowan, MD. I just want to point out that vaccines have many different toxins in them—they are listed on the package inserts, so ask your doctor for it.[9] Most of them will contribute to the "electron-hungry process" that breaks down EZ, damages the artery lining, and initiates an atherosclerotic response.

As Dr. Cowan argues, fighting off the childhood infectious diseases may actually be protective from chronic disease later in life, including cancer.[10] A Japanese study found that people who had measles and mumps in childhood have less incidence of atherosclerosis as adults. Having had one infection or the other was associated with less risk, having had both was associated with even less risk, and the more acute infections that caused fever reduced risk even further. The authors concluded "measles and mumps, especially in case of both infections, were associated with lower risks of mortality from atherosclerotic CVD."[11]

Yes, these are only associational studies and cannot show that having the illnesses was the cause of less disease later in life, but childhood illness, as uncomfortable as it is for the child to have and the parent to watch, is a natural part of life. These studies suggest that they may be a sort of "training" for the child's body and may have a benefit to the child's health in the long run.

Endotoxemia and Gut Health

While acute infection in the form of childhood illness may help prevent atherosclerosis later in life, having chronic low levels of bacteria in our bloodstream, termed *endotoxemia*, is not a good idea. Endotoxemia is the presence of excess gram-negative bacteria in the blood, and it contributes to oxidative stress in the body. I briefly noted that a damaged digestive tract (or leaky gut) and poor dental health are sources of endotoxemia when we discussed the relationship of endotoxemia and atherosclerosis. Although endotoxins are frequently overlooked, they contribute significantly to many chronic diseases. To combat endotoxemia, it is essential that we protect the health of our gut and our mouth. Luckily, an animal-based diet helps with both of these. By excluding sugars from the diet, an animal-based diet significantly reduces the risk of gum disease and cavity formation. This ensures that the mouth stays healthy and that no bacteria will leak from the mouth into the bloodstream. An animal-based diet is also rich in fat-soluble vitamins like vitamin D and vitamin K, which are essential for the strength of the teeth.

I have already discussed how an animal-based diet will eliminate the plant toxins that contribute to leaky gut. But there are a few additional aspects of an animal-based diet that will help us avoid a porous digestive system that leaks bacteria. A well-constructed animal-based diet will include connective tissue protein from collagen, and this collagen plays an essential role in the health of the gut lining. When the gut lining becomes leaky, it is because of a breakdown of what are called tight junctions that bind cells together in the gut lining. This breakdown is caused by inflammation. One study that tested a few different proteins found that collagen peptides had the "most effective activity in protecting the tight junction barrier function against [the potent inflammatory marker] TNF-α stimulation."[12] Collagen has even been shown to be able to repair the lining of the digestive tract of mice who had damage induced through burns on their digestive-system lining.[13] Adequate collagen protein in the diet will help keep our gut sealed off so that bacteria cannot leak into the bloodstream and cause oxidative stress. The discovered benefits of connective tissue proteins in the diet just keep growing.

Another aspect of an animal-based diet that will keep our gut healthy is that it helps us avoid the toxin glyphosate. Glyphosate is an herbicide used on genetically modified crops. If you go to a home improvement store, you can buy it right off the shelf in the form of Roundup weed killer. Glyphosate is widely sprayed on crops, and it has been shown to cause damage to the cells lining our intestines.[14] In Dr. Pollack's lab they directly tested the effects of glyphosate on the EZ barrier protecting the arterial lining. They found that "the weed killer, Roundup, which impairs health, steadily diminished EZ with increasing concentration."[15] If we don't eat the sprayed crops, and instead choose an animal-based diet, ideally of 100 percent grass-fed or pastured animal foods, we will not allow glyphosate to create a leaky gut, contribute to oxidative stress, and deplete the EZ water of our bodies. Some would say that the animals we eat are bound to be exposed to glyphosate and therefore by ingesting the animals we are also exposed, but that is not necessarily true. It has been shown that mammals do not bioaccumulate glyphosate.[16] If an animal is exposed to glyphosate directly, it will harm the animal's gut on the way through, but it does not seem to build up in the body. We are much safer from the harms of glyphosate on an animal-based diet.

AGEs and Hormetic Stress

Finally, I have already discussed how advanced glycation end products (AGEs) can be caused by higher blood glucose over time and that the excess sugar damages tissues in the body. The obvious solution here is to maintain stable blood sugars. An animal-based diet that is void of blood-sugar-spiking processed carbohydrates will help us, but unstable blood sugar is not the only way we can be exposed to AGEs. They can also be created by cooking or processing foods.[17] For example, AGEs largely occur when a food, such as a crust of bread, is burned while cooking. While we don't have to worry about bread crust or processed foods on an animal-based diet, we do have to worry about burnt animal foods. We need to be cautious about how we cook our animal foods so that we don't consume too many AGEs. Boiling, pan frying with a little water in the pan, steaming, or poaching are better options than baking, grilling, roasting, frying, deep frying, or broiling.

There is another way to decrease the effect of the harmful compounds that are formed while cooking. In chapter 11, we discussed how ingesting antioxidants in fruits and vegetables has no real effect on antioxidants or oxidative stress. However, some studies show that adding antioxidant-rich spices to meat while cooking it can have a mitigating effect.[18] A 2013 study published in *Diabetic Medicine* compared eating cooked meat with and without an antioxidant-rich spice mix and found that the spice mix was associated with increases in nitric oxide and "improvement in postprandial endothelial function."[19]

That said, there may actually be some benefit to having a little exposure to toxic molecules created while cooking. This benefit is called hormesis. When exposed to a little bit of a toxin, the body responds by upregulating its antioxidant production, resulting in a net-positive effect because more antioxidants are produced than are needed to take care of the small toxic stress. There are many things that can have a hormetic effect in the body. Much of the benefit of the phytochemicals in plants that are said to be good for us (like resveratrol and curcumin) is due to their toxins creating a hormetic stress. Personally, I would rather get my hormetic stressors in other ways. For example, I can ingest a small amount of AGEs as heterocyclic amines and polycyclic aromatic hydrocarbons when eating meat that is burned a small amount. Even healthier generators of hormetic stress are exercise, sunlight, and exposure to hot and cold environments. While we want to keep these compounds to a minimum, we are well equipped to handle small amounts of plant toxins and harmful compounds created while cooking; it is when they become overwhelming that we get into trouble.

We may never be able to get AGEs in our diet down to zero, but making an effort with a diet low in AGEs has been shown to decrease oxidative stress. In one study, researchers randomized sixty-one obese people with metabolic syndrome (which includes insulin resistance, a risk factor for type 2 diabetes) into two groups: half ate a diet low in AGEs (they were told, for instance, to avoid baking, grilling, or frying food), while the other half had a standard American diet that was high in AGEs. After one year, the low-AGE group had lower blood levels of AGEs, a reduction in insulin resistance, a decrease in markers for inflammation and oxidative stress, and a small amount of weight loss.[20]

To review, to minimize oxidative stress and help prevent heart disease, we want to limit vegetable oils, avoid common toxins in our everyday lives, keep our mouths and guts healthy to prevent endotoxemia, be conscious of AGEs, and create hormetic stresses in the least harmful and most natural ways possible. An animal-based diet is a great baseline to achieve all of these things.

CHAPTER 13

Achieving Autonomic Balance

A few months after I had moved to Ireland, I found myself pretty stressed. It was my first job after chiropractic school and I had a grace period before I had to start paying off my student loans. It felt like the grace period was evaporating quickly. I wasn't making much money starting out because I was trying to build up a patient base at the clinic, and chiropractic isn't as utilized in Ireland as it is in the United States. It seemed that each time I got paid it was all used up on bills and food and little was left for savings.

On top of that, I had moved to an entirely new country where I knew no one. Aside from the other chiropractor I was working with, I didn't have much of a social support system. Until this point, I had been in school and good friends had always been easy to find among my classmates. Going out in a foreign country and striking up conversations with strangers to make new friends was not my forte. Plus, I was living in the city center of Dublin, and while I had lived in Portland, Oregon, for chiropractic school, I never lived right in the center of a city. I'd grown up in a small town, and the hustle and bustle, constant noise, and 24/7 lights of the city were different for me. Living in this new environment with few social relationships and financial difficulty was leading to an ever-increasing state of stress. I could feel that I was more anxious than my usual self; I was becoming irritable more easily and, despite improvements I felt from adding animals back into my diet, my digestive health was declining once again.

So I joined a group of guys who played soccer every Sunday morning (and ended up playing with them up until the day I left Ireland), and signed up for a kayaking trip through Meetup. The event page said to meet in Skerries, which was north of Dublin right on the coast, so I caught the train and I joined up with ten other people and a guide who outfitted us with two-person kayaks and the necessary equipment. We paired up and carried the kayaks to the beach. The waves were small, and it was easy to paddle out into the surf. The guide led us off into the ocean, but we didn't go far. Our goal was to explore three little islands that were visible from the beach. The farthest one, St. Patrick's Island, was about a mile off the shore. Closer in were Colt Island and Shenick Island. All three were rocky and barren islands with a few little trees.

My kayak partner was from Oman and had taken an IT job in Dublin, but it was hard to get to know him much more than that. It was windy and started raining on the way out to St. Patrick's Island, and he was not a strong paddler; we mostly paddled in silence battling the wind and rain, me in the back and him in the front. By the time we got to St. Patrick's Island and carried our kayaks up on shore, everyone was pretty tired. I took a ten-minute walk around the island with one young woman who was still in good spirits, we had a friendly conversation, and then once we returned, she stayed with the group while I took another lap.

On the far side of the island, I sat on the beach and looked out at the ocean. I felt a sense of calm that I had not felt the last few months. I didn't realize it at the time, but on this day trip, my environment had drastically changed. I had a good conversation with a potential new friend, and I was far from the city, facing the ocean with no visible signs of civilization. I sat for a while on the sand, in direct contact with the Earth, and listened to the small waves lap the shore.

It would be years until I understood the mechanisms of how that environment—that idyllic island in Skerries—calmed my ANS. After that moment on the island, I found myself seeking environments away from the city noise. I discovered a coastal hike called Bray to Greystones, spent time in Phoenix Park and St. Stephen's Green, and, when we moved our clinic outside the city, savored my weekday bike rides through the Irish countryside. (My social life improved as well when my socialite sister moved to Dublin a few months later.)

———

Sir E. A. Wallis Budge was the Keeper of Egyptian Antiquities at the British Museum in London from 1894 to 1924. In a 1967 book, he described eight aspects of the soul that Egyptians found important. One of them was the *Ab*, or heart. It was "regarded as the center of the spiritual and thinking life. . . . It typifies everything which the word 'conscience' signifies to us." He went on to discuss how the heart, and what its owner had imprinted upon it by his or her choices in life, is the specific object of judgment in the Netherworld.[1] In this regard the Egyptians understood the connection between our emotional state and the heart, as well as the importance of emotional balance to guide us through life and, according to them, influence ethical decision making that determines our fate in the afterlife. In modern parlance, this connection between the heart and our emotional state is balance in the ANS. This balance can have a huge impact on heart health.

Modern-day research shows that all our organs are connected to our emotional state via the vagus nerve, but the vagus nerve seems to have a deeper relationship with the heart. The ANS (via the vagus nerve) has been shown to heavily innervate and affect the heart.[2] When studying this high vagus nerve innervation of the heart, one group of researchers stated, "understanding the role that the intrinsic cardiac nervous system (ICNS) play in controlling cardiac function and how it interacts with information between central command centers and its integration with sensory information from the myocardium [muscle tissue in the heart] could prove crucial for prophylactic and corrective treatments of heart disease."[3]

Two other organs have very distinct neurological connections as well.[4] Our use of language reflects an intuitive understanding of the connection the vagus nerve makes between the heart, our gut, and our brain. This means that how we feel emotionally is felt through these organs the most, and information from these organs contributes heavily when the brain is deciding if we are in a safe or threatening environment. There is a reason we say things like "I have a gut feeling," and "I love you with all my heart," and not "I have a pancreas feeling," or "I love you with all my spleen."

I could even argue that the heart is *most* connected to our emotional state. Through the vagus nerve, the heart is anatomically connected to the muscles of facial expression, which is how we interpret how others are feeling and express how we are feeling emotionally.[5] Because of the vagus nerve, our emotional state is directly linked to heart health.

Maintaining balance in our ANS is the key here, but it is the hardest aspect of achieving a healthy heart long term because it's hard to control how we feel about something; we feel what we feel. In 1984 by George Orwell, the narrator describes how facts could be tortured out of anyone, but how you feel about something is always yours. "Facts, at any rate, could not be kept hidden. They could be tracked down by inquiry, they could be squeezed out of you by torture. But if the object was not to stay alive but to stay human, what difference did it ultimately make? They could not alter your feelings; for that matter you could not alter them yourself, even if you wanted to. They could lay bare in the utmost detail everything that you had done or said or thought; but the inner heart, whose workings were mysterious even to yourself, remained impregnable."[6]

Since we can't always easily change how we feel, sometimes it's more effective to focus on our environment and make sure it is an environment that creates feelings that lead to balance in our ANS. Some of the best ways to balance the ANS also help ensure that the body has plenty of energy to construct fourth phase water. Here is a list, by no means comprehensive, of some things that create ANS balance and things that both create ANS balance *and* energize the body.

BALANCE ANS

Meditation	Eating enough omega-3s
Healing the digestive tract	Gargling
Deep breathing	Acupuncture
Positive social relationships	Cold therapy
Proper sleep	Satiety
Laughter	Maintaining serotonin
Massage	levels (gut)
Singing	Music
Chewing food thoroughly	Ketogenic diet
Acupuncture	Love
Yoga	Having a positive outlook
Tai chi	Helping others
Prayer	
Fasting	

BALANCE ANS AND ENERGIZE BODY

Sunlight	Being in nature
Infrared sauna	Avoiding electromagnetic field
Grounding/earthing	(EMF) exposure
Pulsed electromagnetic field	
(PEMF) therapy	

Energizing the body is reasonably simple: The body gets energy from the Earth and other living things. So being in contact with those things will keep the body energized. Drinking energized water can also contribute. You can purchase a water-energizing device for your drinking water, and also take care with the food you eat: Fresh food is best because the cells of the food we eat are full of fourth phase water.

Heart Rate Variability

As you know, the best measure of balance in the ANS is called heart rate variability (HRV). Respiratory sinus arrhythmia (RSA) is a biometric similar to HRV in that it also measures the state of balance in the ANS. To get a sense of RSA, find a quiet place and take a seat. Now find the pulse on the thumb side of your wrist (radial pulse) and just feel it for a little bit to notice its rhythm. Now take a slow deep breath in through your nose and then breathe it out through your mouth slowly. What you should feel is that your pulse quickens when you breathe in and slows when you breathe out. This is a normal physiologic process, and it reflects the adaptability of our ANS; it illustrates how easy it is for our bodies to go back and forth between sympathetic and parasympathetic signaling.

While RSA measures the difference between the fastest our heart rate gets when inhaling and the slowest our heart rate gets when exhaling, HRV measures the variation in the time interval between heartbeats. These are different ways of measuring the same thing—balance in our ANS—but HRV is the more commonly used measurement. In general, we want to have a high HRV, which means the body has a stronger ability to adapt to different situations in our environment. Adaptability in any part of our physiology is a sign of health. We want to be metabolically flexible so that our bodies can adapt to burning fat or carbohydrates when they need to, neurologically flexible and able to use different brain waves in different situations, and flexible in our nervous systems so that we experience the proper body-wide responses to what is happening in our environment.

The general range for "normal" HRV is said to be anywhere from twenty to one hundred, which is a wide range (but take care to not compare your HRV with other individuals, because there is no better or worse within the range). Generally, the higher your HRV score the better balance of your stress response. If your HRV is too low, your parasympathetic nervous system is either not being stimulated enough or is overwhelmed by an overactive sympathetic nervous system. The best way to use the HRV number is to get a baseline and then work to improve it from there with the strategies listed above. There are many HRV measuring devices. They come in the form of wristbands, rings, and finger sensors. I have a ring from the company Ōura Ring. I don't really like wearing rings, so I put it on at night and it measures my HRV while I sleep.

Nature

It makes sense that time in nature helps balance our ANS. After all, this is much closer to the environment that the physiology of our human ancestors evolved in during the millions of years of evolution that resulted in us modern humans. The irony is that we have become so far removed from our natural habitat that being immersed in nature actually creates stress for some people, mainly as a result of our minds convincing us to fear something we are unfamiliar with. While the psychology of some people may have an adverse reaction to nature, our physiology tells a different story.

One aspect of nature that we can access without having to immerse ourselves in nature is the sun. Unfortunately, the sun has gotten a bad rap in modern times because of skin cancer. While burning your skin too often from sun exposure is not a good idea, it's counterintuitive that something we humans evolved getting exposure to every day would be bad for us. The toxic ingredients in sunscreens, lotions, and cosmetics we put on our skin pose a greater risk to the health of our skin by causing oxidative stress.

There are many benefits to sun exposure when it comes to preventing heart disease. The first is it is the original source of radiant energy that will help us maintain fourth phase water in our bodies to ensure blood flow and protection of the arterial lining. This benefit has been proven by Zheng Li, a graduate student at University of Washington (see chapter 6). In his PhD thesis, he tested the effects of UV light on blood flow and found that "when UV light was turned on, the flow velocity could be boosted by up to five times." The sun is also a source of infrared light, which also promotes blood flow. A study in rats looked at this by first controlling for vasodilation from nitric oxide (NO) by inhibiting the enzyme that produces it. (Infrared light also increases NO, which dilates the blood vessels.) Even when they inhibited the NO, however, the researchers still saw an increase in blood flow velocity with infrared light exposure.[7]

NO itself is also a good thing. Remember, it is essential for the proper signaling of the ANS to heart cells and it can act like an antioxidant, helping us lower oxidative stress. Both sunlight and infrared light therapy have been shown to increase the production of NO. Infrared light therapy has been shown to increase NO in mice and rats, and infrared sauna therapy has been shown to increase NO in humans.[8] While these artificial sources of light can deliver, the original source has always been the sun. One study concluded that "UVA irradiation of human skin caused a significant drop in blood pressure even at moderate UVA doses. The effects were attributed to UVA induced release of NO from cutaneous photolabile NO derivates."[9] The production of NO takes place in the lining of the arteries, and infrared light will increase the production of fourth phase water to protect the lining of the arteries so that they can synthesize it.

The benefits of sunlight don't stop there. Infrared light exposure balances the ANS, including a "drastic increase in parasympathetic nerve activity and continuous suppression of sympathetic nerve activity."[10] Exposure to plenty of natural light during the day also helps us regulate our circadian rhythm, which is associated with higher HRV. An imbalance in circadian rhythm as indicated by decreased HRV at night, when it is supposed to be higher, can be a risk factor for cardiovascular problems.[11]

Sunlight is just one aspect of nature that can help prevent heart disease. The research into other aspects is fascinating. A 2010 study looked at the impact of sound in autonomic recovery after a stressor. It compared "nature sounds" to "noisy environments" and concluded that "these results suggest that nature sounds facilitate recovery from sympathetic activation after a psychological stressor."[12] Meanwhile a 2013 study looked at how ample green spaces in underprivileged urban Scottish neighborhoods affected perceived stress and levels of cortisol, the hormone we secrete in response to stress. The researchers found that people with more green spaces in their neighborhoods had lower levels of cortisol throughout the day and reported being less stressed.[13]

Putting our skin in direct contact with the ground—termed *grounding* or *earthing*—also helps with both ANS balance and energizing our bodies, because the Earth gives off radiant energy. In his book *The Fourth Phase of Water*, Dr. Pollack stated that "lightning strikes so frequently around the Earth that the Earth's surface cannot dissipate the accumulating negative charge leaving it electronically negative. Standing on the ground, your nose is about 200 volts more positive than your toes." Soaking up energy in this manner energizes the water in our bodies.

Grounding also has a positive effect on ANS balance. When infants are born preterm, they are often characterized by low vagal tone because they are in distress; without intervention, the outcomes are often poor. A 2017 study used a patch electrode and a wire connected to a grounding outlet to expose preterm infants to the energy from the Earth, also known as electrical grounding. This exposure increased vagal tone as measured through HRV by 67 percent.[14] A study in adults looked at the effect of a grounding technique, skin contact on the Earth, on healthy adults and found that "grounded subjects had improvements in HRV that go beyond basic relaxation (P<.01). Since improved HRV has such a positive impact on cardiovascular status, it is suggested that simple grounding techniques be utilized as a basic integrative strategy in supporting the cardiovascular system, especially under situations of heightened autonomic tone [ANS balance]."[15] Grounding can be a powerful way to energize our bodies and balance our ANS, but the benefit is inhibited by shoes. Simply take off your shoes and spend some time barefoot in the yard or in the woods, and reap the benefits.

The reduction in stress and the ANS balance created by being in nature have been directly investigated. Although this study is only associational, the results are interesting: Scientists looked at elderly individuals living in various neighborhoods in Florida and compared the amount of green space in their neighborhoods to the amount of heart disease they suffered. They found that, compared with the people living near the lowest amount of green space, the people living in the greener neighborhoods had 25 percent reduced odds of acute myocardial infarction, 20 percent reduced odds of ischemic heart disease, 16 percent reduced odds of heart failure, and 6 percent reduced odds of atrial fibrillation.[16]

Whether it is what we see, hear, or feel, nature has a positive effect on our physiologies through energizing our bodies and balancing our ANS. As these two things play a key role in whether we develop heart disease, nature is a powerful tool in the creation of heart health.

Being Social

In part 1, I discussed how the development of a stress response is part of what enabled mammals to evolve from reptiles. I then discussed how eating primarily animals enabled our prehuman ancestors to grow in stature and brain size, leading them to develop into humans as we know ourselves today. From the time when one species split into two different lineages—one that became us and one that became our closest living ancestors (what we think of as the great apes), there were many different selection pressures on the way to becoming human. Many of them led to physical changes, like our digestive system adapting to eating meat, but many of them led to behavior changes as well. These changes are just as relevant to heart disease as the dietary ones.

If we look at our closest relatives in the animal kingdom (chimps and bonobos), it is clear that they live in groups, but it is also clear that they are not nearly as cooperative as humans are. Among chimps and bonobos, there is fierce competition for food, reproductive opportunities, and territory. While we humans also compete for these, we are more civil about it and generally aim for equal opportunity, at least within our immediate social groups. Our social nature stems from a change in landscape that happened long ago.

At some point prior to 6 million years ago, the Earth went through a drastic change. One of the most affected areas was the East African Rift Valley. Prior to this massive change, this area was dense rain forest, a perfect home for our distant tree-dwelling ancestors. Then, tectonic plates started moving and slowly started raising portions of this rain forest to a high plateau. This caused the rain forests to slowly start to dry up and become the African savannah that we know today.

At this point our ancestors still looked very much like the apes we think of today, and they were uncooperative as well. However, in order to find enough food, they were forced to come down out of the small number of trees that were left. Many predators were waiting on the ground, so how did our ancestors defend themselves? I have always found it interesting that humans are the only species in the world that can throw a football so accurately, or pitch a 100-mile-per-hour fastball. It seems that this unique characteristic came about during this time. Our ancestors who could pick up a rock and throw it with precision and force had an advantage. Not only could they defend themselves from a predator, but they could do so from a distance. There are many animals out there today that are good at killing or defending themselves, but there are few that can do so from a distance.

Still, one ape throwing a rock was not that big of a threat, especially when the throwing mechanics of the shoulder were still evolving. However, ten or twenty apes stoning a predator, or perhaps their next meal, was more of a match. Because of this, evolution favored those apes that could work together to fend off predators so they could eat the berries and leaves on the savannah; this throwing of stones likely killed some of those predators and also gave our ancestors a way to hunt. Hunting in this way was dependent on cooperation, and it sparked the evolution of this unique human characteristic.

Over the millions of years that followed, our ancestors made and used tools, began dividing labor to achieve tasks, developed the ability to conceive that someone else might be thinking something different than they were (termed *theory of mind*), and eventually developed the skills of teaching and learning. These are all incredible social characteristics that are more or less unique to humans, especially in the capacity that we can do them. In his book *The Social Conquest of Earth*, Edward O. Wilson sums up how important being social was to human evolution: "To play the game the human way, it was necessary for the evolving populations to acquire an ever higher degree of intelligence. They had to feel empathy for others, to measure the emotions of friend and enemy alike, to judge the intentions of all of them, and to plan a strategy for personal social interactions."

These evolutionary adaptations allowed us to be unbelievably successful in our climb to domination of the Earth. For example, if you put one human in the middle of the jungle to survive, that human probably would not make it. However, if you put one hundred people in the jungle to survive, there is a far better chance of their survival as a group. In addition to the advantages our social characteristics have given us, they also made us the most socially dependent species on the planet. The state of our social environment has far-reaching impact in our lives; so much so that many aspects of our health are dependent on it, including our heart health.

Our social environment is important from day one. When we are born, our ANS is incomplete. In order to alert us to an unsafe environment, our ANS essentially needs to learn what a baseline of safety feels like. A baby's ANS is trained by watching its parents' faces: Loving looks and comforting noises teach babies what it means to be safe. While this is learned throughout all of childhood development, researchers have found that the first three months of life are most critical.[17] If a child is not given this baseline, their ANS is at a disadvantage. Research has shown that improper ANS development in infancy or childhood leads to social behavioral problems later in life.[18]

Given all we have discussed about the heart and its connection with the ANS and our emotional states, it should come as no surprise that improper social development or a prolonged, unhealthy social environment can decrease balance of our ANS and negatively impact the heart. Humans are evolved to have close social relationships with up to 150 people. This may seem like a lot to some and not enough to others. Regardless of how extensive one's social network is, all of us are dependent on some amount of positive social support to maintain proper ANS balance and robust heart health.

People who are socially isolated have worse health outcomes.[19] A 2012 study of patients with heart failure found that the stronger their social support group, the more likely they were to take an active role in their self-care, and the better the outcomes.[20] Perhaps a strong social network increases our desire to be present for others and motivates us to care for ourselves. Another study showed that the quality of social relationships had an effect on heart outcomes in cardiac patients. If someone reported having more strained relationships, that person was more likely to have a worse health outcome. Conversely, the reporting of more positive relationships was associated with better health outcomes.[21] So it is not just the amount of social connectivity and support we have, it is the quality of those relationships as well.

According to one study, within thirty days of the loss of a spouse, both men and women between the ages of sixty and eighty-nine are at increased risk of stroke or a heart attack.[22] Another study looked at outcomes, based on their social status, in people who had already had heart disease. They found that men who had experienced a heart attack were four times more likely to die in the next three years if they were socially isolated. They also found that both men and women who had heart operations were three times more likely to survive for five years if they were married or had a close friend.[23] Once someone's health starts to decline, it seems that having people around to live for and to give social support—maybe as simple as a sense of purpose—is a predictor of long-term success.

Other humans are not the only source of social health protection. "Dog ownership is associated with a lower risk of cardiovascular disease in single households and with a reduced risk of cardiovascular and all-cause death in the general population." Interestingly, a hunting dog offers the most risk reduction.[24] Aside from the social effects, pets can also have a positive influence on our lives by stimulating heart healthy activity. One study found that "pet owners, and specifically dog owners, were more likely to report physical activity, diet, and blood glucose at ideal level, and smoking at poor level, which resulted in higher cardiovascular health score than non-pet owners."[25]

Humans also enjoy giving, and having people around provides us with recipients. A survey of one thousand adults between the ages of thirty-four and ninety-three assessed how much stress the participants experienced in their lives based on major stressful events, as well as how much time they spent giving back to their communities. The researchers then tracked participants through public health records and found that every major stressful event reported was associated with a 30 percent increased risk of death. However, among those who also reported helping others, the risk of death dropped to 0 percent.[26] Pretty amazing. Given this information it is not surprising that giving to others has also been shown to decrease sympathetic activation and contribute to ANS balance.[27]

A systematic review of all the literature on loneliness and social isolation as risk factors for heart disease and stroke found poor social relationships were associated with a 29 percent increased risk of coronary heart disease and a 32 percent increased risk of stroke.[28] Our social nature has the power to balance our ANS and affect our susceptibility to heart disease and death. In a world that is more connected than ever through technology, it is important to make sure that our relationships are plentiful and positive. Not connecting with others, or connecting with the wrong people, can have negative impacts on our health and can contribute to heart disease. So reach out to the long lost friends and family that you have positive feelings about and do not allow toxic relationships into your life for any longer than you have to.

Attitude and Outlook

There is another evolutionary event that occurred after our ancestors split from apes and evolved for survival on the savannah, and it involves the capacity to think and plan ahead. Modern-day chimps do not have much capacity to think into the future and take steps to prepare for what may come. They might take time to look for an ideal stick that they can manipulate into a tool for sticking into a termite mound so that termites will gather on it, making for easy and efficient eating. But once they are done, they don't take the stick with them. At other termite mounds, even shortly after a successful "hunt," they don't seem to have the capacity to anticipate needing the stick they carefully crafted. They have to make a new one.

At some point after the split from our human ancestors and apes, this changed. Archaeologists first notice evidence of forethought in our ancestor *Homo erectus*. Along with *Homo erectus* fossils, they have found stone tools that did not originate anywhere near the archaeological site. This meant that *Homo erectus* made these tools and then carried them for future use. *Homo erectus* had the ability to anticipate needing the tool. This ability is unseen anywhere else in the animal kingdom and is tied with our social evolution as well. Edward O. Wilson said it best: "As a result, the human brain became simultaneously highly intelligent and intensely social. It had to build mental scenarios of personal relationships rapidly, both short-term and long-term. Its memories had to travel far into the past to summon old scenarios and far into the future to imagine the consequences of every relationship. Ruling on the alternative plans of action were the amygdala and other emotion-controlling centers of the brain and autonomic nervous system."[29]

While the ability to anticipate the future gave us a huge advantage in the evolutionary success game millions of years ago, it has proven slightly problematic when it comes to our ANS in the modern day. Fast-forward from the birth of our species to the 1950s, and a story of two cardiologists, Meyer Friedman and Ray H. Rosenman, with a busy practice. Over time they noticed that they were often having to replace or reupholster the chairs in their waiting room because they were wearing out quickly. One day, an upholsterer arrived and made an interesting observation. He had never seen such wear patterns on chairs. In most every chair, the front edge of the seat cushion and the front of the arm rests were heavily worn.

At the time, Dr. Friedman didn't think too much of it. It wasn't until years later that he started putting the pieces together. He found that doctors of other specialties did not experience this strange furniture phenomenon to the extent cardiologists did. In his research he started to illuminate the connection between heart disease and an anxious personality, which caused many of their patients to sit on the edge of their chairs in the waiting room. In fact, the term "Type A personality" came from his work. Early on, these people were characterized as being competitive, overachieving, always hurried, impatient, and hostile. The work of Friedman and others showed an association between these personality characteristics and heart disease.[30]

Since those early studies, the Type A personality has gotten a bad rap, but newer research shows that Type As are likely to have a better outcome once they are diagnosed with heart disease.[31] Could it be that attention to detail and drive make Type As more likely to take charge and take control of their health? Being Type A is not a bad thing, it is just not always well suited for our modern-day environment.

Our ANS, as it is in all mammals, is well evolved to deal with an in-the-moment stressor. If we had evolved like the chimp, we would react to that stress, get away from it to safety, and then forget about it. When our human ancestors evolved the ability to anticipate the future, this ability to let go of stress was thrown off. This adaptation was largely because our way of life became so cerebrally demanding that our ANS could not evolve fast enough to keep us from the ill effects of our mind's ability to think about the future.

Humans worry so much about things that we have the ability to think our way into a stress response. Because of this, our outlook on the future is extremely important to maintaining balance in our ANS.

Unfortunately, having the ability to so efficiently think into the future, especially in the context of our unnaturally demanding modern world, can give us a pretty negative outlook. It's hard not to be negative when life constantly seems to be confronting you with sources of stress and worry. However, we should be careful not to let this way of thinking become our norm and turn into a state of chronic cynicism or hostility. Research has shown a link between cynical or hostile reactions to social situations and the development or worsening of heart disease.[32] When we are put in situations such as chronic job stress or unpredictable situations, studies show these increase the risk of heart disease.[33] And these situations often lead to anger, social dominance, repression of emotions, and harassment, all of which have also been linked to increased risk of heart disease and other ailments.[34]

The real question is this: What should we do to ensure we do not succumb to negative thinking? As I have discussed, our ANS is poorly adapted to the modern world and this makes it very difficult to avoid being sucked into a negative-thinking mentality. It is impossible to avoid all negative thoughts, but balancing them by focusing on the positives in life can have huge impacts on health and the heart.

There have been a number of studies looking at the effects of attitude in patients who are recovering from heart procedures or heart disease. One study looked at people who were scheduled for heart transplants. These people were about to undergo a major procedure and were full of anxiety. However, those who had a more optimistic outlook on the surgery and life after surgery had much better outcomes with their operation and lives afterward.[35] Similarly, a study of patients who received coronary angioplasty found that those who had higher self-esteem and a more optimistic outlook had better recovery and long-term success than those who scored lower in these measures.[36] Lastly, a study that assessed individuals who had suffered a heart attack and were in a cardiac rehab center found that those with a more positive outlook who were "choosing to live," as the study said, had much better recovery and long-term health than those who did not have as bright of an outlook for their health.[37] A positive outlook seems to make a huge difference.

Another strategy to combat chronic negative thinking is to express gratitude. Again, there have been a number of studies that have assessed the effect
of gratitude on people who have had cardiac events or cardiac procedures.
One showed that a daily gratitude practice improved the patients' overall
gratitude scores, reduced inflammatory markers, and increased HRV during
the gratitude task.[38] Another had similar results, showing that an assessed
higher ability to express gratitude resulted in better sleep, less depressed
mood, less fatigue, better self-efficacy to maintain cardiac function, and
lower levels of inflammatory biomarkers in heart failure patients.[39]

All of this may sound a little "woo-woo," but the fact is that our thoughts
matter, especially when it comes to heart health. In fact, the heart and the
brain have more nerve connections to each other than any other two organs
in the body.[40] And the kicker is that 90 percent of the fibers between these
two organs communicate from the heart to the brain.[41] This means the
emotions we feel with our heart will have a dramatic effect on how we think
about and see the world with our brain.

An interesting phenomenon has been observed in people who receive
heart transplants. In the decades since heart transplants have been performed,
personality changes in the recipients have been reported, including accounts
of recipients acquiring the personality characteristics of their donor.[42] One
study, where researchers conducted interviews of forty-seven heart transplant
patients and their families during their last postsurgery checkup appoint-
ment, showed that many of the patients had changes in their personalities.
"It has become evident that heart transplantation is not simply a question of
replacing an organ that no longer functions," the researchers concluded.[43]
A study of ten heart transplant patients found anywhere from two to five
changes in personality in the recipients that paralleled the personalities of
the donors, including "changes in food, music, art, sexual, recreational, and
career preferences, as well as specific instances of perceptions of names and
sensory experiences related to the donors."[44]

This makes sense when we look at how our thoughts can influence our
biochemistry. If we are expressing gratitude, a sense of well-being, and feel
safe in our environment, then our body sets off a cascade of biochemistry
that produces 1,400 biochemical changes that promote growth, repair, and
health. Conversely, when we feel hurt, angry, frustrated, hostile, cynical,

or jealous, our body sets off a cascade of biochemistry that produces about 1,200 biochemical changes that reflect these feelings in our body.[45] It has even been shown that our thoughts can positively or negatively affect our genes and influence the expression of them.[46]

All of this means that we need to strive for balance, to achieve coherence between our thoughts and our emotions. There is no way to be perfect at this, but implementing strategies like consciously pointing out the positives, expressing gratitude, keeping a gratitude journal, and ridding ourselves of as much negativity as we can are extremely important for achieving ANS balance in our modern world.

Dopamine Fasting

Another strategy for trying to achieve balance in our ANS is called dopamine fasting. Dopamine is the feel-good neurotransmitter. It is released in our brain when we do something that satisfies us. It can be released when we eat, accomplish something, receive a notification on our phone, have sex, check something off a list, hear our favorite song, and so on. There are many things that cause a release of dopamine. While dopamine itself is not a bad thing, many things that stimulate it in today's world also put us in a stress state. And since the release of dopamine can feel a bit addicting, all the various stimuli can create an overstimulated stress response.

One solution is dopamine fasting. This involves removing as many dopamine stimuli as possible for a twenty-four-hour time period. To achieve balance in the ANS, sometimes people assume that they need to add a bunch of activities to their daily routine (meditation, gratitude journal, nature time, breathing exercises, etc.). This is similar to assumptions about supplements. Sometimes people think that they can just take a bunch of supplements to get all the nutrients they need and then eat whatever they want. But that is not how it works, because poor food choices will cause damage and steal nutrients from the body. While meditation, a gratitude journal, and so forth are good strategies, sometimes we simply need to remove the problem causing stimuli for a while.

To do a dopamine fast, pick a day where you can just sit around and literally do nothing. Food fast for that day. Only use your cell phone if it is an emergency and don't talk to anyone. Only do light exercise, do not watch movies or TV, and unplug from music. It sounds quite hard, and it is. You will soon find out how addicted to dopamine you really are. Obviously, with our busy modern-day lives and all our responsibilities, it would be hard to do something like this for more than a day. But a day seems to do the trick for me. I usually take a pen and paper and lay in my hammock in the woods in my backyard, reflect on things, and write them down. I have found that of all the things I do to increase my HRV, this has the biggest impact.

Breathing and Meditation

In a book that calls into question the idea that the heart is a pressure propulsion pump, I need to discuss another sort of pump in the body that has implications for blood flow and for balance in the ANS. This is what researcher Stephen Elliot has coined the "thoracic pump," and it has to do with the diaphragm.

The diaphragm is a muscle that divides the thoracic cavity and the abdominal cavity. Every time we breathe the diaphragm moves up and down. It moves down when we breathe in, increasing volume in the thoracic cavity, which creates a negative pressure, and it moves up when we breathe out, decreasing volume in the thoracic cavity, which creates a positive pressure. This rhythmic increase and decrease of pressure as we breathe plays a key role in the movement of air in the body but also aids in the movement of blood.

Responses to the changes in volume and pressure as we breathe also change the effects of the ANS on the heart and the intestines. Due to the nature of how the diaphragm moves, when we breathe in, the increased volume and negative pressure created in the thoracic cavity and the decreased volume and positive pressure created in the abdominal cavity results in an increase in sympathetic activity in both areas. The opposite is true when we exhale. The decreased volume and positive pressure created in the thoracic cavity and the increased volume and negative pressure created in the abdominal cavity results in an increase in parasympathetic activity in both areas.[47] Considering that we breathe around fifty thousand times a day, you can imagine that how we choose to breathe can have an effect on balance in our ANS.

Unfortunately, the average adult uses as little as 10 percent of the range of the diaphragm when breathing. This can result in too much sympathetic stimulation and not enough parasympathetic stimulation throughout the day. Practicing how to engage more of the range of the diaphragm can have huge impacts on our health through balancing our ANS. In fact, researchers have found that breathing at a rate of 5.5 to 6 breaths per minute (which forces us to use more of the range of our diaphragm by exhaling longer) has been shown to create balance in our ANS more than any other breathing pattern they tested.[48]

Learning how to breathe for health and use our breath to help create balance is an extremely cheap and effective way to help create balance in our ANS. I believe this is one reason why meditation has been found to be so effective at help with ANS balance.[49] A study that looked at the effects of meditation on cardiovascular risk factors found that after sixteen weeks of a meditation practice, heart disease patients showed "improved blood pressure and insulin resistance components of the metabolic syndrome as well as cardiac autonomic nervous system tone compared with a control group receiving health education."[50]

I have previously stated that health is the ability of the body to adapt to different situations. I heard a good description of meditation that reminded me of this. The body knows two things really well: (1) that everything changes, and (2) that our real identity is deeper than all that change. Meditation is a path for discovering how to stay true to ourselves while everything around us is changing. To me, this means that despite all the craziness that may be going on around us, we learn how not to react to it, but to adapt to it and stay in our calm, steady state. Training myself to adapt to everything that may happen to me by maintaining a calm, steady breathing pattern is one of my main goals in meditation, and in life.

Electromagnetic Field Exposure

In chapter 9, I discussed how the body gives off an electromagnetic field (EMF) and that the heart gives off the strongest EMF of any part of the body. I discussed how this characteristic of the heart helps maintain structured water in its cells and plays a role in protecting the heart from cancer. The sun and experiencing direct contact with the Earth (grounding) expose us to electromagnetic energy that has similar wavelengths to our bodies, which is healthy. But there are many forms of energy in the modern world that are not the same wavelength and can do our bodies harm.

These energy sources come from our electronics and wireless signals. They include everything from a cordless house phone to wireless speakers/ headphones, cell phone towers and cell phones, and wi-fi, to name a few. Humans today are bombarded with energy signals with wavelengths that are not compatible with our electromagnetic physiology, especially our hearts.

Back in the 1950s, '60s, and '70s, researchers in the Soviet Union found that subjects experienced physical symptoms and changes in their electrocardiograms (EKGs) when exposed to radio waves. The EKG changes indicated both conduction blocks and oxygen deprivation to the heart.[51] They concluded that the radio waves interfered with mitochondrial function and therefore the ability of the cell to make ATP (energy) through oxidative phosphorylation. Later, these scientists' experiments showed that activity of the electron transport chain (part of the mitochondrial process of making ATP in our cells) is diminished in animals exposed to radio waves and to the EMFs from regular power lines.[52] This finding has major implications for healthy oxidative phosphorylation in cells.

For a long time, we have known that these electromagnetic exposures could do some harm, but we weren't sure how exactly. It had been observed that the blood pressure medications called calcium channel blockers seemed to mitigate the damage that could be caused by EMFs. One researcher, Dr. Martin Pall, used that information and discovered that one way these EMFs cause damage is by triggering an opening up of calcium channels in the membranes of our cells. This causes calcium to flood into the cell. Too much calcium in the cell causes dysfunction and DNA damage.[53]

In chapter 8, I discussed how dysregulation of calcium in heart cells due to buildup of lactic acid causes issues that can lead to ischemia—and heart attack without a blockage. But altering calcium physiology in heart cells has another consequence. Dr. Pall discussed some of his alarming findings: "Pacemaker cells have very high densities of VGCCs [voltage-gated calcium channels] in them and may, therefore, be particularly susceptible to EMF activation. In the heart hyperactivity of the VGCCs produces tachycardia and arrhythmias, leading in some cases to sudden cardiac death. There are studies, in two cases going back to the 1960s, showing that isolated animal hearts exposed to microwave EMFs (again, well within current safety standards) developed tachycardia and arrhythmia and have shown that some electromagnetic hypersensitive (EHS) individuals developed instantaneous tachycardia when unknowingly exposed to an activated cordless phone"[54]

There was even a study done on humans that showed the direct impacts of electromagnetic energy from cell phones on heart rhythm. The researchers studied 356 people, some with heart disease and some without, and observed their echocardiograms (ECGs) with a cell phone in different places on the body—near the hip as well as over the heart. They observed the ECGs both while the phones were off and while they were on and receiving a call. They found that whether the phone was at the hip or over the heart, "prolongation of QTc interval was significantly observed" in both the subjects with and without existing heart disease.[55]

While it is clear that inappropriate forms of electromagnetic signals can affect calcium physiology and alter heart rhythm, the effects on heart rhythm could be due to effects on the ANS as well. A study of the effects of magnetic resonance imaging (MRI) testing on forty-two patients found that "MRI may affect the HRV most likely by changing the sympathetic-parasympathetic balance."[56] Another study looked at the effects of EMF exposure on HRV in seventy-one workers at a radio broadcast station. The researchers concluded that "occupational exposure to EM fields brings about impairments in the neurovegetative regulation of the cardiovascular function" and that those with the highest exposure saw the most significant negative changes.[57]

I have discussed the role of fourth phase water, or EZ water, in the body. As far as keeping it healthy, I have mainly discussed the effects of oxidative stress on EZ water. However, just like the right type of energy (sunlight, earthing) can help build EZ, the wrong type can tear it down. Early unpublished results of experiments out of Dr. Pollack's lab have suggested that EMFs decrease the size of EZ.[58]

A research article discussing all the research on the effects of EMFs on the cardiovascular systems of humans and animals found evidence to support that EMFs cause increases in lactate production, decreases in plasma calcium levels, decreases in total antioxidant capacity, degeneration of heart muscle fiber, distortion and irregular structure of cardiac myocytes, rupture of muscle cells, and damage to mitochondria. The authors concluded by saying that

EMFs have "a negative effect on the heart and blood vessels by causing a histopathological changes and disturbances in the functions of the organs of the cardiovascular system."[59] Given what we know about EZ water and its role in the protection of the arterial wall as well as in the structure of the cytoplasm of the cells, I find it unsurprising that these issues would be seen in the cardiovascular system after exposure to EMFs.

All of that can seem pretty scary. But we need to remember that people are not dying of a heart disease just from sitting next to the wi-fi router all day. This is just another hurdle to maintaining the correct body energy. Most of us have lives and jobs that depend on this technology, so it is impossible to completely avoid it. But you can make small changes to reduce your EMF exposure, like using your phone on speaker rather than holding it next to your brain, avoiding wireless devices when one with a cord will work, turning off the wi-fi at night, and not putting your phone in a chest pocket or tucking it into a bra. You can even hire a building biologist to assess your home and give you strategies to reduce your EMF exposure.

As I discussed at the beginning of this chapter, there are many ways to encourage balance in our ANS and get adequate energy to the body. In my opinion, loss of exposure to nature, a less than optimal social network, a chronically cynical outlook on life, and a rapidly changing electromagnetic environment are four of the biggest contributors to these imbalances. The best strategies for creating ANS balance and optimal energy are getting nature exposure, maintaining positive social relationships while avoiding negative ones, consciously working to achieve a positive outlook, and avoiding or limiting EMF exposure whenever you can.

CHAPTER 14

Heart Healthy Exercise

During my final year of chiropractic school, my friend Kaylie, a class-mate of mine, asked me for a favor. She was dating a mutual friend of ours, Ian, who had graduated a year ahead of us, and he was going to run the Portland Marathon that weekend. He had asked her to track him on her bike so he could calculate his pace, as well as give him drinks at specific mile markers. I cycled around Portland all the time and knew the city well by bike, so she asked if I would help her out.

It was fun. I felt like part of a pit crew. He was tracking his own mileage in minutes, but sometimes he asked us to ride beside him and give him his actual speed. At one point, about halfway through the race, I was looking down at the speedometer on my bike and didn't see the train tracks ahead of us, set into the pavement. My front tire got stuck in a train track rut at a 45-degree angle and, to this day, I don't know how I stayed up. My rear tire lifted off the ground and all my momentum headed over the handlebars. But just as I felt that momentum, I twisted the handlebars and my body in such a way that righted my front tire. The bike stayed underneath me, but I came off the pedals and landed on my feet, straddling the bike. My friend ran by—in a pack of the leaders—all of us shocked that I didn't go over. All our hearts jumped a little, and they asked if I was okay, and kept right on running. They were all within reach of winning.

Kaylie and I delivered a few more drinks before heading to the finish line in the middle of downtown Portland to wait. We were excited because Ian was still among the leaders, and we kept hearing reports that they were get-ting closer. Finally, Ian rounded the corner of a building. He was all on his own and running faster than I had seen him run all day. He got halfway to the finish line from that corner he rounded and still no one else had come around the corner yet. It was clear that he had broken away from the other runners and was going to win.

I suddenly got very excited and started cheering him on. The crowd was getting loud as well. I have never been very interested in running, but to be part of Ian's pit crew and then watch him win was thrilling. He crossed the finish line, having run a personal best of two hours and twenty-something minutes. Kaylie ran out to him and they celebrated. My job now was to take pictures, so I was snapping shots of everything, as the others crossed the finish soon after.

I could see how much winning meant to Ian after all his hard work, and it was rewarding to feel like I played a small part in his success. We celebrated there on the finish line, and it was quite a joyous moment. Looking back, however, I find the moment a touch ironic: I was feeling positive emotions that boost heart health through ANS balance while celebrating a friend who triumphed at an intense form of "cardio" often touted as heart healthy. Later, I came to believe that this form of long-distance "cardio" is actually not particularly good for the heart.

There is so much information about exercise that it can be confusing to the average person who is just trying to stay fit. Recommendations often revolve around what type of exercise and how much of it we should be doing. There are obvious benefits to exercise, and people who regularly do it can attest to having more energy and feeling better overall, but what is the best way to exercise, especially for a healthy heart?

Endurance or long-distance training, many times called "cardio," or chronic cardio implies cardiovascular benefit, but marathons or endurance triathlons are not activities I recommend doing often for heart health. A study presented at the Canadian Cardiovascular Congress in 2010 showed a two- to threefold reduction in cardiovascular risk with regular moderate "cardio" exercise, but they also found that the intense exercise of a marathon *increased* cardiac risk sevenfold. In a 2011 study, researchers recruited a group of one hundred elderly men who belonged to the 100 Marathon

Club—which requires completing a minimum of one hundred marathons. Researchers found that half the men, especially the half that trained the hardest and longest, had significant heart muscle scarring as a result of their training.[1] If endurance cardiovascular exercise is the best thing you can do for your heart—like we are often told—then these men should have all had some of the healthiest looking hearts. Yet half of them had severe damage to their hearts.

Another study showed that endurance athletes had decreased right ventricle function and elevated markers for heart injury after a long-distance race.[2] On top of that, research has shown that endurance runners had more calcified plaque in their arteries compared to nonendurance athletes.[3] Research conducted by Dr. Arthur Siegel, director of Internal Medicine at Harvard's McLean Hospital, also found that long-distance running led to prolonged high levels of inflammation and a twofold increase in clotting factors that "may trigger acute cardiac events associated with strenuous exercise."[4]

I find this conclusion intriguing. A few case studies provide additional context. In one, a forty-one-year-old man had been running marathons for two years and then died of a heart attack, but not during a race. Prior to his death, he had seen a doctor and the evaluation showed that he had complete occlusion of the left circumflex coronary artery and a 50 percent stenosis of the right coronary artery. Against the advice of his doctor, he ran a fifty-kilometer race, a forty-two-kilometer race, and three marathons before he died. Autopsy revealed complete occlusion of the left circumflex coronary artery and the right coronary artery, as well as an 80 percent stenosis of the left anterior descending artery. In a second case study, a forty-four-year-old man ran eight forty-two-kilometer marathons, a fifty-six-kilometer race, and a ninety-kilometer race in the span of fourteen months. Shortly after, he visited a doctor complaining of lack of energy, but then he decided to run a twenty-four-kilometer race. During the race he lost consciousness and died instantly. Autopsy showed that he had a grade 4 (75–100 percent) stenosis in his left anterior descending coronary artery, as well as another significant stenosis in the left circumflex branch. Autopsy also showed no evidence of infarction and a normal heart conduction system.[5]

The thing I find most curious is that these men were able to run these endurance races with many of the major arteries severely compromised.

This goes to show the power of the collateral arteries that form around stenoses and how capable they are of supplying the heart tissue with blood despite full or partial blockages. The other thing I find interesting is that since they were running with these severe stenoses, we know it was not the stenoses that suddenly killed them. It must have been something else.

There is a famous case of someone dying during a long run, and it will help us theorize as to what could have caused the heart attacks in these men. In 2009 a book called *Born to Run* by Christopher McDougall hit the shelves. It is a thrilling tale and it sold well. In it, McDougall argued that humans are designed to run long distances, largely based on reports from the Tarahumara tribe in Mexico, whose people are incredibly adept at running long distances. The book also chronicled the lives of many well-known professional long-distance runners, including Micah True, a long-distance runner who lived a life of relative solitude in the deserts of Mexico among the Tarahumara tribe.

Unfortunately, True's story did not end well. After the book was published, True was found dead in the desert, presumably having died on one of his long runs through the desert hills. Although the autopsy was inconclusive about his cause of death, the medical examiner found that True had idiopathic cardiomyopathy, a disease characterized by an enlarged left ventricle. Other cardiologists who have looked at the report believe that True developed the cardiomyopathy from his long-distance running, a pathology termed Phidippides cardiomyopathy by researchers.[6]

I do not know exactly how Micah True died, but my speculation is from heart complications, possibly induced by his habits. If you will remember back to the three imbalances that can trigger a heart attack without a blockage, I believe True may have had all of them. McDougall described some of True's dietary habits, saying, "he started eating *pinole* for breakfast (after learning to cook it like oatmeal with water and honey), and carrying it dry with him in a hip bag during his rambles through the canyons."[7] Pinole is roasted ground corn, a high-carbohydrate food. If this was indeed what True was eating, then it is very likely that ketosis was a rarity for him, and his heart may have had less fatty acids and ketones than it would have liked. Running on carbohydrates likely also increased oxidative stress and depleted nitric oxide. True was also socially isolated and this isolation could have affected his ANS balance.

Curiously, it has also been found that a runner's HRV suffers during marathon runs, with one study noting "a progressive decrease in vagally-mediated HRV in conjunction with an increase in sympathetic drive" among study participants.[8] In former endurance cyclists, researchers found that heart conduction abnormalities "occurred significantly more often compared with age-matched controls" in the former athletes, and that "there is trend towards more frequent ventricular tachycardias."[9] Could the combination have led to the unfortunate death of Micah True? What if he had been on a more metabolically flexible diet? Unfortunately, there is no research, as far as I can find, that has assessed the heart health outcomes of long-distance running while on a metabolically flexible diet. A 2016 study looked at the effects of a ketogenic diet on long-distance athletes' performances and how their bodies handled the workload metabolically, and while it determined that fat-adapted endurance athletes could perform just as well metabolically as those on a carbohydrate-based metabolism, it did not look at markers of cardiac risk during their exercise.[10]

Another study looked at hormones in males during a marathon and found that not only did stress hormones rise, but testosterone decreased significantly.[11] It has also been shown that male endurance athletes have smaller testes and decreased release of hormones from the testes.[12] Lastly, a study that looked at sperm quality divided runners into three groups: a high-mileage group that ran an average of 108 miles a week, a moderate-mileage group that ran around 54 miles a week, and a sedentary control group. Compared to the moderate-mileage group and the control group, the high-mileage group had lower total motile sperm count and density, decreased sperm motility, and increased population of immature sperm; sperm penetration was also decreased.[13] And males are not the only ones affected, studies have shown that irregular or absent menstrual cycles in female collegiate endurance athletes is common.[14] Some people argue that humans evolved to run long distances to chase our prey until the prey got tired. But evolution is ultimately about being fit enough to pass on our genes, and it's hard to imagine why we would have evolved to do something that, as this research suggests, compromises this gene-passing ability.

Why am I dwelling on long-distance athletes? Because it's common these days for people with unhealthy diets and lifestyles to decide they want to get healthy and set a goal of running a marathon. While this may not be inherently dangerous as far as dying of a heart attack, it does happen. A review of data from all marathons from 2000 to 2009 found that twenty-eight people died while running a marathon and that 93 percent of those deaths were from a heart attack.[15] Even regular marathon runners are at risk. When researchers looked at segments of heart tissue among twenty recreational marathon runners, they found that 36 percent developed edema, 53 percent showed decreased function, and 59 percent showed decreased perfusion following a marathon. They concluded that "completing a marathon leads to localized myocardial edema, diminished perfusion, and decreased function occurring more extensively in less trained and fit runners."[16]

If people want to run marathons or other forms of endurance exercise events for reasons other than health—maybe it is their way to clear their mind or it is a life goal—then by all means they should. My argument is that if you want to get healthy, especially heart healthy, there are much better ways to do it. For example, running short distances. Running even five to ten minutes a day and at speeds under six miles per hour is associated with markedly reduced risks of death from all causes and cardiovascular disease.[17] No one should feel like they have to be able to run a marathon to be healthy. Research also shows that "cardio"—which I define here as a run of no more than five miles—has positive effects on your *brain*. It makes you smarter by increasing levels of brain-derived neurotrophic factor, makes you happier and more creative, and increases your lung capacity.[18] These benefits can be attained with shorter distances, and other forms of less intense "cardio" like hiking or walking, so there is no need to risk running longer distances to achieve health.

There are other options for improving heart health through exercise as well. I usually recommend a combination of resistance exercise, some sort of stretching or lengthening movement, and burst exercise, also called high-intensity interval training (HIIT). Resistance exercise means using your muscles against some resistance or force, like weights or exercise bands. Weightlifting is the most popular form of resistance exercise, but it can be as simple as squatting into a chair. Research has shown many, many benefits to resistance training. It increases strength and makes nerve signals stronger and travel faster, helps you detoxify by increasing lymphatic flow 300–600 percent, makes you happier, and increases bone density.[19] It is also an effective way to increase muscle mass, an important predictor of longevity as we age.

Many people think that they have to exercise for a long time to burn fat because you burn fat while you work out and the longer you do it the more fat you will burn. However, this is not true. Resistance exercise will increase your metabolic rate, improve your insulin sensitivity, and enable you to burn more fat while you are *not* working out.[20] This means that resistance exercise will make you better at burning fat while not working out than you are when you are working out. Resistance exercise for the win!

I am also an advocate of some sort of stretching or lengthening movement. This can be yoga, foam rolling, or a general stretching routine. In today's society, we spend a lot of time in static seated positions. Over time seated postures can result in microtears in muscles that result from the body trying to sustain this unnatural position. Eventually these tears will develop into scar tissue, shortening of muscles, and pain. Rolling out tight muscles and stretching should be a daily activity. Yoga is particularly helpful because it not only lengthens muscles; it has also been shown to regulate hormones, mitigate depression, reduce stress, and stabilize blood sugar.[21] Yoga is also great for calming the mind and moving our joints through a full range of motion. Joints do not have a direct blood supply and rely on motion to push nutrients in and out of them so that they can stay healthy. If we do not move our joints fully every day, they start to degenerate.

Lastly, in burst training or HIIT, you alternate very short periods of rapid and intense movement with rest, repeating the train–rest cycle for twenty to thirty minutes. You can do this with any resistance exercise or any movement in general. Even in running, you can do sprints. Heavy resistance exercise can transiently increase human growth hormone in men and women by 200–700 percent, helping to burn fat and gain strength, but HIIT can transiently increase human growth hormone in men and women by a whopping 2,000 percent.[22] HIIT is the most useful way to burn fat. Ultimately, health is the ability of the body to adapt in certain situations. Burst exercise is like a signal to the body that it's not adept enough adapting to increased demand and that it needs to get better for next time. Burst training tells the body that it needs more muscle mass, more oxygen saturation, more mitochondria, and a more efficient metabolism.

So, my recommendations for weekly exercise are as follows. First and foremost, even if you do some form of exercise every day, try not to stay sedentary in between those workouts. Get up from your workstation often or get a standing desk. As far as a workout routine, I think resistance exercise or strength training one or two times per week, burst training one or two times per week, and a daily stretching routine with maybe one longer yoga or stretching session per week is a great plan for a heart healthy exercise schedule.

CHAPTER 15

The Dental Health–Heart Health Connection

When I was living in Ireland I got motivated about my health and wanted to do everything I could to protect it. One of the things I had wanted to do for a while was get the amalgam fillings (which contain toxic mercury) from my childhood taken out and replaced with a less toxic filling. For this I needed to find a dentist in my area who would take them out the correct way, a way in which my body wouldn't be overly exposed to mercury.

I found one up in Dundalk, so I had to travel a little way out of Dublin to get to him. He seemed knowledgeable in holistic dentistry, and over two appointments he extracted all my amalgam fillings and replaced them with something less toxic. However, on the very last one, he said that when the filling was originally placed, the entire cavity was not removed and so he had to drill a tiny bit into the root to get it all. There was a chance the tooth would become infected, so he put a temporary filling in and told me to let him know how the tooth was feeling in about two weeks.

A few days later I was pretty sure the tooth was infected. I was having sensitivity to hot and cold and the tooth was starting to ache. By this time in my life, I had educated myself a little on dental health and knew that my options were a root canal or an extraction. I did not want a root canal (for reasons I will soon discuss), but I didn't want to lose the tooth either. I decided to do a deep dive into the research and try to heal the tooth in other ways. I had read it was impossible, but I wanted to try.

I did all kinds of things, from diet changes to essential oils. I definitely had good days and bad days with the tooth, but it did not heal. However, I learned more about dental health during this time than I ever thought I would. After about a month, I was having one of the bad days, and I ended up going to a dentist in Dublin the same day. They did an x-ray and showed that the tooth was infected. The only option they offered was a root canal. I told them that I would rather have it taken out, and they sort of laughed at me and asked why. When I told them I didn't want a dead tooth that would develop infection in my mouth, they rolled their eyes. I left without getting anything done.

At this point I didn't know what to do. I didn't want a root canal or to get a tooth extracted, nor could I really afford either. I was leaning toward an extraction, but I wanted to find someone who would extract it the proper way so a cavitation would not form. I looked for a dentist who was knowledgeable about how to do this but couldn't find one. Even the "holistic" dentist who had replaced my amalgam fillings didn't impress me when I asked him about it. The clinic I really wanted to go to was in the United Kingdom; it was run by a couple who literally wrote the book on dental health and systemic health, *Toxic Dentistry Exposed*. But of course, I could not afford to fly to the United Kingdom to get the tooth pulled properly and get an implant to replace it.

I ultimately had that infected tooth for over a year. It hurt, but it wasn't unbearable. It wasn't until I moved back to the United States and was working in South Carolina that I decided to get it taken out, mainly because the chiropractor I was working with was friends with a good dentist who knew all about the things I had discovered in my research during this time. He extracted the tooth and properly cleaned it out so that I would not get a cavitation. After it healed, I asked about an implant and he told me that it wasn't necessary if I didn't want one. While I don't recommend this for everyone, because teeth can shift around without all of them there, this has worked out for me and I still don't have a tooth there.

My tooth "adventure" lasted over a year. I learned a lot about dentistry; of particular interest was the fact that the state of one's oral health can have an impact on the health of the entire body, including the heart.

I have been researching heart disease for quite some time now and I have come across some fascinating things. After all that I have found, I was not surprised to find a connection between heart health and dental health. When I went through my own dental health issues, I already had some insight into dental health and how it relates to heart health.

I was already familiar with the work of Dr. Weston A. Price, a dentist who traveled around the world in the 1930s studying traditional people, their diets, and the source of their good health, but there was another story of his I wasn't so familiar with. This was an investigation he conducted after he lost his son, Donald Price. Dr. Price had performed a root canal on his son when he was sixteen years old. Soon after, his son suddenly died of a heart attack. This drove Price to search for answers.

Dr. Price began placing pieces of his son's infected tooth under the skin of rabbits. Each time he did this, the rabbit would die of a heart attack in about ten to fourteen days. He repeated this on one hundred rabbits and the same thing happened in each one. Price was a meticulous researcher and documenter. In addition to the research he conducted for his book *Nutrition and Physical Degeneration*, he also experimented on over sixty thousand rabbits to understand the health of the mouth and its relationship to the health of the body.[1]

The research linking dental health to overall systemic health is plenty.[2] As I investigated this, I was impressed but not surprised to encounter this statement in the *Compendium of Continuing Education in Dentistry*: "we caution clinicians not to recommend extracting infected teeth, based on the periodontal-systemic disease associations, if the teeth do not warrant extraction otherwise, because loss of teeth and edentulousness are associated with increased risk of systemic diseases."[3]

Though the effects of poor dental health can be widespread, I want to specifically discuss the connection between the health of the mouth and the health of the heart. When someone has an infected tooth, due to, as Price found when studying traditional peoples, a processed carbohydrate diet, a dentist will typically recommend a root canal. This procedure consists of drilling out the root of the tooth where the infection is and filling it in with a sealing paste. All good right? Not really. As much as any dentist may try, it is actually impossible to clean out all the bacteria from the infected tooth. There are many dental tubules in the tooth where bacteria can hide. Once you seal off the root canal, the bacteria are still in there festering. Since drilling out the root of the tooth removes the nerve and blood supply of the tooth, what we are left with is a piece of dead infected tissue in our mouth. If you ask any surgeon if they would ever leave dead infected tissue in a body, they will tell you absolutely not. Yet this is what happens with root canals.

What's worse is that because the process of a root canal removes the nerves and blood vessels that supply the tooth, the body cannot detect the infection because there are no nerves, nor could it get the immune system to it because there is no blood supply. What happens is a slow drainage of these infectious bacteria into the body through tissues and into the bloodstream. This leads to what is called endotoxemia, which I earlier defined as the leaking of bacteria into the bloodstream from within the body. Endotoxemia can happen any time we have a breakdown of a barrier the body has put up, including when we get severe gum disease, when our digestive tract is damaged and causes leaky gut, and of course when we undergo a root canal.

It is not a good idea to have unintended bacteria floating around in the body. Diving into the research on this is quite scary as well. Endotoxemia has been shown to cause systemic inflammation and atherosclerosis.[4] Summarizing the effect of endotoxins on the blood vessels, a 2004 paper published in *Arteriosclerosis, Thrombosis, and Vascular Biology* stated that "bacterial endotoxin is a potential source of vascular inflammation" and "an important risk factor for atherosclerosis."[5] Another paper published in *Atherosclerosis* looked at the effects of endotoxins on endothelial progenitor cells, which are cells the body uses to repair injured blood vessels and contribute to the formation of new blood vessels. The study found that when the researchers introduced endotoxins there was a 62 percent decrease in endothelial progenitor cells. The researchers even considered the amount of endotoxin they used to be a low dose.[6] Infection of this nature has been shown to significantly increase the risk of a heart attack.[7]

The fact that poor dental health causes endotoxemia is well established in the research, and textbooks have been written on the subject. One textbook states that the evidence was "strong enough to establish oral infections as an independent risk factor for CVD."[8] Yet, when a cardiology patient sees their doctor, it is rare that they are urged to take care of the health of their mouth and to choose a dentist who is knowledgeable about these issues.

It's interesting that the causes of gum disease and infected teeth that lead to root canals are the same causes of leaky gut, including a low-fat, high-processed-carbohydrate diet. In fact, as the percentage of calories from fat in the diet decreases, prevalence of gum disease tends to increase.[9] Eating foods filled with plant toxins, such as gluten, that prevent mineral absorption and cause leaky gut can also contribute to these poor outcomes as well.[10] That is, when people eat these foods, they can suffer endotoxemia from a leaky gut, which can cause an autoimmune condition, and they can get cavities that can lead to an infected tooth. The dentist's solution for the tooth is to do a root canal, which creates more endotoxemia. One study of 6,651 people found that people who still had most of their teeth but reported two or more root canals were much more likely to also have coronary heart disease.[11] Obviously, the best approach is to change the diet and prevent these things from happening. But infected teeth and root canals are not the end of the heart health–dental health story.

There is another way that we can get an infection in our mouths that can produce endotoxemia. This happens when we have teeth pulled, including wisdom teeth. Again, dentists may think they clean the socket well, but that is often not the case. In records of five thousand surgical debridements (cleanings) of cavitations (infections left after removal of a tooth), only two were found to be healed. This persistent infection in the jaw happens if the dentist pulling the tooth does not fully scrape out the periodontoid ligament and then sterilize the socket with ozonated water. These things are not done the majority of the time a tooth is pulled. Then an infection, called a cavitation, can develop within the jaw. Infection in the jaw happens because if the periodontoid ligament is left in, the body never gets the signal to come in and sterilize the area. The situation is similar to a root canal. Since the tooth is gone, the nerves and blood vessels of the tooth are gone as well. Over time the body cannot detect or fight off the cavitation. This will result in toxic bacteria leaking into the body.

Figuring out what to do if you have had, or are facing, any of these procedures done on your teeth can be tricky. When faced with needing a root canal or tooth extraction, or the cleanup of poorly done treatment, I recommend getting to a dentist who is knowledgeable (most are not) about all these pathologies and the connection between oral health and systemic health. He or she can help you with the overall health of your mouth and body. I have found that if you do an internet search for dentists in your area and also include words like endotoxemia, cavitations, or ozone that you will have a good chance of finding a dentist who can help you.

Once you are under the care of one of these dentists, I suggest getting all cavitations opened up and cleaned out properly and all root canal teeth removed, cleaned out, and replaced with a nontoxic implant. These can be expensive procedures and not everyone can afford to do them, but there is something we can do to help protect ourselves from the endotoxic bacteria until we are able to get our dental health in order. We have already discussed the many benefits of cholesterol in our body. One of the most amazing things it can do is protect from infection. This is why those with genetically high cholesterol, known as familial hypercholesterolemia, have been shown to have a protective advantage from infection. This happens because LDL can bind and neutralize infectious bacteria.[12] If you can't afford to get proper dental care for removal of cavitations or root canals, maintaining adequate cholesterol can help mitigate the damage from potential endotoxemia.

Now I must move to the other side of dental health that is so pertinent when it comes to heart health, that is, heavy metals. The danger of using amalgam (mercury) to fill cavities was first exposed in 1840, yet there are still dentists who place these filling in people today. In 1975, the "state of the art" high-copper fillings were implemented into practice. Aside from observations like those of Dr. Hal Huggins, who noticed an increase in auto-immune incidence in his practice after using these, research has shown that the high-copper fillings release fifty times more mercury into the body than the previous amalgam that was used.[13]

Heavy metals like lead, mercury, aluminum, cadmium, and arsenic have been shown to cause all kinds of damage and dysfunction in the body.[14] They were deposited in the Earth billions of years ago and our physiology evolved without their presence. It is only in the last few hundred years that we started mining them out of the ground and exposing ourselves (even putting them in our mouths!). Chapter 7 details how mercury in the body has been linked to atherosclerosis.

If you have silver-looking fillings in your mouth, it is best to get them removed and replaced. You must go to a dentist who is certified to do this in a safe way, as drilling out mercury in teeth can lead to high mercury exposure, and steps need to be taken to avoid that exposure. Huggins Applied Healing (www.hugginsappliedhealing.com) can help you find a knowledgeable dentist near you.

Talk of lipid panels, saturated fat, and cholesterol has dominated the discussion of heart disease for a long time. But this breakdown in normal physiology is not caused by one thing—no disease is. In fact, I argue that cholesterol on its own does not contribute to heart disease at all.

The health of the mouth is essential to the health of the body. This makes sense because the body is not made up of isolated compartments but is one deeply interconnected entity. Eating a whole-food, animal-based diet will keep your heart healthy and protect you from developing the issues in the mouth that contribute to heart disease.

CHAPTER 16

Chiropractic and Heart Health

My first experience with chiropractic was before I could really remember much. I was two years old when my parents noticed that I was coughing and wheezing. They took me to a doctor, who diagnosed me with asthma and provided various interventions. But desperate to pursue anything that might help manage this tricky condition, they also took me to a chiropractor. To this day, my parents are convinced that chiropractic helped control my asthma, but I was too young at the time to understand. So when I began seeing a chiropractor in college, it was just for the health of my spine, to prevent aches and pains, and to keep me able to play intramural sports. Indeed, most people think of chiropractic as a form of medicine that treats back pain, without realizing that it can also dramatically improve the health of the nervous system. Even as I began my own chiropractic education, I was very focused on neuromusculoskeletal conditions and tended to ignore the anecdotes I heard about nonmusculoskeletal benefits it had on the professors and fellow students who surrounded me.

I spent my final year of school as an intern in the various student clinics in and around Portland, Oregon. While working in the on-campus clinic, I treated the wife of a first-year student. Aside from minor aches and pains, I learned during intake that she and her husband had been trying to conceive for the last year without success. They were optimistic that starting chiropractic care, which she had never received before, would help. I admit, I was skeptical.

To my surprise, a few months after I had been treating her, she came in for a visit and told me that she was pregnant. I wrote it off as a coincidence, despite hearing my attending physician tell them she had seen this many times in her career. I asked them if they had made any other changes. They had not. But then a year later, I was visiting some friends—a couple who had gotten married a few years before—and as we were catching up, they mentioned they had been trying to start a family for eight months. Despite my doubts, I told them about my experience and invited her to come to my clinic so I could adjust her.

A month later they called and told me that they were pregnant. To this day they jokingly call their first born a "chiropractic miracle." Again, I was skeptical, since I had only given her one adjustment. Infertility is just as likely to stem from something gone awry in the man's body, and I didn't treat her husband. All the same, I found it interesting that I had seen this twice now. About five years later, a young woman came to my clinic for the sole purpose of getting care to help her carry a pregnancy to full term. She and her husband had already had three miscarriages and she found in her research that chiropractic could help. I told her of my two previous experiences but let her know I couldn't promise anything. By this point I felt it was worth a shot.

After assessing her, I put her on a treatment plan to help correct the structure of her spine and restore normal joint function. By the end of the treatment plan, she reported that she was not pregnant. I discussed the benefits of wellness care throughout pregnancy in case she did get pregnant, but that day was the last treatment she received and she did not return. Two weeks later, however, a longtime patient of mine came in and told me two things. First, she had referred the woman struggling with miscarriages to me, and second, the woman was again pregnant. We all crossed our fingers. A year later I learned her friend had given birth to a baby boy.

I don't tell you these anecdotes to make you think that chiropractic can always help with conception and pregnancy. While there are a few case studies and reviews in the literature that discuss possible mechanisms behind what I have observed clinically in this regard, I cannot make those claims based on anecdotes and a small amount of research.[1] But I do want to draw attention to the fact that chiropractic affects the nervous system in a substantial way that has the potential to affect the body in more ways than just the reduction of pain.

As a chiropractor, it would be hard to finish this book without saying at least a little something about chiropractic when it comes to heart disease. The practice of spinal manipulation has been performed for a long time, with evidence of it as a healing art as far back as ancient China and ancient Greece.[2] As a formal profession, it was established in 1895 by D.D. Palmer in Port Perry, Ontario, and since then, it has been fighting for legitimacy, possibly due to the threat it posed, and continues to pose, to allopathic medicine.[3] In the early 1900s chiropractors began to face stringent licensing laws and accusations of practicing medicine without a license; some were even wrongly imprisoned.[4] The American Medical Association (AMA) encouraged medical doctors to accuse chiropractors of ethical violations.[5] Even after states started establishing their own state chiropractic boards that regulated the profession, there was still constant pressure and ridicule from state medical boards and the AMA.

Things came to a head in 1963 when the AMA established the Committee on Quackery. They developed what they called their "Iowa Plan" that strategized the "containment of the chiropractic profession" that "will result in the decline of chiropractic." It offered that members should "encourage ethical complaints against doctors of chiropractic," "encourage chiropractic disunity," "oppose chiropractic inroads in health insurance," and "oppose chiropractic inroads into hospitals."[6] Despite all of this, the profession persevered (presumably because people found it helpful), and in 1976 a group of chiropractors sued the AMA.[7]

After an eleven-year trial, the AMA settled three lawsuits, and in 1980 it changed its position on referral so that medical doctors could refer to whatever type of practitioner they felt was in the best interest of the patient. In 1987, United States District Judge Susan Getzendanner found the AMA and its codefendants guilty of violating the Sherman Antitrust Act. In her decision, Getzendanner asserted that "the AMA decided to contain and eliminate chiropractic as a profession" and that it was the AMA's intent "to destroy a competitor."[8]

One of the many accusations against chiropractic was that an adjustment of the cervical spine could lead to a kind of stroke known as vertebrobasilar artery (VBA) stroke. The thinking goes that a cervical spine adjustment puts too much strain on the vertebral artery in the neck, which can cause an embolus to form. However, there is scant evidence to support a causal association. The researchers in one study stated that, "VA [vertebral artery] strains obtained during SMT [spinal manipulative therapy] are significantly smaller than those obtained during diagnostic and range of motion testing, and are much smaller than failure strains. We conclude from this work that cervical SMT performed by trained clinicians does not appear to place undue strain on VA, and thus does not seem to be a factor in vertebro-basilar injuries."[9] There are some reports of doctors seeing patients in the emergency room presenting with a stroke after seeing a chiropractor, but these are observed associations, not necessarily causation.

In 2008 researchers analyzed 818 cases of VBA stroke and found that those younger than age forty-five were approximately three times more likely to see a chiropractor or primary care physician (PCP) before the onset of their stroke than the control group. They concluded that "the increased risks of VBA stroke associated with chiropractic and PCP visits is likely due to patients with headache and neck pain from VBA dissection seeking care before their stroke."[10] A 2015 study looked at the association between 1,829 stroke cases among people on Medicare and seeking chiropractic or PCP care prior to the stroke. "We found no significant association between exposure to chiropractic care and the risk of VBA stroke. We conclude that manipulation is an unlikely cause of VBA stroke. The positive association between PCP visits and VBA stroke is most likely due to patient decisions to seek care for the symptoms (headache and neck pain) of arterial dissection."[11]

In 2016, researchers studied 1,157,475 visits that Medicare patients made to chiropractors or PCPs, complaining of neck pain. They then looked for either VBA stroke or any stroke at seven and thirty days after the visit. At seven days, the risk of stroke was "significantly lower" for those who saw a chiropractor than for those who saw a PCP; at thirty days there was a slight elevation in risk for those who saw a chiropractor compared to those who saw a PCP. The researchers concluded by saying, "Among Medicare B beneficiaries aged 66 to 99 years with neck pain, incidence of vertebrobasilar stroke was extremely low. Small differences in risk between patients who saw a chiropractor and those who saw a primary care physician are probably not clinically significant."[12] A systematic review concluded, "there is no convincing evidence to support a causal link between chiropractic manipulation and CAD [cervical artery dissection]."[13]

What this all means is that the small observed association between chiropractic care and stroke is also observed between PCP care and stroke. Someone starts having neck pain or a headache from a stroke and then goes to a doctor—sometimes their PCP and sometimes a chiropractor. Whichever practitioner they see misses the stroke (because they can be hard to diagnose) and treats them for the neck pain and/or headache, but regardless of what practitioner they see or what treatment is given, their stroke symptoms naturally progress, and they later end up in the emergency room diagnosed with the stroke they were having from the beginning.

Chiropractic Benefits for Cardiovascular Health

Before I launch into the benefits of chiropractic for cardiovascular health, it might be helpful to tackle what chiropractic *is*. Most people think of chiropractors as back pain doctors, and it's correct that chiropractic can be very effective for the alleviation of back pain, neck pain, and headaches.[14] However, chiropractic is mainly the treatment of any condition of the neuromusculoskeletal system. I think of it as ensuring proper structure of the skeletal system and proper motion in the joints for proper function of the nervous system. While chiropractic adjustments reduce pain, the most impactful thing they do is create an optimally functioning nervous system.

Chiropractors mainly look for individual joints in the spine that are not moving as well, these are often called subluxations or simply joint restrictions. When joints are not moving well, this can have a negative impact on the nervous system. Research has shown that "areas of reduced or restricted spinal motion causes spinal degeneration and changes in neurological communication between the brain and body."[15] The thing about the nervous system is that it's connected to everything, including our organs.

In 1965, a German cardiologist named W. Kunert noted that "records of numerous cases including myocardial ischemia showed lesions of the spinal column are perfectly capable of stimulating, accentuating, or making a major contribution to (organic) disorders. There can, in fact, be no doubt that the state of the spinal column does have a bearing on the functional status of the internal organs."[16] Plenty of research has shown that issues with spinal motion can cause issues in many different organs, but naturally I will focus on the heart.

In his 1985 book, *Manipulative Therapy in Rehabilitation of the Locomotor System*, neurologist and expert in musculoskeletal medicine Karel Lewit stated, "The following pattern of disturbances of locomotor system (spinal subluxation) seems characteristic of ischemic heart disease. Blockage affecting the thoracic spine from T3-5 most frequently between T4-5, movement restriction most noticeable to the left, at the cervical thoracic junction, and the third to fifth rib on the left side." Concerning paroxysmal tachycardia (the sudden onset of a rapid heartbeat), he said that "the changes found in the spinal column are linked with tachycardia in such a way that when we normalized the function of the spinal column, heart rhythm also became normal and remained so as long as there is no relapse in the spinal column."[17]

Dysfunction in spinal joints contributes to heart issues due to the effect of joint restrictions on the ANS. An article published in the *Journal of Manipulative and Physiological Therapeutics* put it plainly: "Destabilizing neural input to the vagus and cardiac sympathetic nerves may originate from mechanically irritated intervertebral joints. Asymptomatic spinal joint dysfunction can affect the autonomic nervous system and may activate potent somatocardiac reflexes."[18] But how exactly does restriction of joint motion in the spine cause stimulation of the sympathetic nervous system, ultimately contributing to imbalance in our stress response? To find the answer, we need to discuss a little neurology.

When an individual joint of the spine stops moving—which can happen from improper movement patterns, traumas, and just normal wear and tear of life—this can lead to connective tissue degeneration and local changes in the chemical composition of that tissue.[19] This happens because joints don't have a direct blood supply like other tissues do. In order to maintain health, a joint relies on motion to push nutrient-rich fluid in and out of its tissue. If the joint stops moving, it doesn't get adequate nutrition for maintenance and it starts to break down.[20]

In the case of the discs of the spinal cord, the first fibers to start to break down are the annular fibers that surround the nucleus of the disc. The nerves that go to the annular fibers of the disc have nociceptors that detect pain and mechanoreceptors that sense motion. The nociceptors are stimulated by joint restriction and chemical changes in the joint tissue and then relayed via C fibers from the joint to the spinal cord. C fibers are sensory nerve fibers that help us sense pain, and they are the most numerous sensory fibers in mammals.[21] These C fibers go into the spinal cord in the area known as lamina 1, and then convey the signal up the spinal cord through the spinoreticular, spinohypothalamic, and spinomedullary tracts to the brain stem, where they end up in regions of the brain stem that control autonomic homeostatic processing.[22]

When a spinal joint is not moving well, it can create overstimulation of the C fibers that will trigger a sympathetic response in our brain. If this is not addressed, it can contribute to imbalances in our ANS, including chronic sympathetic activation contributing to hypertension, congestive heart failure, cardiac arrhythmias, myocardial infarction, and ischemic stroke.[23]

I've discussed extensively how HRV is the single best marker of balance in our ANS. At least ten studies showed that chiropractic manipulation of the spine created balance in the ANS and increased HRV. One study showed that spinal manipulation of the neck in young healthy adults resulted in an "increase in the ratio of low-frequency (LF)-to-high-frequency (HF) components of the power spectrum of heart-rate variability, which may reflect a shift in balance between sympathetic and parasympathetic output to the heart."[24] Another study showed that spinal manipulative therapy of the neck "enhances dominance of parasympathetic."[25]

Because of the nature of chiropractic and its focus on the nervous system, it would naturally benefit the ANS, but remember that my approach to heart disease is three pronged: We also have to worry about reducing oxidative stress and sustaining metabolic flexibility that prevents the heart from being forced to burn more glucose. Chiropractic adjustments may even help us with these as well. When twenty-three individuals with neck pain received chiropractic adjustments twice a week for five weeks, researchers found that the antioxidants glutathione peroxidase and superoxide dismutase increased after the course of care. They concluded, "High-velocity, low-amplitude spinal manipulation twice weekly for 5 weeks increases the SOD and GPx activities."[26]

When it comes to keeping our bodies burning more fatty acids and making ketones, chiropractic admittedly has less impact, but there are a handful of compelling studies that look at this. In one, researchers assessed the glucose utilization in certain areas of the brains of twelve volunteers before and after a chiropractic adjustment. They found that adjustments did shift the metabolism of certain areas and stated that "the results of this study suggest that CSM [cervical spine manipulation] affects regional cerebral glucose metabolism related to sympathetic relaxation and pain reduction."[27] A similar study examined this in brain and skeletal muscle and found that after spinal manipulation, "glucose uptake in skeletal muscles showed a trend toward decreased metabolism."[28] To be clear, this does not mean that an adjustment of the spine can keep you in ketosis and burning fatty acids; the studies suggest that by having an influence on the nervous system through chiropractic, we can influence cellular metabolism and maybe help maintain a metabolism that keeps us metabolically flexible.

Chiropractic is more than just a way to alleviate back and neck pain. It is a way to have a profoundly positive impact on the body and can help us achieve balance in the three imbalances that drive heart disease. This does not mean that chiropractic alone will prevent heart disease—prevention requires a diversity of different healthy lifestyle strategies. And while chiropractic is not for everyone, it can be a powerful part of an overall strategy to achieve heart health and overall health for those who choose it.

CHAPTER 17

Aspirin and Ouabain

In his book *Travels*, Michael Crichton writes, "Whenever things got bad, whenever my life really wasn't working, I'd get on a plane and go far away. Not to escape my problems so much as to get perspective on them. I found that this strategy worked. I returned to my life with a new sense of balance. I was able to get to the point, to stop spinning my wheels, to know what I wanted to do and how to go about doing it. I was focused and effective."[1] I identify so strongly with this. The opportunity to backpack through Central America in the summer of 2011 gave me many experiences that shaped the way I saw the world and, in some cases, changed my entire approach to life.

While I was there, I spent a few days with my friend Amy in the small mountain town of Boquete, Panama. We were planning on hiking up the 11,398-foot Barú Volcano the next day, and decided to take a short, guided hike through the jungle to tune up for it. At that point, we had only been in Central America for about a week, so this was our first jungle trek. To my surprise, our guide was a young German named Max who worked at the hostel, a fellow traveler like us, not a native Panamanian. Max had traveled to Boquete a few months earlier and liked it so much that he got a job at the hostel.

Once on the trail, Max seemed very concerned that something would happen to our hiking group. He constantly pointed out caterpillars, flowers, and leaves of plants that he claimed were poisonous, as well as unsteady rocks and rough spots. Sometimes he would point something out and then stand guard as we all walked by. He even cleared the path with a large machete, and from the way he was swinging it, I gathered we were more at risk from him than anything we came across on the trail.

I was disappointed that we didn't stop much to look at the jungle sights. I was used to the forests of the Southeastern United States and the Pacific Northwest and there were many differences to explore in this jungle. Because of our overprotective guide, I felt I missed out. A bit later on my jaunt through Central America, I came across Crichton's *Travels*. One passage stood out: "Cut off from direct experience, cut off from our own feelings and sometimes our own sensations, we are only too ready to adapt a viewpoint or perspective that is handed to us, and is not our own."[2]

While I'm sure that some of the things Max did were truly protective, the experience of the hike was not my own; it was based on Max's two-month experience in Boquete and his fear of the jungle harming any of the hikers he was guiding. I was determined not to miss out on our hike up the volcano the next day. Our goal was to get to the top of the volcano at sunrise, so a group of ten to fifteen of us from various hostels in Boquete, all donning headlamps, started hiking at midnight. Surprisingly, there was no guide; we were taken up to the trailhead in a large van and pointed in the right direction. It was a little over eight miles to the summit, all uphill.

The sun was rising as we approached the top. As exhausted as we were, we picked up the pace to be sure we would see it. To our disappointment, the mountaintop was dense with fog, and we couldn't see much of anything. Even worse, it was chilly and breezy at elevation, and I wasn't prepared with enough warm clothes. If I couldn't see a sunrise, I at least wanted to see a view, and a group of us stayed on the summit to see if it would clear up, huddling next to a summit building to block the breeze. A coati approached, and we delighted in it, as it was entertaining and comfortable with humans. Suddenly the door of the summit building flew open, startling us, and a surprised-looking man emerged with a bowl in his hand, clearly not expecting to see us either.

The coati ran over, the man set the bowl down and then, seeing how cold we were, invited us in. Although none of us spoke Spanish well, it was clear that he lived or spent significant time there. There were some bunkbeds, a small kitchen, and what looked like a data collection station. To our great relief, it was warm, and we welcomed the warm drinks he offered. By the time we reemerged around 8 a.m., the sun was shining brilliantly, and the sky had cleared. We could look to the Pacific Ocean in one direction and all the way to the Caribbean in the other. This was the experience I'd been seeking—but not finding—on the hike with Max.

In retrospect, I find it amazing how ancient people's direct experiences led to the discovery of the natural world. The things that Max was pointing out in the jungle very well could have been poisonous, and someone probably learned this the hard way through direct experience. But other direct experiences have offered new and sometimes beneficial uses for elements of the natural world, including compounds used in pharmaceuticals. Two, in particular, aspirin and ouabain, have profound implications for heart health.

I want to discuss these two compounds: aspirin, which is well known and often taken with the belief that it prevents heart attacks; and ouabain, which is not so well known and not often prescribed for the prevention of heart attacks but shows compelling promise. Aspirin, or acetylsalicylic acid, was discovered in the bark of the willow tree and first used therapeutically in the late 1800s. (I wonder what direct experience someone had to figure out its supposed medicinal properties.) It is used in many products today and is the most commonly taken drug in the world. Aspirin works by eliminating prostaglandins, which are chemical messengers released by cells when the cells are damaged or in need of repair. The release of prostaglandins is the natural and appropriate response of the body in a "need of repair" situation, but it can be painful, so people reach for aspirin to suppress it. Although aspirin reduces pain, it suppresses a response that the body wants to happen. The body would not initiate this response if it weren't beneficial; by taking aspirin we override a natural need and process.

Because aspirin is derived from a plant, I sometimes wonder if its effects are due to a plant toxin interfering with a natural process, as many plant toxins do. Thinking about it in this way shifts the way we see the medication: Aspirin is not something that helps our bodies work better, but instead is something that inhibits a natural process. I understand that pain is uncomfortable, and aspirin can help us deal with pain, but it is important to be aware that if we suppress this process, we may in fact delay recovery.

Most of the time the symptoms we see from sickness or cell damage are from the body fighting the sickness or repairing the damage, not from the agent causing the sickness or damage. For example, a bacterial infection does not cause the fever, headache, coughing, sneezing, runny nose, or fatigue that you experience when you are sick; it's the body mounting a defense that causes those symptoms. If you suppress the symptoms, it takes longer for the body to rid itself of the sickness. In a study of people who contracted the flu, those who took aspirin to suppress the fever were sick for an average of 8.8 days; those who didn't take aspirin were sick an average of 5.3 days.[3]

Even in the absence of sickness from infection, prostaglandins are a way for the body to send messages that something needs repair or defense. If we destroy those messages, the repair takes longer, or never even happen. This interference with a normal physiologic response is characteristic of plant toxins; even if the effect appears "beneficial" in the short term, it may not be ideal long term.

Yet aspirin is touted as a blood thinning, harmless drug that will help prevent heart attacks if taken in small amounts daily, a recommendation mainly based on research conducted by the Physicians Health Group on *buffered* aspirin, which contains magnesium. This is an important detail because higher blood levels of magnesium are associated with lower risk of death from heart attack.[4] So is it the aspirin or is it the magnesium? I don't claim to know, but given that injections of magnesium have also demonstrated "dramatic clinical improvements" in heart disease patients, which one is most helpful at least warrants investigation before such pronouncements are made.[5] When I was in the hospital after my stent placement and had concerns about the long-term use of aspirin, I asked about magnesium and the attending doctor told me it was not a blood thinner. I didn't push it at the time because I was unsure if magnesium would be enough to prevent clotting after a stent, but intravenous magnesium has actually been shown to help prevent reocclusion after a heart attack and to be just as effective as pharmaceutical blood thinners at preventing acute clot formation after stent placement in dog and pig models.[6]

As for the notion that aspirin will prevent heart attacks, a clinical trial of 3,350 healthy men and women found that "the administration of aspirin compared with placebo did not result in a significant reduction in vascular events."[7] Some even argue that we attribute a reduced risk of heart attack from taking aspirin because sometimes people don't even realize they're having a heart attack, due to the pain-relieving effect of the aspirin.[8] Only later did they realize they had a heart attack. So, the aspirin wasn't preventing the heart attack; it was making it harder for the person to feel the effects of the heart attack.

The case for aspirin doesn't look good for heart health and looking at the side effects of aspirin and other nonsteroidal anti-inflammatory drugs (NSAIDs) does not strengthen the case for taking them. Many studies have shown an increased risk of upper and lower gastrointestinal bleeding with the use of NSAIDs.[9] A Danish study found that "during periods of NSAID use without use of other drugs associated with UGIBs [upper gastrointestinal bleeds], we observed 365 UGIBs, a number 3.6 times higher than expected . . . all types and formulations of NSAIDS appear to increase the risk of UGIBs."[10] The lining of our digestive tract is constantly being sloughed off and then repairing itself, so if we destroy the prostaglandin signals that tell the body to repair it, no repair happens and our gut lining gets thinner and thinner, eventually leading to bleeding. An estimated 16,500 people die every year in the United States from NSAID-induced gastrointestinal bleeding, not only from high doses—one third of that figure is from daily low doses.[11]

Use of NSAIDs and acetaminophen (Tylenol) is also associated with kidney disease. A nationwide, population-based, case-control study of early-stage chronic renal failure in Sweden that was published in the *New England Journal of Medicine* concluded, "Regular use of either acetaminophen (Tylenol) or aspirin, or of both, was associated, in a dose-dependent manner, with an increased risk of chronic kidney failure." Both acetaminophen and aspirin use was associated with a 2.5 times greater risk for chronic kidney failure compared to nonusers, and the risk was 3.3 times greater for aspirin and 5.3 times greater for acetaminophen when use reached 500 grams or more per year.[12]

Like so many other recommendations related to heart disease, the advice about aspirin is backward. The public is told that taking an aspirin a day could help prevent heart attacks and that taking aspirin is harmless, neither of which is true. To be fair, there are studies that show that aspirin can help improve insulin resistance, likely because inflammation is a factor in insulin resistance and aspirin is anti-inflammatory.[13] Of course, there are far better ways of correcting insulin resistance.

There is also research suggesting that aspirin can reduce the risk of cardiovascular events in patients with hypertension and chronic kidney disease better than in patients with normal kidney function. This, again, is all about insulin resistance. We have discussed how insulin resistance is the main culprit in hypertension and kidney disease, so people who have kidney disease are insulin resistant and people who don't have kidney disease are not. If aspirin improves insulin resistance, which is a major factor in cardiovascular events, this explains why aspirin has been shown to help people with kidney disease prevent heart attacks and to not help people who did not have kidney disease; there was no insulin resistance for the aspirin to mitigate in the people with normal kidney function. The abstract concluded, "an increased risk of major bleeding appears to be outweighed by the substantial benefits."[14] Well, not if those "substantial benefits" can be achieved by the correction of insulin resistance through the strategies discussed in this book without the risks related to long-term aspirin use.

If you are concerned about a heart attack, then, of course, consult with your doctor about what to do; however, if they recommend aspirin, you might consider bringing this information to their attention, and asking their opinion. There is also evidence that other, safer interventions such as CoQ10 (see chapter 7) and magnesium decrease the risk of heart attack more effectively than aspirin (likely because of the role these nutrients play in heart muscle contraction and fatty acid metabolism).[15]

There's another a substance, however, that in some ways is the opposite of aspirin. Ouabain, also known as G-strophanthin, is an extract from the seeds of the blooming liana plant, a vine that grows on trees in the African rain forest. Its effects were first noted through the direct experience of a doctor, botanist, and explorer named John Kirk. It is said that while on an expedition his toothbrush accidently came in contact with the liana plant's seeds and he noticed some effects after brushing his teeth. Ouabain seems to affect the heart by increasing levels of the neurotransmitter acetylcholine in the heart, which improves parasympathetic signaling to the heart.[16]

I'm typically cautious of plant-derived substances, especially those derived from seeds, which are the part of plants most defended by plant toxins. However, ouabain deserves some discussion, in part because an endogenous form is synthesized in the body, and has been found in many of the body's tissues.[17] There is a saying in traditional Chinese medicine that "the kidneys nourish the heart," and in fact this endogenous form of ouabain is released from the adrenal glands, which lie right on top of the kidneys. Long before the advent of modern medicine, the Chinese somehow knew that some substance secreted from the area of the kidney had a positive influence on the heart. The liana plant contains a similar substance to that which is released from our adrenal glands.

It's no coincidence that the excess stress leading to autonomic imbalance can also cause adrenal fatigue, which occurs when our adrenal glands are constantly secreting hormones in response to chronic stress, to the point that they get worn out. This, in turn, can lead to a less functional stress response from these glands. The very organ that is supposed to release ouabain to help with adequate signaling of the parasympathetic nervous system to our heart is no longer able to do so because of chronic stress, which itself creates a lesser parasympathetic signal to the heart. You can see how this can create a vicious cycle and, in really severe situations, the use of exogenous ouabain could be helpful. In fact, the research on its use is promising.

Scientists have been looking at the effects of ouabain for a long time. In 1937, a German pharmacologist named Hans Gremels showed that ouabain increased the effects of the parasympathetic nervous system on the heart up to one thousand times within a few minutes of administering it. He also found the effects of the sympathetic nervous system were reduced.[18] There have been many studies in Germany looking at ouabain use in patients with heart disease. One study, conducted on 150 patients with angina in West Berlin, took patients off all their medications and put them on ouabain. After one week, 122 reported no symptoms and after two weeks 146 reported no symptoms. Improvements were also seen on ECGs.[19] A study in Rhineland, Germany, found similar results.[20] Recall that when sympathetic signaling to the heart is too great and not balanced by parasympathetic signaling, the heart tissue can be forced to burn too much glucose, resulting in a buildup of lactic acid and angina (see chapter 8). These German studies showed that the use of ouabain can help restore normal parasympathetic signals so the heart can return to burning primarily fatty acids and ketones.

Another study done in Freiburg, Germany, looked at ouabain and heart function and found that thirty minutes after subjects took ouabain, their stroke volume (the amount of blood that moved through the heart during a single contraction) and heart performance increased significantly. Three-quarters of the patients also saw improvement on their ECGs.[21] When the heart is not constantly getting a stress signal it is able to balance itself and perform its function much more efficiently. Clinically, a few doctors have also noticed profound impact on the lives of their patients when they recommended ouabain and their patients took it. Dr. Knut Sroka stated: "Most patients say that they feel better after a few days, that their chest feels freer, they feel less anguished and have greater physical capacity. This is also regularly reported by patients who had never before heard about ouabain and who did not have exaggerated expectations due to their research on the internet. Ouabain reduces high blood pressure, and, in my opinion, it has clear psychological effects: it calms, patients have more vitality and their moods are often improved."[22]

Dr. Thomas Cowan has also reported significant benefits to his patients with the use of ouabain: "I have uniformly recorded a decrease in angina episodes, improved exercise tolerance, and thus far, no MI's [myocardial infarction]. . . . I have seen huge improvements in the lives of patients with this otherwise devastating condition."[23]

I have been taking ouabain since my heart attack because I knew that it could help prevent cardiac remodeling and heart failure. One study, done in rats, looked at the effects of taking ouabain on blood pressure and cardiac remodeling. They concluded that "a significant neuroendocrine hormone, such as EO [ouabain], may be used as a target for the clinical treatment of hypertension to reduce blood pressure and myocardial remodeling."[24] Another study, this one done in mice, showed that "safe doses of ouabain prevent or delay cardiac remodeling of pressure overloaded mouse heart." The authors also stated that "potential prophylactic use of digitalis [ouabain] for prevention of heart failure in man deserves serious consideration."[25]

The background and research on ouabain are incredibly compelling, and based on its underlying mechanisms, ouabain could offer a much better option than aspirin for preventing heart attacks and aiding healing after heart attacks. Of course, the best way to prevent heart attacks is by eating a whole-foods, animal-based diet and living a healthy lifestyle with exercise, time outdoors, and loving relationships. However, in those who already have advanced heart disease, ouabain could prove to be a game changer. I encourage anyone in that situation to present this information to their doctor and discuss whether it merits investigation.

CHAPTER 18

Biometrics

Tracking Your Risk

A few weeks after climbing the volcano in Boquete, Panama, Amy and I were crossing from Panama into Costa Rica at Sixaola, a small northern crossing where the border runs along a narrow river. Amy and I queued up in Panama to show our passports, and crossed the river separately via two narrow foot bridges with loose wooden planks. When I approached the Costa Rican border patrol agent and handed her my passport, she looked at me expectantly. I shrugged my shoulders indicating I didn't understand until she grew agitated, glanced through the pages of my passport, and began issuing demanding instructions in Spanish before waving me away.

I wasn't sure what had just happened, but I walked out of the building and into Costa Rica. I asked Amy if she had had any trouble and she said no. I continued to mull this over as we waited for a bus to our hostel in Puerto Viejo de Talamanca. Once we arrived and checked in, I asked, "Don't you think it's weird they didn't stamp our passports for entering Costa Rica?" Amy said they had stamped hers, and when I asked what she gave them besides her passport, she said she presented her flight itinerary. I understood. They wanted to see proof that we had plans to leave.

I was now in Costa Rica without a travel visa, so I asked the front desk for the nearest internet café and walked across town to pull up my flight itinerary and print it off. Then I found a cab, got in, and explained that I need to get to Sixaola. The driver nodded and off we went. But nothing is ever as simple as it seems. My driver said he knew a short cut, and we turned off down a road through the jungle. I was a little worried as we drove along a bumpy jungle road, and endless plantations of banana trees, but we finally turned onto a main road and soon arrived at the border crossing in Sixaola. I rushed in, and found the same agent who had been so agitated with me the day before. I triumphantly handed her my passport and flight itinerary: She rolled her eyes, stamped my passport, and I sprinted back out to the cab, and headed back to Puerto Viejo de Talamanca. Whew, crisis averted!

While I was traveling through Costa Rica, I was asked for my passport multiple times: every time I checked into a hostel and twice by Costa Rican officials. No one, however, ever looked for the stamp with the Costa Rica travel visa on it. They only looked at the page with my picture and information. Even when Amy and I were leaving Costa Rica for Nicaragua, the border patrol agent didn't look for that visa, he just stamped my passport and sent me on my way. I was very concerned about my passport being in order while in Costa Rica, even though, as luck would have it, I could have passed through without it. This is sort of the way I view medical tests. We think we need them, we go out of our way to get them, and it can relieve our minds to have them, but the documentation is not always as important as we think it is.

———————

Before I go into different biological markers, including blood work, that can be useful in assessing risk of heart disease, I want to offer some perspective on medical testing in general, especially in the context of eating a species-appropriate, animal-based diet. People have been scientifically looking at blood since the 1600s when the first blood transfusions are said to have been done. But advanced blood testing was not developed until the 1900s, and it really came along after the push for blood lipid testing in the 1950s. Since then, we have been testing more and more things in blood, and we can look at everything from blood-borne pathogens to red blood cell counts and characteristics to levels of certain vitamins and minerals. Blood testing has become one of the most relied upon ways that doctors assess health and investigate disease. However, while blood testing can be useful, it doesn't make sense to focus on it myopically in assessing our health. There are many other factors, and biometric testing has its limits.

Humans have been around for at least 300 thousand years, yet blood testing has only become prevalent in the last century or so. If we think about the determined normal ranges of certain blood markers, we have to take into account that we have only established "normal ranges" of these for people living in the modern day. We have no idea what the normal ranges were for the very first humanoids, for the hunting and gathering humans that roamed the Earth for 280 thousand years, or even for the first farmers.

Let's say we take an animal out of the wild and place it in a similar but still not natural habitat, feed it an unnatural diet, and place it in an unnatural social environment. After leaving it in that unnatural environment for a while, we then decide to do blood work on this animal and determine what its normal ranges are. Do we think that the levels of blood markers on the animal in this unnatural environment would be truly "normal"? I don't. Yet, this is essentially what we are doing.

As I have discussed, there is evidence that early modern humans were high-level carnivores, perhaps even more so than other carnivores of the time. There is also evidence for early humans doing a lot of hunting, including a substantial die-off of large mammals during the time of the first modern humans. This lifestyle was likely the way of life until about ten to twelve thousand years ago when humans started farming and living in cities. For nearly 280 thousand years, humans lived in small social groups in nature, where they had little exposure to toxins and plentiful access to meat and animal fat. Of course, we have no idea what the blood work of those humans would have looked like. If we did, it might give us a better idea of the numbers we *should* be aiming for.

Finding normal ranges in our modern population and then obsessing over keeping our results within those normal ranges strikes me as a bit short-sighted. This is not to say that there is not useful information in blood work. For example, it can inform us of urgent problems that call for acute interventions. The problem with depending on blood work arises when someone who is in excellent health or in the process of lifestyle changes for better health goes out of the "normal ranges." Should we stick to the conventional wisdom and attempt to correct these numbers, or should we consider that while the person's health is changing (for the better) some markers may actually get "worse"? The question is ultimately this: Which observation is false, how healthy a person is feeling or the potential for an out-of-range number on the blood test?

I am more inclined to believe the blood test is a false indicator of health. I know many people who have become frustrated with symptoms, yet they are told by their doctors that nothing is wrong because their blood tests are normal. I also get messages from people who change their diet in a certain way and experience vast improvements in health but are concerned because certain numbers on their blood work go "out of range." This is not uncommon when people transition to an ancestrally appropriate animal-based diet.

Take blood sugar, for example. While most people on animal-based diets experience in-range blood sugar levels that stay stable, some people develop slightly elevated, but stable, blood sugar levels. This could be due to a glucose-sparing effect, which can happen when people don't consume carbohydrates at all for a long time and the body downregulates the mechanisms for burning glucose. This situation isn't really metabolic flexibility, and in this case it could be a good idea to eat some whole-food carbohydrates every once in a while, so the body doesn't downregulate those glucose-burning mechanisms. However, it's the big fluctuations in blood sugar that drive damage more so than higher but stable blood sugar, so slight elevation should not be a huge concern on a low-carbohydrate, animal-based diet.[1]

Next up: white blood cells, which help us battle inflammation and infection. Some people on an animal-based diet have lower levels of white blood cells, possibly because these diets tend to result in low inflammation, and also because cholesterol can bind and neutralize pathogens. White blood cells are simply not needed as much. On the other hand, kidney tests such as blood urea nitrogen (BUN) and creatinine can be slightly elevated on high-protein diets; the concern is that too much protein may damage the kidney. Multiple studies already discussed and cited in this book show this to be false (see chapter 17). The slight elevation in BUN and creatinine may actually be the "normal range" for humans, given that we ate a high-protein animal-based diet for thousands of years before we started farming.

While most people on animal-based diets see normal levels of liver enzymes, sometimes there are slight elevations. Elevated liver enzymes indicate stress on the liver, but diet is not the only possible cause. Any toxin overload can cause it, alcohol being the most common and well known. But even intense exercise can slightly elevate liver enzymes for about a week. Doctors will also sometimes measure morning cortisol, a stress hormone that always spikes in the morning to wake us up. Some people on an animal-based diet see a higher spike than others do. Because a huge problem in society is feeling sluggish in the mornings and taking a while to get going, I would argue that the "normal" spike in morning cortisol may not be getting the job done. People on animal-based diets tend to report no issues waking up in the morning, so maybe a slightly higher spike is a good thing. Curiously, cortisol has been shown to slightly elevate blood sugar, so perhaps this effect contributes to the elevated but stable blood sugar we see in some people on animal-based diets.[2]

The last biomarker is everyone's favorite: cholesterol. While the other tests discussed above only show slight elevations for people on ketogenic or animal-based diets, some people see huge jumps in their total and LDL cholesterol. The body starts making ketones and, since the process of making ketones is similar to the process of making cholesterol, we get more cholesterol, too. Plant fats also compete for absorption with animal fats in the intestines, so if we eliminate or greatly reduce plant fats and eat mainly animal fats, we get much more animal fat (cholesterol) absorption. I have already discussed the benefits of higher cholesterol, which include a boost to immune defense, energy delivery, delivery of fat-soluble vitamins, cell repair, hormone production, and atherosclerosis prevention; therefore, in the right context (low inflammation and insulin sensitivity), there is no issue with higher cholesterol. There are clear benefits to having cholesterol in circulation, and research shows that higher levels have no negative impact on life span and do not cause heart disease.

It's also important to understand that the "normal ranges" of LDL cholesterol have changed over the years. In 1984, the National Institutes of Health held a conference with the goal of coming to a consensus on whether cholesterol was good or bad.[3] As a result of their incorrect conclusion that it was bad, an organization called the National Cholesterol Education Program (NCEP) was created to educate doctors on how to define and treat their at-risk patients. Unfortunately, the NCEP's definition of "normal" was heavily influenced by drug companies who profit from doctors using LDL-lowering drugs.[4] As the recommendation for what is considered a healthy LDL became lower and lower at subsequent meetings of the NCEP, the bigger the market for LDL-lowering medications became. At first, it was supposed to be no higher than 250. Then they lowered it to 200. Then 150, then 100, and at present they say it needs to be under 100. To me this suggests we have lost a true understanding of what "normal" is. For what it's worth, a 2020 study looked at the association of cholesterol levels and all-cause mortality and found that having LDL cholesterol between 117 mg/dL and 137 mg/dL (above the recommendation of lower than 100) associated with the lowest all-cause mortality and that lower than 84 mg/dL associated with the highest all-mortality.[5]

This scenario seems to be playing out with blood pressure as well. For some reason, in 2017 it was decided that the recommendations for what constitutes high blood pressure needed to be redefined. A change in the guidelines lowered what constitutes high blood pressure from 140/90 to 130/80, making almost half of all American adults eligible for pharmaceutical intervention.[6]

Since we're defining "normal" out of the context of a healthy environment for humans, we shouldn't always allow "abnormal" or "out of range" blood work results to scare us. I think about blood work in the same way I think about Western medicine: It is excellent in an emergency. Western medicine may well save lives in times of life-threatening infection, trauma, or other acute situation. But it is proving to be terrible for preventing and fighting chronic disease. Blood work is similar: If there is a serious imbalance in the body, blood work can be an excellent way to detect it and determine how to correct it. But micromanaging blood work is not a good approach to health. It may even have a negative effect because obsessing over blood work and attempting to overcorrect numbers can lead to high levels of anxiety.

It's misguided to think that a momentary snapshot of one component of the body (the blood) can illuminate the whole complex biological ecosystem that is the human body. I will always take blood work into account, and I do so with all my patients and clients, but we humans became the most dominant species on Earth by listening to our bodies and doing what made us feel strongest so we could pass on our genes and ensure the survival of our species. The time-tested, deep-rooted approach of trying something new and seeing if we feel better, perform better, or otherwise improve can play a powerful role in our quest to achieve health. We should use modern medicine for emergencies, but allowing modern medicine tests and assessments to undermine how we actually feel can be a mistake.

When it comes to heart attacks specifically, it seems testing for the standard risk factors is becoming less and less useful. It is well established in medical literature that a growing number of people had their first heart attack when they were generally fit and healthy, were not overweight, did not smoke or drink excessively, and had normal blood pressure and cholesterol levels. Aside from the risk that type 1 diabetes gives me and my at times moderately elevated cholesterol, I am fit and healthy, not overweight, do not smoke or drink, and have normal blood pressure, and I had a heart attack. A 2017 study in the *European Journal of Preventive Cardiology* concluded that "the proportion of STEMI [heart attack] patients with STEMI poorly explained by SMuRFs [standard modifiable cardiovascular risk factors] is high, and is significantly increasing" and called for an effort to discover "new mechanisms and markers for early identification of these patients." A 2019 study published in the *Journal of the American Heart Association* concluded with similar statements.[7] I would agree. I also think that testing used to measure risk is often incomplete and that results of the testing that is done are oftentimes not interpreted in ways that give us the best picture of someone's risk.

Despite believing that we should not put all our eggs in the medical-testing basket when it comes to heart health, I also believe that there is testing and tracking that is valuable in assessing risk of heart disease, or any disease, and it involves the three imbalances that drive it: not being fat-adapted (or metabolically flexible), having lots of free radicals resulting in oxidative stress, and having an imbalance in ANS signaling to the heart.

People refer to being fat-adapted as being in a state of ketosis, for which you eat so that the primary fuel source for your body is fatty acids and ketones. To do this you must restrict carbohydrates to less than 20–30 grams per day for about four to six weeks, after which you can start including more whole-food carbohydrates. This process will allow your body to become adapted to burning fat and ketones. Fat and ketones are the most efficient fuel source for the body and, as I have discussed, the heart has been shown to prefer ketones for fuel even in the presence of glucose. Providing the heart with enough ketones to thrive is essential for preventing heart attacks.

As I have said, to do this you have to restrict your consumption of carbohydrates and over time your body will become a fat-burning machine. A pretty cool thing happens when the body starts making and burning ketones. Since the body starts relying on fat and protein and not carbohydrates (glucose), it has a much lower spike in insulin. When the body has much less insulin around, it doesn't store energy, and it ends up wasting it. It can waste energy in the form of heat or in the form of ketones. Measuring wasted ketones is one way to tell if the body is in a fat-burning, ketogenic state.

So how do we measure ketones? We waste ketones through our urine and through our breath. You can get urine testing strips to measure ketones in urine or you can buy a device that you breathe into and measure ketones that way, but these are not the most accurate methods. The most accurate way to measure ketones is through the blood. You can buy a relatively inexpensive ketone blood test kit (although the test strips can become costly). A blood ketone level of 0.5–1.5 millimoles per liter (mmol/L) indicates mild ketosis and a level of 1.5–3.0 mmol/L is in the optimal range. It is important to note that ketosis is very different than ketoacidosis, which is sometimes seen in people with uncontrolled diabetes. Ketoacidosis happens when blood ketone levels get above 10 mmol/L.

There are ways other than testing to tell that you are likely in ketosis. Ketosis can cause what is called keto breath. It is often described as a fruity, acidic, or metallic taste in your mouth. You may also have smelly urine or smelly sweat. These things are more common when you first become fat-adapted and tend to fade away the longer you are metabolically flexible. Once the body becomes well adapted to burning fat and ketones, many people find it is possible to have higher amounts of whole-food carbohydrates and still easily retain their metabolic flexibility.

Next up is measuring your oxidative stress. This one is not as straightforward or as easy to measure on your own, and you will probably need to have a knowledgeable health care provider order these tests for you. Remember that oxidative stress's relevance to heart attacks is that high amounts will damage the fourth phase water that lines the arteries and then will damage the arteries, as well as deplete nitric oxide. So, measuring NO levels can offer some indication that high oxidative stress is depleting NO. The best way to do this is probably a blood test for serum NO. You could also get blood tests measuring symmetric dimethylarginine (SDMA) and asymmetric dimethylarginine (ADMA) to get an indication of the health of your arteries, which is where NO is made. NO saliva test strips are another method, but generally they are not as accurate.

There are many other markers we can look at for oxidative stress, and they are all done by blood test. Gamma-glutamyl transferase (GGT) is a liver enzyme that can be elevated in a state of oxidative stress. You can also look for F2-isoprostanes, which measure arachidonic acid damage from oxidative stress; lipid peroxides, which measure damage to unsaturated fatty acids from oxidative stress; and 8-hydroxy-2'-deoxyguanosine, which measures DNA damage from oxidative stress. I think it would also be wise to look at markers of inflammation like hs-CRP, serum ferritin, homocysteine, and various interleukins. Markers of inflammation can be elevated when there is high oxidative stress, though that is not the only reason they can be elevated.

Next, we can measure balance in our autonomic nervous system. The best way to do this is through heart rate variability (HRV) and respiratory sinus arrhythmia (RSA). As I described in chapter 13, if you find your pulse on your wrist and then calmly take slow deep breaths, you will find that when you breathe in your heart rate quickens and when you breathe out your heart rate slows. This is your RSA. The difference between the fastest the heart rate gets on the inhale and the slowest it gets on the exhale is an indication of how balanced the ANS is. When you breathe in, your sympathetic nervous system is stimulated. When you breathe out, your parasympathetic nervous system is stimulated.

HRV measures the same thing, and it tells you how readily you can go from one state to the other and the balance you have between the two. The most common question I get when it comes to HRV is what the "normal range" is supposed to be. There is actually no truly normal range. When you start tracking your HRV, you should get a good idea of your baseline after a few weeks and then can work to improve your score from there. As far as devices to measure HRV, there are many. My two favorites are Elite HRV finger sensor and the Ōura ring. With the Elite HRV sensor, you can test your HRV at certain times during the day. The Ōura ring is an actual ring that tracks your HRV and other biomarkers throughout the day. There are many other devices, most of them wristbands. Most of them will have an app for your phone so you can track your markers.

How you sleep is also a good marker of your risk for cardiovascular disease, and your health in general. If you sleep well on a consistent basis, it is a great indicator of balance in the ANS. Unfortunately, the research on sleep and cardiovascular disease is mostly associational so it cannot prove that poor sleep causes all these things, but sleep is still worth mentioning and considering. For example, researchers found that people who slept well but for less than six hours a night had a 23 percent increased risk of coronary heart disease compared to those who slept more than seven hours. Short sleepers who had poor quality sleep had a 79 percent increased risk.[8] Messing with our day/night cycle and sleep schedule doesn't bode well either; one study found a 70 percent increased risk of having a heart attack in men the morning after the biannual time change.[9] Poor sleep is also associated with elevated markers of inflammation. The more inflammation, the greater the risk of heart disease.[10]

Lastly, I will list the general baseline blood work that I think will give you a good idea of where you stand on your health. While many of these markers can be ordered on your own through independent labs, it is important to discuss them with a knowledgeable provider before taking any action. Preferably, that provider will be trained in functional medicine and familiar with animal-based diets.

BASIC LIPID PROFILE

Lp(a)

Lp-PLA2

Glucose control—fasting insulin, HbA1c, fasting glucose

Comprehensive metabolic panel + GGT

CBC w/diff

Markers of inflammation—Hs-CRP, myeloperoxidase, homocysteine

Full thyroid panel—TSH, free T4, free T3, total T4, total T3, reverse T3, and thyroid antibodies (TPO, TgAb)

Hormone panel (cortisol, free testosterone, total testosterone, SHBG, estradiol, DHEA, LH, FSH, DHT, prolactin)

Iron panel (TIBC, serum Fe, ferritin, transferrin)

25-hydroxy vitamin D

It is important to always assess cholesterol in the context of inflammation. I have discussed at length how cholesterol does not cause issues on its own, but there is plenty of evidence to suggest that when LDL becomes damaged it leads to increased risk of clotting.[11] This damage can be assessed through markers like Lp(a) and oxLDL. High triglycerides and having diabetes or metabolic syndrome have also been shown to cause an increased in hypercoagulability.[12]

Unfortunately, no one tested my general inflammation levels or my Lp(a) and oxLDL upon my admittance to the hospital after my event. However, I am diligent about tracking these numbers on myself, and all my markers that would suggest inflammation and damage to LDL or an artery, like Lp(a), oxLDL, homocysteine, hs-CRP, Lp-PLA2, and myeloperoxidase, had been consistently low for me prior to the event. My triglycerides are consistently in the normal to optimal range as well. Even my coronary artery calcium (CAC) score was zero when I had it tested six months prior to my event, which suggests no calcified atherosclerosis in my coronary arteries.

While assessing the lipid panel in the context of inflammation is important, it is more important to use blood work to assess your metabolic health using measures like the triglyceride/HDL ratio, which should be less than 1.5, and the HOMA-IR score (fasting insulin × fasting blood sugar, divided by 405), which should also be less than 1.5. These two numbers have been shown to be excellent indicators of risk for heart disease because they tell us if we have become insulin resistant, which can happen well before we look or feel unhealthy or have any formal diagnosis of disease.[13] For example, when 147 normal, healthy nonobese individuals were tested for insulin resistance, one in five of the most-insulin-resistant group would go on to have a "serious clinical event" within the next five years.[14] Another study stated that "insulin resistance is likely the most important single cause of CAD [coronary artery disease]."[15] Insulin resistance is also associated with premature development of atherosclerosis.[16] When it comes to blood work, understanding how to assess for insulin resistance is critical for assessing risk of heart disease. The CAC score, which tells you how much older calcified plaque is in your coronary arteries, is another great measure for health of the endothelial lining of the main arteries in the heart.

By tracking these markers, you can get a sense of where you stand on your overall health as well as on the three imbalances that cause heart disease. But remember: Do not get too caught up in tracking and testing, especially if it starts to stress you out. While these markers can help you cover all your bases to prevent heart disease, they are not perfect. Sometimes a proper philosophy of health is more important than obsessing over biomarkers.

Conclusion

We have come a long way in understanding what causes heart disease, from the beginning of life, to the evolution of the first mammals, to the first humans. We saw how those humans drastically changed their way of life through civilization and ultimately used modern science to attribute a cause to heart disease before all the data was really in. We have explored the true role of the heart in the body, detailed the pathogenesis of atherosclerosis, and addressed some mysteries about heart attacks. We have considered diet and lifestyle to help combat the development of heart disease in the modern world. I hope you have started to see that we modern humans have not only misunderstood the human heart, we have also somewhat misunderstood the world and our place in it.

I have argued in this book that, from a health perspective, it is best to see our place in this world as right alongside other animals in the natural world that we have far removed ourselves from. Our heart gives us another example of how different we have become from animals in the natural world. Animals share about the same number of heartbeats during their lifetime, about 800 million, even though the average life span of different animals varies greatly. For example, the average life span of an elephant is quite a bit longer than a mouse. While a steady 30 beats a minute gets the elephant to around 800 million by the end, the mouse's heart beats around 600 times a minute to get it to 800 million. Eight hundred million is astoundingly consistent for all animals; humans are the exception.

The average healthy human heart beats around 60 times a minute. This means we would reach 800 million after about twenty-five years. But our hearts keep on going for another forty to sixty years. Modern medicine has no answer for why this is, and neither do I, but we don't need an answer in order to gain insight from this curious information. All we need is a sound health philosophy on which to base our path to health.

Unfortunately, there are many popular ideas about health that are driven more by dogma than by truth. Rather than having sound reasons for a health practice, oftentimes modern medical practices and conventional wisdom only persist because "that is how we were taught" or because it's the standard of care. These practices sometimes lack the foundation of a cogent philosophy, which is part of why they don't always lead to good outcomes.

When we make decisions about our health, it's important to do so from the basis of a concrete philosophical construct about human beings and our place in the world. The proper lens, in my opinion, is an evolutionary lens. It makes sense to understand humans within the context of the natural world, which is where we've been for the vast majority of our time on this planet. In my first book, *The Health Evolution*, I discuss how the removal of humans from the natural environment in such a short time has led to the chronic disease epidemic we have today, including and especially heart disease. We cannot hope to successfully understand and address modern chronic diseases without evaluating them in the context of a toxic modern world.

Once we accept this, we also begin to see that there is an illusion to medical science. A medical science lab is diametrically opposed to nature. Labs are sterile and strictly controlled environments, whereas nature is a complex biological ecosystem that is far from sterile and is uncontrolled. Of course, our medical science labs need to be the way they are for accurate and untainted experimental results. At the same time, can we really expect to get a grasp on the uncontrolled, complex biological ecosystem that is the human body by only studying certain aspects of it in such an isolated environment?

For example, much of the research on human cells is done in sterile Petri dishes. But humans are not sterile; we are covered in dirt and bacteria. Studying cells in sterile Petri dishes is not going to give us an accurate account of what happens in real human physiology. Further, a lot of research done on heart cells is conducted in a glucose-based solution. We have discussed how the heart prefers fatty acids and ketones for fuel. Perhaps conducting experiments on heart cells in a glucose solution offers a poor understanding of how a heart cell operates in the body, where it has surrounded itself with fatty acids and ketones.

One characteristic of modern science forces us to take it all with a grain of salt: trying to eliminate all variables to ascertain a causal relationship. This characteristic makes sense in some disciplines of science, and as steps used as intermediaries to greater scientific discovery, but because the human body is a complex biological ecosystem that never experiences one variable at a time, how far can eliminating all variables take us in the quest to understand what creates health in a human?

I used to work in a chiropractic clinic more or less across the street from Virginia Tech Carilion School of Medicine and Research Institute. I had many medical researchers and PhD students as patients in the clinic. One of my favorite things to do was ask them what they were working on. While explaining their research, many would describe how they were trying to understand a specific biochemical pathway in some aspect of human physiology, as well as how they could affect it in order to develop a drug. They were all trained in this reductive approach. Not only is the idea that a drug can truly fix something awry in the body fundamentally flawed, but so is the method of trying to understand human physiology by eliminating all variables but one specific biochemical pathway.

I have said before that modern medicine can do amazing things in an emergency life-or-death situation. But that doesn't mean that modern medicine has the human body completely figured out. I don't believe it ever will. I once heard a mathematician give a public lecture, and in it, he described how in mathematics, you can easily describe how two things interact with each other—two planets in space, for example. If you add a third planet, their interactions become more difficult to describe and predict, as the effect of one planet on another can further alter the effect of the second on the third (and so on). With, say, four or five planets, it becomes extremely difficult to describe or predict how they will interact with each other. There are not only four or five things happening in a living cell; there are hundreds of thousands of things happening.

Trying to understand the body by studying individual mechanisms is fundamentally flawed; the body doesn't operate by turning on and off different mechanisms in a nice, neat way. It is arrogant to think that we can fully understand the complexity of the human body. It is even more arrogant to think that we can control it with drugs that force changes in single biochemical pathways. This approach will never result in health. We cannot continue to construct a simplistic view of nature in our heads and use that simplistic view to try and understand a system that is not simple.

Michael Crichton is one of my favorite authors, most well known for *Jurassic Park* and *The Lost World*. What's largely left out of the theatrical versions of these books is how he weaves complex ethical and philosophical concepts into his fictional adventures through his characters. In *Jurassic Park*, humans have tried to control nature to such an extent that they have re-created dinosaurs in the modern world. Of the concepts Crichton includes, the most relevant to the scientific approach to health is the idea of inherited wealth. When someone inherits wealth, they often don't respect that wealth or where it came from. They did not have to work for it, and so they missed out on any wisdom they would have gained in the journey of earning it.

There is a sort of inherited wealth today in the scientific community. There is so much documented and easily accessed scientific information for scientists to build on that a person can easily learn a multitude of information without being required to understand it within a broader context. The Virginia Tech medical researchers, for example, were searching for the next biochemical mechanism they could alter in order to make a drug. They had learned many things without necessarily mastering the bigger picture: how altering that specific biochemical mechanism changes its interaction with other reactions in a particular cell, how that cell then changes its interactions with the tissue as a whole, how that tissue changes its interaction with the organ, how that organ changes its interaction with that human's body as a whole, and how that human being then changes its interaction with its social network of other humans.

We must understand the implications of powerful scientific knowledge being used without discipline, or we will never understand what creates health, and may actually do damage. Science has helped us build a world with so many wondrous things. These things have made our lives easier and more enjoyable. But within the world that science has built, science cannot tell us what to do with all we have achieved or how to ethically live within this world. This is especially true for health. Medical science strives to tell us how a system in the body works, but it cannot tell us how best to create health in that system. We create more and more technologically advanced medical therapies, but medical science cannot tell us when to use them and when not to use them. Modern medical science is always inventing new drugs and medical procedures, but it cannot tell us when it is best to use them.

This makes medical care consumers (patients) dependent on a whole new level of inherited wealth. While medical doctors and researchers at least undertake rigorous training—inadequate though it may be—most of us as patients more or less blindly consume the medical technology that comes out of the medical sciences, with even less of an understanding of how the human body works and the effects of the medical therapies. As a society we have outsourced our health to our modern medical system. So much so that most of us don't know what it takes to achieve health and are entirely dependent on the medical system. The yearly checkups, lab tests, and medical assessments are supposed to tell us if we are healthy or at risk of disease. This system gives us a false sense of health.

In the Allegory of the Cave, Plato describes a group of individuals who have been imprisoned in a cave since infancy and are taught about the world through shadows on a wall that are created by people who are not imprisoned passing objects in front of the light of a fire behind the prisoners. One day, a prisoner is allowed to leave the cave. Life outside the cave is so alien to what he has known for his entire life, that he at first does not think the real world is actually real. He can only see shadows. In such a situation, many people will prefer to return to the comfort of the cave.

From the time we are born, we are told that our bodies are not good enough and that we need some external force to help them achieve health. We are told that our immune system is not good enough and therefore we need vaccines to make it better. We are told that our genes are programmed to give us disease and we need medicine to fight that disease. We are told that diet and lifestyle may keep us fit and thin but have little effect on whether or not we will get a disease. Society's messages are like those shadows in the cave; those notions are so ubiquitous that they have become more real than the truth of what really creates health. Those messages have become more real to us than how we feel in our bodies.

I say all this to illustrate how we as a society have ended up with such poor health and why we are plagued by a disease like heart disease. Modern medicine misunderstands the heart because it has never taken into account the natural science of evolution, which positions humans within their rightful context of the natural world. Modern medicine has progressed too fast for its own good, divorcing practitioners from the discipline of firsthand, holistic knowledge acquisition in the context of the natural world from which humans came.

At this point you may be confused. I have just given you reasons why modern medical science is not the answer to our health woes, but you have also just read a book that made an argument using a lot of modern medical science. I do not dismiss modern medical science altogether, but I try to remain consciously aware of its flaws. For the sake of your health journey, I want to share with you how I determine if something is a good health practice or not.

I developed a habit of putting ideas through a set of steps before I will consistently implement them into my health routine or recommend them to others: First, if the health strategy is relevant to me, or won't cause me harm if it is not relevant to me, I try it on myself. I have always been my first patient. If I see evidence that it benefits me I move on to the next step. Second, the strategy needs to make sense from an evolutionary perspective, or at least an evolutionary perspective within our modern world. If the strategy mimics something we would have done or been exposed to throughout our millions of years of evolving in nature, it passes step two. Third, I start trying the strategy with some of my clients and patients, and I need to see that it works for a majority of them.

The fourth and final step can come at any time, but it is not a requirement for implementation, so I have put it last. The last step is research: I see if I am able to identify some research that reinforces the strategy, or at least determines that there is no high-quality research saying that it is harmful. (That said, it's rare for a health strategy to pass the first three steps that doesn't have research to back it up.) This research step is last because of the shortcomings and political capture of medical research. As Dr. Marcia Angell, former editor-in-chief of the *New England Journal of Medicine* put it: "It is simply no longer possible to believe much of the clinical research that is published, or to rely on the judgment of trusted physicians or authoritative medical guidelines. I take no pleasure in this conclusion, which I reached slowly and reluctantly over my two decades as an editor of the *New England Journal of Medicine*."[1]

Unfortunately, corporate influence, through funding, on researchers and research institutions has resulted in the failure of "evidence-based medicine." A 2014 article in the *Journal of Evaluation in Clinical Practice* described the situation well: "We argue EBM's [evidence-based medicine's] indiscriminate acceptance of industry-generated 'evidence' is akin to letting politicians count their own votes. Given that most intervention studies are industry funded, this is a serious problem for the overall evidence base. Clinical decisions based on such evidence are likely to be misinformed, with patients given less effective, harmful or more expensive treatments. More investment in independent research is urgently required."[2]

Because of this, I will implement a health strategy in my life and the lives of my clients and patients even if there is no research backing it up, as long as it passes the other three steps. I understand the shortcomings of modern medical research and, as I have discussed, no single study, or group of studies, can ever fully account for all the complexities in the biological ecosystem that is the human body.

The strategies put forth in this book have been put through these steps and have passed all four. For example, first, ketone availability provided by a metabolically flexible diet gave me levels of health I had not experienced before; second, this diet makes sense evolutionarily, as processed carbohydrates and vegetable oils did not exist through the vast majority of time in which humans have lived; third, adjusting my clients and patients to this strategy has changed their lives from a health perspective; and, finally, there is plenty of research demonstrating the benefit to having ketones around, especially for the heart. The same goes for reducing oxidative stress and achieving balance in our ANS—all four steps have been passed.

The key is to use this approach to push medicine forward. To do this, practitioners need to share their successes and failures with various treatments in patients to accumulate a database of what works and what doesn't. Dr. Ralph Horwitz and Dr. Burton Singer proposed something encouragingly different to evidence-based medicine in a 2017 paper: "We propose Medicine-based evidence (MBE), based on the profiles of individual patients, as the evidence base for individualized or personalized medicine. MBE will build an archive of patient profiles using data from all study types and data sources, and will include both clinical and socio-behavioral information. The clinician seeking guidance for the management of an individual patient will start with the patient's longitudinal profile and find approximate matches in the archive that describes how similar patients responded to a contemplated treatment and alternative treatments."[3]

I can imagine how useful a resource that would be when working with clients/patients, and there are good models of less formal ways to do this. For example, www.meatheals.com offers a large collection of anecdotes on how a carnivore diet has helped people improve their health. While it is not formal research, it is useful and powerful data, and should be considered as such.

Most of what we think are scientific facts are really only theories, and theories can be disproven. Two hundred years from now, people may look back and laugh at what we believed scientifically valid today. I hope they are looking back and laughing at what the conventional medical wisdom currently says causes heart disease. New theories will always come along and make old ones look silly; it has been happening since the dawn of science. What's important is that we keep our eyes on why we humans seek new knowledge in the first place: because we want to create the best lives for ourselves, our families, and all of humanity.

I love reading modern research and searching for answers to our complex biology, but I do not think it is essential that we find those answers. I know that it is quite possible that we may never find the exact mechanisms that cause arteries to form atherosclerosis, or the exact mechanism that causes heart muscle to die in heart attack fashion, or why the human heart beats billions of times more on average during a normal life span compared to other animal hearts. Perhaps we should view the fact that we far outlive our heartbeat life span as a gift, one that should not be taken for granted. With that in mind, I believe it is important we start using the time given to us by those extra heartbeats to ask research questions in the context of our appropriate environment so that we can find a way of living that prevents heart disease, creates excellent health, and leads to a better future for ourselves, our families, and our world. This will help ensure that humans are included in that future. Heart disease aside, isn't that what we all really care about?

Aside from the personal connection I have with the heart because of my own health journey, the heart is my favorite organ for another reason. While my mind may get frustrated with all the conflicting research and tell me that we will never understand the complexities of the body, my heart enables me to accept that we aren't meant to, and it helps me understand that knowing all those details is not necessary to achieve the kind of heart health that leads to a brighter, healthier future for us all.

Acknowledgments

Gratitude is very important, especially for heart health, and there are many people to thank. First off, my parents. My mother has taught me how to have a positive outlook even in the worst situations, and my father taught me curiosity of the world and how to question the status quo and think on my own. Secondly, my editor. Her insight is always tremendous, and she improves how I am able to convey my message more than I could have ever imagined. Lastly, I want to thank all those who like and follow my work. Your interest and positive feedback are what make it all worth the effort.

Resources for a Heart Healthy Lifestyle

I t can be hard to extract all the recommendations out of a book and boil it down to what you need to do. It can also be hard to find the right resources to get started. To get you on the right track, here are some resources.

Diet

The most important thing is to eat whole foods. The majority of your nutrients should come from (nonprocessed) animal food and the majority of your energy should come from animal fats. For protein, aim for at least 1.1 gram per kilogram of ideal body weight of animal protein per day. I recommend the following sources for animal foods:

- USwellnessmeats.com
- Whiteoakpastures.com
- Belcampo.com
- Nosetotail.org
- Eatwild.com

I like the Weston A. Price Foundation for general health and nutrition information.

All produce should be organic and as fresh and local as possible. Avoid the Environmental Working Group's Dirty Dozen. Avoid packaging when you can. Find your nearest farmers' market.

Boiling, pan frying with a little water in the pan, steaming, or poaching animal foods are better options than baking, grilling, roasting, frying, deep frying, or broiling.

Do not eat vegetable oils (corn oil, soy oil, canola oil, sunflower oil, safflower oil, palm oil). Instead, use animal fats such as lard, beef tallow, butter, bone marrow, ghee, or suet.

Do not eat processed sugars (white sugar, fruit juice, high fructose corn syrup, etc.).

Eat little, if any, grains (wheat, barley, rye, oats, etc.).

Eat little, if any, legumes (beans, peas, lentils, peanuts, cashews, etc.).

Water

The best water comes from a natural spring that you go and collect. You can search for a spring in your area at www.findaspring.com.

Collecting water from a spring may not be realistic for many people, so the next best option is filtered tap water that has been restructured with a water-structuring device (e.g., www.pHPrescription.com) and then remineralized. Or bottled spring water. My favorites are Mountain Valley and Topo Chico.

Exercise

Even if you do some form of exercise every day, try not to stay too sedentary in between those workouts. Get up from your workstation often or get a standing desk.

Try to do resistance exercise or strength training one to two times per week, burst training one to two times per week, and a daily stretching routine with one additional longer yoga or stretching session per week.

Reducing Oxidative Stress

Many of the recommendations in this appendix will reduce oxidative stress; review others—such as ways to reduce toxicants you take in via air and through your cleaning products—in chapter 12.

Energizing the Body

Get into nature often. Get sunlight and walk barefoot on the Earth. Use an infrared sauna or red light in the winter. I like Sunlighten (www.sunlighten.com). Drink structured water. Eat the freshest, most locally raised food that you can.

Dental Health

Find a dentist that recognizes how the health of the mouth affects the entire body. I have found that searching for a dentist in your area by typing the words "dentist" and "cavitations" is a good way to find a knowledgeable dentist. "Ozone" and "toxic root canals" can also surface some good search results. If their website discusses the harmful effects of mercury, root canals, and jaw cavitations, then you've likely found a good choice. For more information on biological dentistry, I suggest Huggins Applied Healing (www. hugginsappliedhealing.com).

Autonomic Nervous System Balance

Track your ANS health using a heart rate variability device (options and what to look for are discussed in chapter 18). Neurofeedback can also be a good tool.

The best strategy for ANS balance is to remove all the stimuli in your life, that you can, that are contributing to imbalance. From there you can use tools like spending time in nature, dopamine fasting, meditation, and cultivating meaningful loving relationships (including with furry companions) to help maintain balance. For a longer list, refer to chapter 13.

Recommended Reading

Part I

Behave by Robert Sapolsky

Why Zebras Don't Get Ulcers by Robert Sapolsky

The Big Fat Surprise by Nina Teicholz

Catching Fire by Richard Wrangham

The Social Leap by William von Hippel

The Polyvagal Theory by Stephen Porges

Sapiens by Yuval Noah Harari

Part II

Cells, Gels, and the Engines of Life by Gerald Pollack

The Fourth Phase of Water by Gerald Pollack

Human Heart, Cosmic Heart by Thomas Cowan

Cancer and the New Biology of Water by Thomas Cowan

Tripping Over the Truth by Travis Christofferson

Cancer as a Metabolic Disease by Thomas Seyfried

The Heart and Circulation: An Integrative Model by Branko Furst

The Etiopathogenesis of Coronary Heart Disease: A Heretical Theory Based on Morphology by Giorgio Baroldi and Malcolm Silver

Natural History of Atherosclerosis by Constantin Velican and Doina Velican

Part III

Eat Rich, Live Long by Ivor Cummins and Jeffry Gerber

Eat Like a Human by Bill Schindler

The P:E Diet by Ted Naiman and William Shewfelt

Deep Nutrition by Catherine Shanahan

The Salt Fix by James DiNicolantonio

Sacred Cow by Diana Rodgers and Robb Wolf

Becoming Supernatural by Joe Dispenza

Toxic Dentistry Exposed by Graeme Munro-Hall and Lilian Munro-Hall

The Invisible Rainbow by Arthur Firstenberg

Notes

Introduction

1. Benjamin, E. J., Virani, S. S., & Calloway, C. W. (2018). Correction to: Heart disease and stroke statistics—2018 update: A report from the American Heart Association. *Circulation, 137*(12). doi:10.1161/cir.0000000000000573

2. Dou, M., Ma, A. G., Wang, Q. Z., Liang, H., Li, Y., Yi, X. M., & Zhang, S. C. (2009). Supplementation with magnesium and vitamin E were more effective than magnesium alone to decrease plasma lipids and blood viscosity in diabetic rats. *Nutrition Research, 29*(7), 519–524. https://doi.org/10.1016/j.nutres.2009.07.001; Ruttmann, T. G., Montoya-Pelaez, L. F., & James, M. F. (2007). The coagulation changes induced by rapid in vivo crystalloid infusion are attenuated when magnesium is kept at the upper limit of normal. *Anesthesia & Analgesia, 104*(6), 1475–1480. https://doi.org/10.1213/01.ane.0000261256.88414.e4

Chapter 1. Order and Energy: The Purpose of Life

1. Pace, N. R. (1991). Origin of life-facing up to the physical setting. *Cell, 65*(4), 531–533. https://doi.org/10.1016/0092-8674(91)90082-a

2. England, J. L. (2015). Dissipative adaptation in driven self-assembly. *Nature Nanotechnology, 10*(11), 919–923. doi:10.1038/nnano.2015.250

3. Krasnovsky, A. A. (1974). Pathways of chemical evolution of photosynthesis. *Cosmochemical Evolution and the Origins of Life*, 397–404. doi:10.1007/978-94-010-2239-2_32

4. Ochman, H. (2001). Genes lost and genes found: Evolution of bacterial pathogenesis and symbiosis. *Science, 292*(5519), 1096–1099. doi:10.1126/science.1058543

5. Al Amir Dache, Z., Otandault, A., Tanos, R., Pastor, B., Meddeb, R., Sanchez, C., ... Thierry, A. R. (2020). Blood contains circulating cell-free respiratory competent mitochondria. *The FASEB Journal*. doi:10.1096/fj.201901917rr

6. Parris, K. M. (1997). Glutathione: Systemic protectant against oxidative and free radical damage. https://pdfs.semanticscholar.org/36b6/ea59e3a30c66ca83cd0aa05a64ada6007f50.pdf

7. Ruiz-Ramírez, A., Ortiz-Balderas, E., Cardozo-Saldaña, G., Diaz-Diaz, E., & El-Hafidi, M. (2014). Glycine restores glutathione and protects against oxidative stress in vascular tissue from sucrose-fed rats. *Clinical Science, 126*(1), 19–29. doi:10.1042/cs20130164; Sekhar, R. V., McKay, S. V., Patel, S. G., Guthikonda, A. P., Reddy, V. T., Balasubramanyam, A., & Jahoor, F. (2010). Glutathione synthesis is diminished in patients with uncontrolled diabetes and restored by dietary supplementation with cysteine and glycine. *Diabetes Care, 34*(1), 162–167. doi:10.2337/dc10-1006

8. Nuran Ercal, B. S., Hande Gurer-Orhan, B. S., & Nukhet Aykin-Burns, B. S. (2001). Toxic metals and oxidative stress part I: Mechanisms involved in metal induced oxidative damage. *Current Topics in Medicinal Chemistry, 1*(6), 529–539. doi:10.2174/1568026013394831

9. Cai, H., & Harrison, D. G. (2000). Endothelial dysfunction in cardiovascular diseases: The role of oxidant stress. *Circulation Research, 87*(10), 840–844. doi:10.1161/01.res.87.10.840

10. Liberti, M. V., & Locasale, J. W. (2016). The Warburg effect: How does it benefit cancer cells? *Trends in Biochemical Sciences, 41*(3), 211–218. doi:10.1016/j.tibs.2015.12.001

11. Seyfried, T. N., Flores, R. E., Poff, A. M., & D'Agostino, D. P. (2013). Cancer as a metabolic disease: Implications for novel therapeutics. *Carcinogenesis, 35*(3), 515–527. doi:10.1093/carcin/bgt480

12. Gonzalez, M. J., Miranda Massari, J. R., Duconge, J., Riordan, N. H., Ichim, T., Quintero-Del-Rio, A. I., & Ortiz, N. (2012). The bio-energetic theory of carcinogenesis. *Medical Hypotheses, 79*(4), 433–439. doi:10.1016/j.mehy.2012.06.015

13. Merkle, S., & Pretsch, W. (1992). A glucosephosphate isomerase (GPI) null mutation in Mus musculus: Evidence that anaerobic glycolysis is the predominant energy delivering pathway in early post-implantation embryos. *Comparative Biochemistry and Physiology Part B: Comparative Biochemistry, 101*(3), 309–314. doi:10.1016/0305-0491(92)90004-b

14. Milder, J., & Patel, M. (2012). Modulation of oxidative stress and mitochondrial function by the ketogenic diet. *Epilepsy Research, 100*(3), 295–303. doi:10.1016/j.eplepsyres.2011.09.021

15. Sinatra, S. T. (2019, May 21). What are mitochondria? HeartMD Institute. https://heartmdinstitute.com/health-and-wellness/what-are-mitochondria/

16. Neely, J., Rovetto, M., & Oram, J. (1972). Myocardial utilization of carbohydrate and lipids. *Progress in Cardiovascular Diseases, 15*(3), 289–329. doi:10.1016/0033-0620(72)90029-1

Chapter 2. The Stress of Becoming Mammals

1. Porges, S. W. (1995). Orienting in a defensive world: Mammalian modifications of our evolutionary heritage. A Polyvagal Theory. *Psychophysiology, 32*(4), 301–318. doi:10.1111/j.1469-8986.1995.tb01213.x

2. Shoubridge, E. A., & Hochachka, P. W. (1980). Ethanol: Novel end product of vertebrate anaerobic metabolism. *Science, 209*(4453), 308–309. doi:10.1126/science.7384807

3. Fagernes, C. E., Stensløkken, K., Røhr, Å. K., Berenbrink, M., Ellefsen, S., & Nilsson, G. E. (2017). Extreme anoxia tolerance in crucian carp and goldfish through neofunctionalization of duplicated genes creating a new ethanol-producing pyruvate decarboxylase pathway. *Scientific Reports, 7*(1). https://doi.org/10.1038/s41598-017-07385-4

4. Nilsson, G. E. (2010). *Respiratory physiology of vertebrates: Life with and without oxygen.* Cambridge University Press.

5. Storz, J. F., & McClelland, G. B. (2017). Rewiring metabolism under oxygen deprivation. *Science, 356*(6335), 248–249. https://doi.org/10.1126/science.aan1505

6. Pamenter, M. E., Dzal, Y. A., Thompson, W. A., & Milsom, W. K. (2018). Do naked mole rats accumulate a metabolic acidosis or an oxygen debt in severe hypoxia? *The Journal of Experimental Biology, 222*(3), jeb191197. https://doi.org/10.1242/jeb.191197

7. Sapolsky, R. M. (2004). *Why zebras don't get ulcers: The acclaimed guide to stress, stress-related diseases, and coping—now revised and updated.* Holt Paperbacks.

8. Roelofs, K., Bakvis, P., Hermans, E. J., Van Pelt, J., & Van Honk, J. (2007). The effects of social stress and cortisol responses on the preconscious selective attention to social threat. *Biological Psychology, 75*(1), 1–7. doi:10.1016/j.biopsycho.2006.09.002

9. Sapolsky, R. M. (2017). *Behave: The biology of humans at our best and worst.* Penguin: p. 126.

10. Väänänen, A., Koskinen, A., Joensuu, M., Kivimäki, M., Vahtera, J., Kouvonen, A., & Jäppinen, P. (2008). Lack of predictability at work and risk of acute myocardial infarction: An 18-Year prospective study of industrial employees. *American Journal of Public Health, 98*(12), 2264–2271. https://doi.org/10.2105/ajph.2007.122382; Bosma, H., Peter, R., Siegrist, J., & Marmot, M. (1998). Two alternative job stress models and the risk of coronary heart disease. *American Journal of Public Health, 88*(1), 68–74. https://doi.org/10.2105/ajph.88.1.68

11. Jabri, A., Kalra, A., Kumar, A., Alameh, A., Adroja, S., Bashir, H., . . . Reed, G. W. (2020). Incidence of stress cardiomyopathy during the coronavirus disease 2019 pandemic. *JAMA Network Open, 3*(7), e2014780. https://doi.org/10.1001/jamanetworkopen.2020.14780

12. George, W. J., Ignarro, L. J., Paddock, R. J., White, L., & Kadowitz, P. J. (1975). Oppositional effects of acetylcholine and isoproterenol on isometric tension and cyclic nucleotide concentrations in rabbit atria. *Journal of Cyclic Nucleotide Research, 1*(5), 339–347.

Chapter 3. Becoming Human

1. Smith, F. A., Elliott Smith, R. E., Lyons, S. K., & Payne, J. L. (2018). Body size downgrading of mammals over the late Quaternary. *Science, 360*(6386), 310–313. doi:10.1126/science.aao5987

2. Stringer, C. (2012). *The origin of our species.* Penguin: p. 73.

3. Jaouen, K., Richards, M. P., Le Cabec, A., Welker, F., Rendu, W., Hublin, J., . . . Talamo, S. (2019). Exceptionally high δ15N values in collagen single amino acids confirm Neandertals as high-trophic level carnivores. *Proceedings of the National Academy of Sciences, 116*(11), 4928–4933. doi:10.1073/pnas.1814087116; Wißing, C., Rougier, H., Baumann, C., Comeyne, A., Crevecoeur, I., Drucker, D. G., . . . Bocherens, H. (2019). Stable isotopes reveal patterns of diet and mobility in the last Neandertals and first modern humans in Europe. *Scientific Reports, 9*(1). doi:10.1038/s41598-019-41033-3

4. Beasley, D. E., Koltz, A. M., Lambert, J. E., Fierer, N., & Dunn, R. R. (2015). The evolution of stomach acidity and its relevance to the human microbiome. *PLOS ONE, 10*(7), e0134116. https://doi.org/10.1371/journal.pone.0134116

5. Cornélio, A. M., De Bittencourt-Navarrete, R. E., De Bittencourt Brum, R., Queiroz, C. M., & Costa, M. R. (2016). Human brain expansion during evolution is independent of fire control and cooking. *Frontiers in Neuroscience, 10.* https://doi.org/10.3389/fnins.2016.00167

6. Gowlett, J. A. (2016). The discovery of fire by humans: A long and convoluted process. *Philosophical Transactions of the Royal Society B: Biological Sciences, 371*(1696), 20150164. https://doi.org/10.1098/rstb.2015.0164

7. Parker, B., Walton, C., Carr, S., Andrus, J., Cheung, E., Duplisea, M., . . . Bikman, B. (2018). β-Hydroxybutyrate elicits favorable mitochondrial changes in skeletal muscle. *International Journal of Molecular Sciences, 19*(8), 2247. doi:10.3390/ijms19082247

8. Neely, J., Rovetto, M., & Oram, J. (1972). Myocardial utilization of carbohydrate and lipids. *Progress in Cardiovascular Diseases*, *15*(3), 289–329. doi:10.1016/0033-0620(72)90029-1

9. Bassenge, E., Wendt, V. E., Schollmeyer, P., Blumchen, G., Gudbjarnason, S., & Bing, R. J. (1965). Effect of ketone bodies on cardiac metabolism. *American Journal of Physiology*, *208*(1), 162–168. https://doi.org/10.1152/ajplegacy.1965.208.1.162

10. Chen, V., Wagner, G., & Spitzer, J. (1984). Regulation of substrate oxidation in isolated myocardial cells by β-hydroxybutyrate. *Hormone and Metabolic Research*, *16*(05), 243–247. doi:10.1055/s-2007-1014756

11. Yurista, S. R., Chong, C., Badimon, J. J., Kelly, D. P., De Boer, R. A., & Westenbrink, B. D. (2021). Therapeutic potential of ketone bodies for patients with cardiovascular disease. *Journal of the American College of Cardiology*, *77*(13). https://doi.org/10.1016/j.jacc.2020.12.065

12. Woodall, B. P., Gresham, K. S., Woodall, M. A., Valenti, M., Cannavo, A., Pfleger, J., . . . Koch, W. J. (2019). Alteration of myocardial GRK2 produces a global metabolic phenotype. *JCI Insight*, *4*(10). doi:10.1172/jci.insight.123848

Chapter 4. The Consequences of Defying Evolution

1. Barker, G. (2009). *The agricultural revolution in prehistory: Why did foragers become farmers?* Oxford University Press on Demand.

2. Allam, A. H. (2009). Computed tomographic assessment of atherosclerosis in ancient Egyptian mummies. *JAMA*, *302*(19), 2091. doi:10.1001/jama.2009.1641

3. Touzeau, A., Amiot, R., Blichert-Toft, J., Flandrois, J., Fourel, F., Grossi, V., . . . Lécuyer, C. (2014). Diet of ancient Egyptians inferred from stable isotope systematics. *Journal of Archaeological Science*, *46*, 114–124. doi:10.1016/j.jas.2014.03.005

4. Hajar, R. (2017). Coronary heart disease: From mummies to 21st century. *Heart Views*, *18*(2), 68. doi:10.4103/heartviews.heartviews_57_17

5. Albinali, H. A. (2012). Majnoon Lila. *Global Cardiology Science and Practice*, *2012*(2), 16. doi:10.5339/gcsp.2012.16

6. Stefansson, V. (1962). *My life with the Eskimo*. Ravenio Books.

7. Stefansson, V. (2019). *Not by bread alone: The all-meat diet classic*. Echo Point Books & Media.

8. Price, W. A. (1945). *Nutrition and physical degeneration: A comparison of primitive and modern diets and their effects*. Author.

9. Osler, W. (1944). *The principles and practice of medicine*. Ravenio Books.

10. Donaldson, B. F. (2017). *Strong medicine*. Pickle Partners Publishing.

11. Pennington, A. W. (1953). A reorientation on obesity. *New England Journal of Medicine*, *248*(23), 959–964. doi:10.1056/nejm195306042482301

Chapter 5. The Infamous Diet–Heart Hypothesis

1. Blasbalg, T. L., Hibbeln, J. R., Ramsden, C. E., Majchrzak, S. F., & Rawlings, R. R. (2011). Changes in consumption of omega-3 and omega-6 fatty acids in the United States during the 20th century. *The American Journal of Clinical Nutrition*, *93*(5), 950–962. https://doi.org/10.3945/ajcn.110.006643

2. Keys, A., Mickelsen, O., Miller, E. V., & Chapman, C. B. (1950). The relation in man between cholesterol levels in the diet and in the blood. *Science*, *112*(2899), 79–81. https://doi.org/10.1126/science.112.2899.79

3. Keys, A. (1970). Coronary heart disease in seven countries. *Annals of Internal Medicine, 73*(2), 356. https://doi.org/10.7326/0003-4819-73-2-356_8

4. Steinemann, N., Grize, L., Ziesemer, K., Kauf, P., Probst-Hensch, N., & Brombach, C. (2017). Relative validation of a food frequency questionnaire to estimate food intake in an adult population. *Food & Nutrition Research, 61*(1), 1305193. https://doi.org/10.1080/16546628.2017.1305193

5. Yerushalmy, J., & Hilleboe, H. (1957). Fat in the diet and mortality from heart disease: A methodologic note. *New York State Journal of Medicine, 57*(14), 2343–2354.

6. Mann, G. V., Shaffer, R. D., Anderson, R. S., Sandstead, H. H., Predergast, H., Mann, J. C., . . . Dicks, K. (1964). Cardiovascular disease in the Masai. *Journal of Atherosclerosis Research, 4*(4), 289–312. https://doi.org/10.1016/S0368-1319(64)80041-7

7. Ramsden, C. E., Zamora, D., Majchrzak-Hong, S., Faurot, K. R., Broste, S. K., Frantz, R. P., . . . Hibbeln, J. R. (2016). Re-evaluation of the traditional diet-heart hypothesis: Analysis of recovered data from Minnesota coronary experiment (1968–73). *BMJ*, i1246. https://doi.org/10.1136/bmj.i1246

8. Ramsden, C. E., Zamora, D., Leelarthaepin, B., Majchrzak-Hong, S. F., Faurot, K. R., Suchindran, C. M., . . . Hibbeln, J. R. (2013). Use of dietary linoleic acid for secondary prevention of coronary heart disease and death: Evaluation of recovered data from the Sydney diet heart study and updated meta-analysis. *BMJ, 346*(feb04 3), e8707–e8707. https://doi.org/10.1136/bmj.e8707

9. Astrup, A., Magkos, F., Bier, D. M., Brenna, J. T., De Oliveira Otto, M. C., Hill, J. O., . . . Krauss, R. M. (2020). Saturated fats and health: A reassessment and proposal for food-based recommendations: JACC State-of-the-Art review. *Journal of the American College of Cardiology, 76*(7). https://doi.org/10.1016/j.jacc.2020.05.077

10. O'Connor, L. E., Kim, J. E., Clark, C. M., Zhu, W., & Campbell, W. W. (2020). Effects of total red meat intake on glycemic control and inflammatory biomarkers: A meta-analysis of randomized controlled trials. *Advances in Nutrition, 12*(1), 115–127. https://doi.org/10.1093/advances/nmaa096

11. Hodge, A. M., English, D. R., O'Dea, K., Sinclair, A. J., Makrides, M., Gibson, R. A., & Giles, G. G. (2007). Plasma phospholipid and dietary fatty acids as predictors of type 2 diabetes: Interpreting the role of linoleic acid. *The American Journal of Clinical Nutrition, 86*(1), 189–197. https://doi.org/10.1093/ajcn/86.1.189; Wang, L., Folsom, A. R., Zheng, Z., Pankow, J. S., & Eckfeldt, J. H. (2003). Plasma fatty acid composition and incidence of diabetes in middle-aged adults: The atherosclerosis risk in communities (ARIC) study. *The American Journal of Clinical Nutrition, 78*(1), 91–98. https://doi.org/10.1093/ajcn/78.1.91; Miettinen, T. A., Naukkarinen, V., Huttunen, J. K., Mattila, S., & Kumlin, T. (1982). Fatty-acid composition of serum lipids predicts myocardial infarction. *BMJ, 285*(6347), 993–996. https://doi.org/10.1136/bmj.285.6347.993; Miettinen, T. A., Naukkarinen, V., Huttunen, J. K., Mattila, S., & Kumlin, T. (1982). Fatty-acid composition of serum lipids predicts myocardial infarction. *BMJ, 285*(6347), 993–996. https://doi.org/10.1136/bmj.285.6347.993; Jakobsen, M. U., O'Reilly, E. J., Heitmann, B. L., Pereira, M. A., Bälter, K., Fraser, G. E., . . . Ascherio, A. (2009). Major types of dietary fat and risk of coronary heart disease: A pooled analysis of 11 cohort studies. *The American Journal of Clinical Nutrition, 89*(5), 1425–1432. https://doi.org/10.3945/ajcn.2008.27124; Volk,

B. M., Kunces, L. J., Freidenreich, D. J., Kupchak, B. R., Saenz, C., Artistizabal, J. C., . . . Volek, J. S. (2014). Effects of step-wise increases in dietary carbohydrate on circulating saturated fatty acids and Palmitoleic acid in adults with metabolic syndrome. *PLOS ONE*, *9*(11), e113605. https://doi.org/10.1371/journal.pone.0113605

Chapter 6. The True Function of the Heart

1. Harvey W. (1952). A second disquisition to John Riolan (Translated by R. Willis). In R. M. Hutchins (Ed.), *Encyclopedia Britannica: Great books of the western world*. Encyclopedia Britannica: pp. 313–328.

2. Thudichum, I. L. (1855). On the cause of the emptiness of the arteries after death. *BMJ*, *s3-3*(110), 122–127. https://doi.org/10.1136/bmj.s3-3.110.122

3. Weber, E. H. (1850). *Ueber die anwendung der wellenlehre auf die lehre vom kreislaufe des blutes und insbesondere auf die pulslehre. Berichte ueber die Verhandlungen, Koenigl.* Sacchsische Gesellschaft der Wissenschaften, Leipzig: pp. 164–204.

4. Barclay, C. J. (2003). Initial mechanical efficiency of isolated cardiac muscle. *Journal of Experimental Biology*, *206*(16), 2725–2732. doi:10.1242/jeb.00480

5. Thompson, S. A. (1948). The effect of pulmonary inflation and deflation upon the circulation. *Journal of Thoracic Surgery*, *17*(3), 323–334. https://doi.org/10.1016/s0096 -5588(20)31907-3

6. Carvalho, P., Hildebrandt, J., & Charan, N. B. (1996). Changes in bronchial and pulmonary arterial blood flow with progressive tension pneumothorax. *Journal of Applied Physiology*, *81*(4), 1664–1669. doi:10.1152/jappl.1996.81.4.1664

7. Manteuffel-Szoege, L., Michalowski, J., Grundman, J., & Pacocha, W. (1966). On the possibility of blood circulation continuing after stopping the heart. *The Journal of Cardiovascular Surgery*, *7*(3), 201–208. https://pubmed.ncbi.nlm.nih.gov/5938806/

8. Chai, B., Yoo, H., & Pollack, G. H. (2009). Effect of radiant energy on near-surface water. *The Journal of Physical Chemistry B*, *113*(42), 13953–13958. doi:10.1021/jp908163w

9. Li, Z., & Pollack, G. H. (2020). Surface-induced flow: A natural microscopic engine using infrared energy as fuel. *Science Advances*, *6*(19), eaba0941. https://doi.org/10.1126 /sciadv.aba0941

10. Pollack, G. H. (2013). *The fourth phase of water: Beyond solid, liquid, and vapor*. Ebner and Sons Publishers: pp. 216–217.

11. Li, Z., & Pollack, G.H. (2020). On the driver of blood circulation beyond the heart. (Unpublished doctoral dissertation). University of Washington, Seattle, Washington: p. Abstract. https://www.biorxiv.org/content/10.1101/2021.04.19.440300v1

12. Manteuffel-Szoege, L. (1960). Energy sources of blood circulation and the mechanical action of the heart. *Thorax*, *15*(1), 47–53. https://doi.org/10.1136/thx.15.1.47

13. Furst, B. (2013). *The heart and circulation: An integrative model*. Springer Science & Business Media: p. 176.

14. Calbet, J. A., Jensen-Urstad, M., Van Hall, G., Holmberg, H., Rosdahl, H., & Saltin, B. (2004). Maximal muscular vascular conductances during whole body upright exercise in humans. *The Journal of Physiology*, *558*(1), 319–331. https://doi.org/10.1113/jphysiol.2003.059287

15. Stene, J. K., Burns, B., Permutt, S., Caldini, P., & Shanoff, M. (1982). Increased cardiac output following occlusion of the descending thoracic aorta in dogs. *American Journal of*

Physiology-Regulatory, Integrative and Comparative Physiology, 243(1), R152–R158. https://doi.org/10.1152/ajpregu.1982.243.1.r152

16. Zocalo, Y., Bia, D., Armentano, R. L., Arias, L., Lopez, C., Etchart, C., & Guevara, E. (2007). *Assessment of training-dependent changes in the left ventricle torsion dynamics of professional soccer players using speckle-tracking echocardiography.* 2007 29th Annual International Conference of the IEEE Engineering in Medicine and Biology Society. https://doi.org/10.1109/iembs.2007.4352888

17. Torrent-Guasp, F., Kocica, M. J., Corno, A. F., Komeda, M., Carreras-Costa, F., Flotats, A., ... Wen, H. (2005). Towards new understanding of the heart structure and function. *European Journal of Cardio-Thoracic Surgery*, 27(2), 191–201. doi:10.1016/j.ejcts.2004.11.026

18. Buckberg, G. D. (2002). Basic science review: The helix and the heart. *The Journal of Thoracic and Cardiovascular Surgery*, 124(5), 863–883. https://doi.org/10.1067/mtc.2002.122439

19. McMurrich, J. P. (1930). *Leonardo da Vinci: The anatomist (1452–1519)*. Published for Carnegie Institution of Washington by the Williams & Wilkins Company.

20. Mayo Clinic. (2020, May 29). Heart failure—Symptoms and causes. https://www.mayoclinic.org/diseases-conditions/heart-failure/symptoms-causes/syc-20373142

21. Wilson, M., O'Hanlon, R., Prasad, S., Deighan, A., MacMillan, P., Oxborough, D., ... Whyte, G. (2011). Diverse patterns of myocardial fibrosis in lifelong, veteran endurance athletes. *Journal of Applied Physiology*, 110(6), 1622–1626. doi:10.1152/japplphysiol.01280.2010

22. Aubert, G., Martin, O. J., Horton, J. L., Lai, L., Vega, R. B., Leone, T. C., ... Kelly, D. P. (2016). The failing heart relies on ketone bodies as a fuel. *Circulation*, 133(8), 698–705. doi:10.1161/circulationaha.115.017355

23. Valayannopoulos, V., Bajolle, F., Arnoux, J., Dubois, S., Sannier, N., Baussan, C., ... De Lonlay, P. (2011). Successful treatment of severe cardiomyopathy in glycogen storage disease type III with D,L-3-hydroxybutyrate, ketogenic and high-protein diet. *Pediatric Research*, 70(6), 638–641. doi:10.1203/pdr.0b013e318232154f

24. Brambilla, A., Mannarino, S., Pretese, R., Gasperini, S., Galimberti, C., & Parini, R. (2014). Improvement of cardiomyopathy after high-fat diet in two siblings with glycogen storage disease type III. *JIMD Reports*, 17(91–95). doi:10.1007/8904_2014_343

25. McCommis, K. S., Kovacs, A., Weinheimer, C. J., Shew, T. M., Koves, T. R., Ilkayeva, O. R., ... Finck, B. N. (2020). Nutritional modulation of heart failure in mitochondrial pyruvate carrier–deficient mice. *Nature Metabolism*, 2(11), 1232–1247. https://doi.org/10.1038/s42255-020-00296-1

26. De Miguel Díez, J., Chancafe Morgan, J., & Jiménez Garcia, R. (2013). The association between COPD and heart failure risk: A review. *International Journal of Chronic Obstructive Pulmonary Disease*, 305. doi:10.2147/copd.s31236

27. Curkendall, S. M., DeLuise, C., Jones, J. K., Lanes, S., Stang, M. R., Goehring, E., Jr., & She, D. (2006). Cardiovascular disease in patients with chronic obstructive pulmonary disease, Saskatchewan Canada cardiovascular disease in COPD patients. *Annals of Epidemiology*, 16(1), 63–70. https://doi.org/ 10.1016/j.annepidem.2005.04.008

28. Miyata, M., Kihara, T., Kubozono, T., Ikeda, Y., Shinsato, T., Izumi, T., ... Tei, C. (2008). Beneficial effects of Waon therapy on patients with chronic heart failure: Results of a

prospective multicenter study. *Journal of Cardiology, 52*(2), 79–85. doi:10.1016/j.jjcc
.2008.07.009

29. Kihara, T., Biro, S., Ikeda, Y., Fukudome, T., Shinsato, T., Masuda, A., . . . Tei, C. (2004).
Effects of repeated sauna treatment on ventricular arrhythmias in patients with chronic
heart failure. *Circulation Journal, 68*(12), 1146–1151. doi:10.1253/circj.68.1146; Kihara,
T., Biro, S., Imamura, M., Yoshifuku, S., Takasaki, K., Ikeda, Y., . . . Tei, C. (2002).
Repeated sauna treatment improves vascular endothelial and cardiac function in patients
with chronic heart failure. *Journal of the American College of Cardiology, 39*(5), 754–759.
doi:10.1016/s0735-1097(01)01824-1; Miyamoto, H., Kai, H., Nakaura, H., Osada, K.,
Mizuta, Y., Matsumoto, A., & Imaizumi, T. (2005). Safety and efficacy of repeated sauna
bathing in patients with chronic systolic heart failure: A preliminary report. *Journal of
Cardiac Failure, 11*(6), 432–436. doi:10.1016/j.cardfail.2005.03.004; Mussivand, T., Alshaer,
H., Haddad, H., Beanlands, D. S., Beanlands, R., Chan, K., . . . Silver, M. A. (2008).
Thermal therapy: A viable adjunct in the treatment of heart failure? *Congestive Heart
Failure, 14*(4), 180–186. doi:10.1111/j.1751-7133.2008.07792.x; Kihara, T., Miyata, M.,
Fukudome, T., Ikeda, Y., Shinsato, T., Kubozono, T., . . . Tei, C. (2009). Waon therapy
improves the prognosis of patients with chronic heart failure. *Journal of Cardiology, 53*(2),
214–218. doi:10.1016/j.jjcc.2008.11.005

30. Sobajima, M., Nozawa, T., Ihori, H., Shida, T., Ohori, T., Suzuki, T., . . . Inoue, H. (2013).
Repeated sauna therapy improves myocardial perfusion in patients with chronically
occluded coronary artery-related ischemia. *International Journal of Cardiology, 167*(1),
237–243. https://doi.org/10.1016/j.ijcard.2011.12.064

31. Sobajima, M., Nozawa, T., Shida, T., Ohori, T., Suzuki, T., Matsuki, A., & Inoue, H.
(2011). Repeated sauna therapy attenuates ventricular remodeling after myocardial
infarction in rats by increasing coronary vascularity of noninfarcted myocardium. *American Journal of Physiology-Heart and Circulatory Physiology, 301*(2), H548–H554. https://doi
.org/10.1152/ajpheart.00103.2011

Chapter 7. Cholesterol and Atherosclerosis

1. Netea, M. G., Demacker, P. N., Kullberg, B. J., Jacobs, L. E., Verver-Jansen, T. J., Boerman,
O. C., . . . Van der Meer, J. W. (1998). Bacterial lipopolysaccharide binds and stimulates
cytokine-producing cells before neutralization by endogenous lipoproteins can occur.
Cytokine, 10(10), 766–772. doi:10.1006/cyto.1998.0364

2. Emancipator, K., Csako, G., & Elin, R. J. (1992). In vitro inactivation of bacterial endotoxin
by human lipoproteins and apolipoproteins. *Infection and Immunity, 60*(2), 596–601.
doi:10.1128/iai.60.2.596-601.1992

3. Famino, R., Famino, G., Cavezzi, A., & Troiani, E. (2021). PCSK9 inhibition, LDL and
lipopolysaccharides: A complex and "dangerous" relationship. *International Angiology:
A Journal of the International Union of Angiology, 40*(3). https://doi.org/10.23736/s0392
-9590.21.04632-0

4. Ingallinella, P., Bianchi, E., Ladwa, N. A., Wang, Y., Hrin, R., Veneziano, M., Bonelli, F., . . .
Pessi, A. (2009). Addition of a cholesterol group to an HIV-1 peptide fusion inhibitor
dramatically increases its antiviral potency. *Proceedings of the National Academy of Sciences,
106*(14), 5801–5806. https://doi.org/10.1073/pnas.0901007106

5. Lee, K. K., Pessi, A., Gui, L., Santoprete, A., Talekar, A., Moscona, A., & Porotto, M. (2011). Capturing a fusion intermediate of influenza hemagglutinin with a cholesterol-conjugated peptide, a new antiviral strategy for influenza virus. *Journal of Biological Chemistry, 286*(49), 42141–42149. https://doi.org/10.1074/jbc.m111.254243

6. Berghoff, S. A., Gerndt, N., Winchenbach, J., Stumpf, S. K., Hosang, L., Odoardi, F., . . . Saher, G. (2017). Dietary cholesterol promotes repair of demyelinated lesions in the adult brain. *Nature Communications, 8*(1). doi:10.1038/ncomms14241

7. Payne, A. H., & Hales, D. B. (2004). Overview of steroidogenic enzymes in the pathway from cholesterol to active steroid hormones. *Endocrine Reviews, 25*(6), 947–970. doi:10.1210/er.2003-0030

8. Traber, M. G., & Kayden, H. J. (1984). Vitamin E is delivered to cells via the high affinity receptor for low-density lipoprotein. *The American Journal of Clinical Nutrition, 40*(4), 747–751. doi:10.1093/ajcn/40.4.747

9. Blom, D. J., Djedjos, C. S., Monsalvo, M. L., Bridges, I., Wasserman, S. M., Scott, R., & Roth, E. (2015). Effects of evolocumab on vitamin E and steroid hormone levels. *Circulation Research, 117*(8), 731–741. doi:10.1161/circresaha.115.307071

10. Simopoulos, A. P., & Meester, F. D. (2009). *A balanced omega-6/omega-3 fatty acid ratio, cholesterol and coronary heart disease.* Karger Medical and Scientific Publishers.

11. Srikanthan, P., & Karlamangla, A. S. (2014). Muscle mass index as a predictor of longevity in older adults. *The American Journal of Medicine, 127*(6), 547–553. doi:10.1016/j.amjmed.2014.02.007

12. Parpal, S., Karlsson, M., Thorn, H., & Strålfors, P. (2000). Cholesterol depletion disrupts caveolae and insulin receptor signaling for metabolic control via insulin receptor substrate-1, but not for mitogen-activated protein kinase control. *Journal of Biological Chemistry, 276*(13), 9670–9678. doi:10.1074/jbc.m007454200

13. El Asmar, M., Naoum, J., & Arbid, E. (2014). Vitamin K dependent proteins and the role of vitamin K2 in the modulation of vascular calcification: A review. *Oman Medical Journal, 29*(3), 172–177. doi:10.5001/omj.2014.44

14. Okuyama, H., Langsjoen, P. H., Hamazaki, T., Ogushi, Y., Hama, R., Kobayashi, T., & Uchino, H. (2015). Statins stimulate atherosclerosis and heart failure: Pharmacological mechanisms. *Expert Review of Clinical Pharmacology, 8*(2), 189–199. doi:10.1586/17512433.2015.1011125; Saito, E., Wachi, H., Sato, F., Sugitani, H., & Seyama, Y. (2007). Treatment with vitamin K2 combined with bisphosphonates synergistically inhibits calcification in cultured smooth muscle cells. *Journal of Atherosclerosis and Thrombosis, 14*(6), 317–324. doi:10.5551/jat.e501

15. Ogbru, O. (n.d.). Top 10 drugs prescribed in the U.S. MedicineNet. https://www.medicinenet.com/top_drugs_prescribed_in_the_us/views.htm

16. Fuhrmeister, J., Tews, M., Kromer, A., & Moosmann, B. (2012). Prooxidative toxicity and selenoprotein suppression by cerivastatin in muscle cells. *Toxicology Letters, 215*(3), 219–227. doi:10.1016/j.toxlet.2012.10.010

17. Kawashima, H., Nakajima, Y., Matubara, Y., Nakanowatari, J., Fukuta, T., Mizuno, S., . . . Nakamura, T. (1997). Effects of vitamin K2 (Menatetrenone) on atherosclerosis and blood coagulation in hypercholesterolemic rabbits. *The Japanese Journal of Pharmacology, 75*(2), 135–143. doi:10.1254/jjp.75.135

18. Langsjoen, P. H., Langsjoen, J. O., Langsjoen, A. M., & Lucas, L. A. (2005). Treatment of statin adverse effects with supplemental coenzyme Q10 and statin drug discontinuation. *BioFactors, 25*(1–4), 147–152. doi:10.1002/biof.5520250116

19. Dirks, A. J., & Jones, K. M. (2006). Statin-induced apoptosis and skeletal myopathy. *American Journal of Physiology-Cell Physiology, 291*(6), C1208–C1212. doi:10.1152/ajpcell .00226.2006

20. Langsjoen, P. H., & Langsjoen, A. M. (2003). The clinical use of HMG CoA-reductase inhibitors and the associated depletion of coenzyme Q10. A review of animal and human publications. *BioFactors, 18*(1–4), 101–111. doi:10.1002/biof.5520180212

21. Rees-Milton, K. J., Norman, P., Babiolakis, C., Hulbert, M., Turner, M. E., Berger, C., . . . Holden, R. M. (2020). Statin use is associated with insulin resistance in participants of the Canadian multicentre osteoporosis study. *Journal of the Endocrine Society, 4*(8). https://doi.org/10.1210/jendso/bvaa057

22. Correction: Statin use and risk of developing diabetes: Results from the Diabetes Prevention Program. (2017). *BMJ Open Diabetes Research & Care, 5*(1), bmjdrc-2017-000438corr1. doi:10.1136/bmjdrc-2017-000438corr1

23. Muscogiuri, G., Sarno, G., Gastaldelli, A., Savastano, S., Ascione, A., Colao, A., & Orio, F. (2014). The good and bad effects of statins on insulin sensitivity and secretion. *Endocrine Research, 39*(4), 137–143. https://doi.org/10.3109/07435800.2014.952018

24. van Bruggen, F. H., Nijhuis, G. B., Zuidema, S. U., & Luijendijk, H. (2020). Serious adverse events and deaths in PCSK9 inhibitor trials reported on ClinicalTrials.gov: A systematic review. *Expert Review of Clinical Pharmacology, 13*(7), 787–796. https://doi.org /10.1080/17512433.2020.1787832

25. Battaggia, A., Scalisi, A., & Donzelli, A. (2018). The systematic review of randomized controlled trials of PCSK9 antibodies challenges their "efficacy breakthrough" and the "lower, the better" theory. *Current Medical Research and Opinion, 34*(10), 1725–1730. https://doi.org/10.1080/03007995.2018.1428188

26. Wang, X., Dong, Y., Qi, X., Huang, C., & Hou, L. (2013). Cholesterol levels and risk of hemorrhagic stroke. *Stroke, 44*(7), 1833–1839. https://doi.org/10.1161/strokeaha .113.001326; Elias, P. K., Elias, M. F., D'Agostino, R. B., Sullivan, L. M., & Wolf, P. A. (2005). Serum cholesterol and cognitive performance in the Framingham heart study. *Psychosomatic Medicine, 67*(1), 24–30. https://doi.org/10.1097/01.psy.0000151745.67285.c2; Huang, X., Abbott, R. D., Petrovitch, H., Mailman, R. B., & Ross, G. W. (2008). Low LDL cholesterol and increased risk of Parkinson's disease: Prospective results from Honolulu-Asia aging study. *Movement Disorders, 23*(7), 1013–1018. https://doi.org/10.1002/mds.22013; Seneff, S., Wainwright, G., & Mascitelli, L. (2011). Nutrition and Alzheimer's disease: The detrimental role of a high carbohydrate diet. *European Journal of Internal Medicine, 22*(2), 134–140. https://doi.org/10.1016/j.ejim.2010.12.017; American College of Cardiology. (2012, March 26). Low LDL cholesterol is related to cancer risk. *ScienceDaily*. Retrieved April 3, 2021 from www.sciencedaily.com/releases/2012/03/120326113713.htm; Brescianini, S., Maggi, S., Farchi, G., Mariotti, S., Di Carlo, A., Baldereschi, M., Inzitari, D., & For The ILSA Group. (2003). Low total cholesterol and increased risk of dying: Are low levels clinical warning signs in the elderly? Results from the Italian longitudinal study on aging. *Journal of the American Geriatrics Society, 51*(7), 991–996. https://doi.org/10.1046/j.1365-2389.2003.51313.x

27. Abramson, J., & Wright, J. (2007). Are lipid-lowering guidelines evidence-based? *The Lancet, 369*(9557), 168–169. doi:10.1016/s0140-6736(07)60084-1

28. Brown, B. G., & Taylor, A. J. (2008). Does ENHANCE diminish confidence in lowering LDL or in ezetimibe? *New England Journal of Medicine, 358*(14), 1504–1507. doi:10.1056/nejme0801608

29. Newman, D. (2015, January 10). Statin drugs given for 5 years for heart disease prevention (without known heart disease). *NNT.* http://www.thennt.com/nnt/statins-for-heart-disease-prevention-without-prior-heart-disease/. Updated November 2017.

30. Casteel, B. (2016, April 3). Evacetrapib fails to reduce major adverse cardiovascular events. *American College of Cardiology.* https://www.acc.org/about-acc/press-releases/2016/04/03/13/02/evacetrapib-fails-to-reduce-major-adverse-cardiovascular-events

31. Downs, J. R., Clearfield, M., Weis, S., Whitney, E., Shapiro, D. R., Beere, P. A., . . . for the AFCAPS/TexCAPS Research Group. (1998). Primary prevention of acute coronary events with Lovastatin in men and women with average cholesterol levels. *JAMA, 279*(20), 1615. https://doi.org/10.1001/jama.279.20.1615

32. Shepherd, J., Cobbe, S. M., Ford, I., Isles, C. G., Lorimer, A. R., Macfarlane, P. W., . . . Packard, C. J. (1995). Prevention of coronary heart disease with pravastatin in men with hypercholesterolemia. *New England Journal of Medicine, 333*(20), 1301–1308. https://doi.org/10.1056/nejm199511163332001

33. Ridker, P., Danielson, E., & Fonseca, F. (2009). Rosuvastatin to prevent vascular events in men and women with elevated c-reactive protein. *Journal of Vascular Surgery, 49*(2), 534. https://doi.org/10.1016/j.jvs.2008.12.037

34. Johannesson, M., Jönsson, B., Kjekshus, J., Olsson, A. G., Pedersen, T. R., & Wedel, H. (1997). Cost effectiveness of simvastatin treatment to lower cholesterol levels in patients with coronary heart disease. *New England Journal of Medicine, 336*(5), 332–336. https://doi.org/10.1056/nejm199701303360503

35. Antonopoulos, A. S., Margaritis, M., Lee, R., Channon, K., & Antoniades, C. (2012). Statins as anti-inflammatory agents in atherogenesis: Molecular mechanisms and lessons from the recent clinical trials. *Current Pharmaceutical Design, 18*(11), 1519–1530. https://doi.org/10.2174/138161212799504803

36. Kelley, B. J., & Glasser, S. (2014). Cognitive effects of statin medications. *CNS Drugs, 28*(5), 411–419. doi:10.1007/s40263-014-0147-5; Davis, R., Reveles, K. R., Ali, S. K., Mortensen, E. M., Frei, C. R., & Mansi, I. (2015). Statins and male sexual health: A retrospective cohort analysis. *The Journal of Sexual Medicine, 12*(1), 158–167. doi:10.1111/jsm.12745; Ganga, H. V., Slim, H. B., & Thompson, P. D. (2014). A systematic review of statin-induced muscle problems in clinical trials. *American Heart Journal, 168*(1), 6–15. doi:10.1016/j.ahj.2014.03.019

37. Genetics Home Reference. (n.d.). Abetalipoproteinemia. Retrieved from https://ghr.nlm.nih.gov/condition/abetalipoproteinemia

38. Sijbrands, E. J. (2001). Mortality over two centuries in large pedigree with familial hypercholesterolaemia: Family tree mortality study commentary: Role of other genes and environment should not be overlooked in monogenic disease. *BMJ, 322*(7293), 1019–1023. doi:10.1136/bmj.322.7293.1019

39. Diamond, D. M., Alabdulgader, A. A., De Lorgeril, M., Harcombe, Z., Kendrick, M., Malhotra, A., . . . Volek, J. S. (2020). Dietary recommendations for familial

hypercholesterolaemia: An evidence-free zone. *BMJ Evidence-Based Medicine*, bmjebm
-2020-111412. https://doi.org/10.1136/bmjebm-2020-111412

40. Velican, C., & Velican, D. (1989). *Natural history of coronary atherosclerosis.* CRC Press LLC:
p. 10.

41. Van Peet, P. G., Drewes, Y. M., De Craen, A. J., Westendorp, R. G., Gussekloo, J., & De
Ruijter, W. (2012). Prognostic value of cardiovascular disease status: The Leiden 85-plus
study. *AGE, 35*(4), 1433–1444. doi:10.1007/s11357-012-9443-5

42. Deary, I. J., Gow, A. J., Taylor, M. D., Corley, J., Brett, C., Wilson, V., . . . Starr, J. M. (2007).
The Lothian Birth Cohort 1936: A study to examine influences on cognitive ageing from
age 11 to age 70 and beyond. *BMC Geriatrics, 7*(1). doi:10.1186/1471-2318-7-28

43. Sung, K.-C., Huh, J. H., Ryu, S., Lee, J.-Y., Scorletti, E., Byrne, C. D., . . . Ko, S.-B. (2019).
Low levels of low-density lipoprotein cholesterol and mortality outcomes in non-statin
users. *Journal of Clinical Medicine, 8*(10), 1571. https://doi.org/10.3390/jcm8101571

44. Ravnskov, U., Diamond, D. M., Hama, R., Hamazaki, T., Hammarskjöld, B., Hynes,
N., . . . Sundberg, R. (2016). Lack of an association or an inverse association between
low-density-lipoprotein cholesterol and mortality in the elderly: A systematic review.
BMJ Open, 6(6), e010401. https://doi.org/10.1136/bmjopen-2015-010401

45. Sachdeva, A., Cannon, C. P., Deedwania, P. C., LaBresh, K. A., Smith, S. C., Dai, D., . . .
Fonarow, G. C. (2009). Lipid levels in patients hospitalized with coronary artery disease:
An analysis of 136,905 hospitalizations in Get with the Guidelines. *American Heart
Journal, 157*(1), 111–117.e2. doi:10.1016/j.ahj.2008.08.010

46. Pollack, G. H. (2013). *The fourth phase of water: Beyond solid, liquid, and vapor.* Ebner and
Sons Publishers: p. 98.

47. Harrison, D., Griendling, K. K., Landmesser, U., Hornig, B., & Drexler, H. (2003). Role
of oxidative stress in atherosclerosis. *The American Journal of Cardiology, 91*(3), 7–11.
doi:10.1016/s0002-9149(02)03144-2; Malhotra, A., Redberg, R. F., & Meier, P. (2017).
Saturated fat does not clog the arteries: coronary heart disease is a chronic inflammatory condition, the risk of which can be effectively reduced from healthy lifestyle
interventions. *British Journal of Sports Medicine, 51*(15), 1111–1112. doi:10.1136
/bjsports-2016-097285

48. Ceriello, A., Esposito, K., Piconi, L., Ihnat, M. A., Thorpe, J. E., Testa, R., . . . Giugliano,
D. (2008). Oscillating glucose is more deleterious to endothelial function and oxidative
stress than mean glucose in normal and type 2 diabetic patients. *Diabetes, 57*(5),
1349–1354. doi:10.2337/db08-0063

49. Mohanty, P., Hamouda, W., Garg, R., Aljada, A., Ghanim, H., & Dandona, P. (2000).
Glucose challenge stimulates reactive oxygen species (ROS) generation by leucocytes.
The Journal of Clinical Endocrinology & Metabolism, 85(8), 2970–2973. doi:10.1210/jcem
.85.8.6854

50. Li, M., Absher, P. M., Liang, P., Russell, J. C., Sobel, B. E., & Fukagawa, N. K. (2001). High
glucose concentrations induce oxidative damage to mitochondrial DNA in explanted
vascular smooth muscle cells. *Experimental Biology and Medicine, 226*(5), 450–457.
doi:10.1177/153537020122600510

51. Schleicher, E., & Friess, U. (2007). Oxidative stress, AGE, and atherosclerosis. *Kidney
International, 72*, S17–S26. doi:10.1038/sj.ki.5002382

52. Vlassara, H. (1996). Advanced glycation end-products and atherosclerosis. *Annals of Medicine, 28*(5), 419–426. https://doi.org/10.3109/07853899608999102

53. Stoll, L. L., Denning, G. M., & Weintraub, N. L. (2004). Potential role of endotoxin as a proinflammatory mediator of atherosclerosis. *Arteriosclerosis, Thrombosis, and Vascular Biology, 24*(12), 2227–2236. doi:10.1161/01.atv.0000147534.69062.dc

54. Carnevale, R., Nocella, C., Petrozza, V., Cammisotto, V., Pacini, L., Sorrentino, V., . . . Violi, F. (2018). Localization of lipopolysaccharide from escherichia coli into human atherosclerotic plaque. *Scientific Reports, 8*(1). https://doi.org/10.1038/s41598-018-22076-4

55. Mayr, F., Spiel, A., Leitner, J., Firbas, C., Sieghart, W., & Jilma, B. (2007). Effects of low dose endotoxemia on endothelial progenitor cells in humans. *Atherosclerosis, 195*(1), e202–e206. doi:10.1016/j.atherosclerosis.2007.04.003

56. Geerts, S. O., Nys, M., Mol, P. D., Charpentier, J., Albert, A., Legrand, V., & Rompen, E. H. (2002). Systemic release of endotoxins induced by gentle mastication: Association with periodontitis severity. *Journal of Periodontology, 73*(1), 73–78. doi:10.1902/jop.2002.73.1.73; Fukui, H. (2016). Endotoxin and other microbial translocation markers in the blood: A clue to understand leaky gut syndrome. *Cellular & Molecular Medicine: Open access, 02*(03). doi:10.21767/2573-5365.100023; Alves, J., Walton, R., & Drake, D. (1998). Coronal leakage: Endotoxin penetration from mixed bacterial communities through obturated, post-prepared root canals. *Journal of Endodontics, 24*(9), 587–591. doi:10.1016/s0099-2399(98)80115-5

57. Nuran, E., Gurer-Orhan, H., & Aykin-Burns, N. (2001). Toxic metals and oxidative stress part I: Mechanisms involved in me-tal induced oxidative damage. *Current Topics in Medicinal Chemistry, 1*(6), 529–539. doi:10.2174/1568026013394831

58. Salonen, J. T., Seppänen, K., Lakka, T. A., Salonen, R., & Kaplan, G. A. (2000). Mercury accumulation and accelerated progression of carotid atherosclerosis: A population-based prospective 4-year follow-up study in men in eastern Finland. *Atherosclerosis, 148*(2), 265–273. doi:10.1016/s0021-9150(99)00272-5

59. Schwartz, J. (1995). Lead, blood pressure, and cardiovascular disease in men. *Archives of Environmental Health: An International Journal, 50*(1), 31–37. https://doi.org/10.1080/00039896.1995.9955010; Simeonova, P., & Luster, M. (2000). Arsenic and atherosclerosis. *Atherosclerosis, 151*(1), 179. https://doi.org/10.1016/s0021-9150(00)80813-8; Tseng, C., Chong, C., Tseng, C., Hsueh, Y., Chiou, H., Tseng, C., & Chen, C. (2003). Long-term arsenic exposure and ischemic heart disease in arseniasis-hyperendemic villages in Taiwan. *Toxicology Letters, 137*(1–2), 15–21. https://doi.org/10.1016/s0378-4274(02)00377-6; Houtman, J. (1993). Prolonged low-level cadmium intake and atherosclerosis. *The Science of The Total Environment, 138*(1–3), 31–36. https://doi.org/10.1016/0048-9697(93)90402-r; Costello, S., Brown, D. M., Noth, E. M., Cantley, L., Slade, M. D., Tessier-Sherman, B., . . . Cullen, M. R. (2013). Incident ischemic heart disease and recent occupational exposure to particulate matter in an aluminum cohort. *Journal of Exposure Science & Environmental Epidemiology, 24*(1), 82–88. https://doi.org/10.1038/jes.2013.47

60. Babu, S., Uppu, S., Claville, M. O., & Uppu, R. M. (2013). Prooxidant actions of bisphenol A (BPA) phenoxyl radicals: Implications to BPA-related oxidative stress and toxicity. *Toxicology Mechanisms and Methods, 23*(4), 273–280. doi:10.3109/15376516.2012.753969

61. Sui, Y., Park, S., Helsley, R. N., Sunkara, M., Gonzalez, F. J., Morris, A. J., & Zhou, C. (2014). Bisphenol A increases atherosclerosis in pregnane X receptor-humanized ApoE

deficient mice. *Journal of the American Heart Association, 3*(2). doi:10.1161/jaha .113.000492

62. Peters, A., Liu, E., Verrier, R. L., Schwartz, J., Gold, D. R., Mittleman, M., . . . Dockery, D. W. (2000). Air pollution and incidence of cardiac arrhythmia. *Epidemiology, 11*(1), 11–17. https://doi.org/10.1097/00001648-200001000-00005; Baccarelli, A., Martinelli, I., Zanobetti, A., Grillo, P., Hou, L., Bertazzi, P. A., . . . Schwartz, J. (2008). Exposure to particulate air pollution and risk of deep vein thrombosis. *Archives of Internal Medicine, 168*(9), 920. https://doi.org/10.1001/archinte.168.9.920

63. Saadeh, A. M., Farsakh, N. A., & Al-Ali, M. K. (1997). Cardiac manifestations of acute carbamate and organophosphate poisoning. *Heart, 77*(5), 461–464. https://doi.org/10.1136/ hrt.77.5.46; Lind, P. M., Van Bavel, B., Salihovic, S., & Lind, L. (2012). Circulating levels of persistent organic pollutants (POPs) and carotid atherosclerosis in the elderly. *Environmental Health Perspectives, 120*(1), 38–43. https://doi.org/10.1289/ehp.1103563

64. Shankar, A., Xiao, J., & Ducatman, A. (2012). Perfluorooctanoic acid and cardiovascular disease in US adults. *Archives of Internal Medicine, 172*(18), 1397. https://doi.org /10.1001/archinternmed.2012.3393

65. Hill, M. A., Yang, Y., Zhang, L., Sun, Z., Jia, G., Parrish, A. R., & Sowers, J. R. (2021). Insulin resistance, cardiovascular stiffening and cardiovascular disease. *Metabolism, 119*, 154766. https://doi.org/10.1016/j.metabol.2021.154766

66. Davies, H. (1990). Atherogenesis and the coronary arteries of childhood. *International Journal of Cardiology, 28*(3), 283–291. https://doi.org/10.1016/0167-5273(90)90310-2

67. Willeit, P., Yeang, C., Moriarty, P. M., Tschiderer, L., Varvel, S. A., McConnell, J. P., & Tsimikas, S. (2020). Low-density lipoprotein cholesterol corrected for Lipoprotein(a) cholesterol, risk thresholds, and cardiovascular events. *Journal of the American Heart Association, 9*(23). https://doi.org/10.1161/jaha.119.016318

68. Lu, H., Cassis, L., & Daugherty, A. (2007). Atherosclerosis and arterial blood pressure in mice. *Current Drug Targets, 8*(11), 1181–1189. doi:10.2174/138945007782403829

69. Nakashima, Y., Fujii, H., Sumiyoshi, S., Wight, T. N., & Sueishi, K. (2007). Early human atherosclerosis. *Arteriosclerosis, Thrombosis, and Vascular Biology, 27*(5), 1159–1165. https://doi.org/10.1161/atvbaha.106.134080

70. Doyle, B., & Caplice, N. (2007). Plaque neovascularization and antiangiogenic therapy for atherosclerosis. *Journal of the American College of Cardiology, 49*(21), 2073–2080. https:// doi.org/10.1016/j.jacc.2007.01.089

71. Subbotin, V. M. (2016). Excessive intimal hyperplasia in human coronary arteries before intimal lipid depositions is the initiation of coronary atherosclerosis and constitutes a therapeutic target. *Drug Discovery Today, 21*(10), 1578–1595. https://doi.org/10.1016 /j.drudis.2016.05.017

72. Levine, D. M., Parker, T. S., Donnelly, T. M., Walsh, A., & Rubin, A. L. (1993). In vivo protection against endotoxin by plasma high density lipoprotein. *Proceedings of the National Academy of Sciences, 90*(24), 12040–12044. doi:10.1073/pnas.90.24.12040; Netea, M. G., Demacker, P. N., Kullberg, B. J., Boerman, O. C., Verschueren, I., Stalenhoef, A. F., & Van der Meer, J. W. (1996). Low-density lipoprotein receptor-deficient mice are protected against lethal endotoxemia and severe gram-negative infections. *Journal of Clinical Investigation, 97*(6), 1366–1372. doi:10.1172/jci118556

73. Smith, L. L. (1990). Yet another cholesterol hypothesis—cholesterol as antioxidant. *Free Radical Biology and Medicine, 9,* 71. doi:10.1016/0891-5849(90)90419-j

74. Grimes, D., Hindle, E., & Dyer, T. (1996). Sunlight, cholesterol and coronary heart disease. *QJM, 89*(8), 579–590. https://doi.org/10.1093/qjmed/89.8.579; MacPherson, A. (2000). Relationship of hair calcium concentration to incidence of coronary heart disease. *The Science of the Total Environment, 255*(1–3), 11–19. https://doi.org/10.1016 /s0048-9697(00)00433-2

75. Wood, A. D., Secombes, K. R., Thies, F., Aucott, L., Black, A. J., Mavroeidi, A., . . . Macdonald, H. M. (2012). Vitamin D3 supplementation has no effect on conventional cardiovascular risk factors: A parallel-group, double-blind, placebo-controlled RCT. *The Journal of Clinical Endocrinology & Metabolism, 97*(10), 3557–3568. https://doi.org /10.1210/jc.2012-2126

76. Seneff, S., Lauritzen, A., Davidson, R., & Lentz-Marino, L. (2012). Is endothelial nitric oxide synthase a moonlighting protein whose day job is cholesterol sulfate synthesis? Implications for cholesterol transport, diabetes and cardiovascular disease. *Entropy, 14*(12), 2492–2530. https://doi.org/10.3390/e14122492

77. Tian, Q., Sun, D., Zhao, M., & Zhang, W. (2007). Inhibition of nitric oxide synthase (NOS) underlies aluminum-induced inhibition of root elongation in *Hibiscus moscheutos. New Phytologist, 174*(2), 322–331. https://doi.org/10.1111/j.1469-8137.2007.02005.x; Alexidis, A. N., Rekka, E. A., & Kourounakis, P. N. (1994). Influence of mercury and cadmium intoxication on hepatic microsomal CYP2E and CYP3A subfamilies. *Research Communications in Molecular Pathology and Pharmacology, 85*(1), 67–72. https://pubmed .ncbi.nlm.nih.gov/7953196/; Samsel, A., & Seneff, S. (2013). Glyphosate's suppression of cytochrome P450 enzymes and amino acid biosynthesis by the gut microbiome: Pathways to modern diseases. *Entropy, 15*(12), 1416–1463. https://doi.org/10.3390 /e15041416; Samsel, A., & Seneff, S. (2013). Glyphosate, pathways to modern diseases II: Celiac sprue and gluten intolerance. *Interdisciplinary Toxicology, 6*(4), 159–184. https:// doi.org/10.2478/intox-2013-0026

78. Seneff, S. (2018, January 30). Cholesterol sulfate deficiency and coronary heart disease. The Weston A. Price Foundation. https://www.westonaprice.org/health-topics /modern-diseases/cholesterol-sulfate-deficiency-coronary-heart-disease/

79. Rasmussen-Lathrop, S. J., Koshiyama, K., Phillips, N., & Stephens, R. S. (2000). Chlamydia-dependent biosynthesis of a heparan sulphate-like compound in eukaryotic cells. *Cellular Microbiology, 2*(2), 137–144. https://doi.org/10.1046/j.1462-5822.2000.00039.x; Schaffer, S. W., Jong, C. J., Ito, T., & Azuma, J. (2012). Effect of taurine on ischemia–reperfusion injury. *Amino Acids, 46*(1), 21–30. https://doi.org/10.1007/s00726-012-1378-8

80. Collins, K. (1997). Charge density-dependent strength of hydration and biological structure. *Biophysical Journal, 72*(1), 65–76. https://doi.org/10.1016/s0006-3495(97)78647-8

Chapter 8. The Three Imbalances of a Heart Attack

1. DeVore, A. D., Yow, E., Krucoff, M. W., Sherwood, M. W., Shaw, L. K., Chiswell, K., . . . Velazquez, E. J. (2019). Percutaneous coronary intervention outcomes in patients with stable coronary disease and left ventricular systolic dysfunction. *ESC Heart Failure, 6*(6), 1233–1242. doi:10.1002/ehf2.12510

2. Boden, W., O'Rourke, R., & Teo, K. (2007). Optimal medical therapy with or without PCI for stable coronary disease. *Journal of Vascular Surgery, 45*(6), 1286. https://doi.org/10.1016/j.jvs.2007.04.027

3. Malhotra, A. (2014). The whole truth about coronary stents. *JAMA Internal Medicine, 174*(8), 1367. doi:10.1001/jamainternmed.2013.9190

4. McIntosh, H. D., & Garcia, J. A. (1978). The first decade of aortocoronary bypass grafting, 1967–1977. A review. *Circulation, 57*(3), 405–431. https://doi.org/10.1161/01.cir.57.3.405

5. Cass Principle Investigators and Their Associates. (1984). Myocardial infarction and mortality in the coronary artery surgery study (CASS) randomized trial. *New England Journal of Medicine, 310*(12), 750–758. https://doi.org/10.1056/nejm198403223101204; Alderman, E. L., Bourassa, M. G., Cohen, L. S., Davis, K. B., Kaiser, G. G., Killip, T., . . . Robertson, T. L. (1990). Ten-year follow-up of survival and myocardial infarction in the randomized coronary artery surgery study. *Circulation, 82*(5), 1629–1646. https://doi.org/10.1161/01.cir.82.5.1629.

6. Rihal, C. S., Raco, D. L., Gersh, B. J., & Yusuf, S. (2003). Indications for coronary artery bypass surgery and percutaneous coronary intervention in chronic stable angina. *Circulation, 108*(20), 2439–2445. https://doi.org/10.1161/01.cir.0000094405.21583.7c

7. Velazquez, E. J., Lee, K. L., Deja, M. A., Jain, A., Sopko, G., Marchenko, A., . . . STICH Investigators. (2011). Coronary-artery bypass surgery in patients with left ventricular dysfunction. *New England Journal of Medicine, 364*, 1607–1616. doi:10.1056/NEJMoa1100356

8. Heron, M., & Anderson, R. N. (2016, August 24). Changes in the leading cause of death: Recent patterns in heart disease and cancer mortality. National Center for Health Statistics. Retrieved from https://www.cdc.gov/nchs/products/databriefs/db254.htm

9. Baroldi, G., Falzi, G., & Mariani, F. (1979). Sudden coronary death. A postmortem study in 208 selected cases compared to 97 "control" subjects. *American Heart Journal, 98*(1), 20–31. doi:10.1016/0002-8703(79)90316-8

10. Baroldi, G., & Silver, M. D. (2004). *The etiopathogenesis of coronary heart disease: A heretical theory based on morphology*, Second Edition. CRC Press.

11. Khouri, E. M., Gregg, D. E., & Lowensohn, H. S. (1968). Flow in the major branches of the left coronary artery during experimental coronary insufficiency in the unanesthetized dog. *Circulation Research, 23*(1), 99–109. doi:10.1161/01.res.23.1.99

12. Schaper, W., & Pasyk, S. (1976). Influence of collateral flow on the ischemic tolerance of the heart following acute and subacute coronary occlusion. *Circulation, 53*(3), 157–162. https://pubmed.ncbi.nlm.nih.gov/1253370/

13. Radhakrishnan, J. (2017, October 1). Renal infarction. Retrieved from https://www.uptodate.com/contents/renal-infarction

14. Bassenge, E., Wendt, V. E., Schollmeyer, P., Blümchen, G., Gudbjarnason, S., & Bing, R. J. (1965). Effect of ketone bodies on cardiac metabolism. *American Journal of Physiology-Legacy Content, 208*(1), 162–168. doi:10.1152/ajplegacy.1965.208.1.162

15. Chen, V., Wagner, G., & Spitzer, J. (1984). Regulation of substrate oxidation in isolated myocardial cells by β-hydroxybutyrate. *Hormone and Metabolic Research, 16*(05), 243–247. doi:10.1055/s-2007-1014756

16. Woodall, B. P., Gresham, K. S., Woodall, M. A., Valenti, M., Cannavo, A., Pfleger, J., . . . Koch, W. J. (2019). Alteration of myocardial GRK2 produces a global metabolic phenotype. *JCI Insight, 4*(10). doi:10.1172/jci.insight.123848

17. Goss, S. P., Kalyanaraman, B., & Hogg, N. (1999). [46] Antioxidant effects of nitric oxide and nitric oxide donor compounds on low-density lipoprotein oxidation. *Methods in Enzymology*, 444–453. doi:10.1016/s0076-6879(99)01108-8; Title, L. M., Cummings, P. M., Giddens, K., & Nassar, B. A. (2000). Oral glucose loading acutely attenuates endothelium-dependent vasodilation in healthy adults without diabetes: An effect prevented by vitamins C and E. *Journal of the American College of Cardiology, 36*(7), 2185–2191. doi:10.1016/s0735-1097(00)00980-3

18. Sapolsky, R. M. (2017). *Behave: The biology of humans at our best and worst*. London, England: Penguin: p. 126.

19. George, W. J., Ignarro, L. J., Paddock, R. J., White, L., & Kadowitz, P. J. (1974). Oppositional effects of acetylcholine and isoproterenol on isometric tension and cyclic nucleotide concentrations in rabbit atria. *Journal of Cyclic Nucleotide Research, 1*(5), 339–347. https://europepmc.org/article/med/178695

20. Blomquist, T. M., Priola, D. V., & Romero, A. M. (1987). Source of intrinsic innervation of canine ventricles: A functional study. *American Journal of Physiology-Heart and Circulatory Physiology, 252*(3), H638–H644. doi:10.1152/ajpheart.1987.252.3.h638

21. Fujii, S., Sawa, T., Ihara, H., Tong, K. I., Ida, T., Okamoto, T., . . . Akaike, T. (2010). The critical role of nitric oxide signaling, via protein S-guanylation and nitrated cyclic GMP, in the antioxidant adaptive response. *Journal of Biological Chemistry, 285*(31), 23970–23984. doi:10.1074/jbc.m110.145441

22. Porges, S. W. (2009). The polyvagal theory: New insights into adaptive reactions of the autonomic nervous system. *Cleveland Clinic Journal of Medicine, 76*(Suppl_2), S86–S90. doi:10.3949/ccjm.76.s2.17

23. Sroka, K., Peimann, C., & Seevers, H. (1997). Heart rate variability in myocardial ischemia during daily life. *Journal of Electrocardiology, 30*(1), 45–56. doi:10.1016/s0022-0736(97)80034-9

24. Kochiadakis, G. E., Marketou, M. E., Igoumedidis, N. E., Simantirakis, E. N., Parthenakis, F. I., Manios, E. G., & Vardas, P. E. (2000). Autonomic nervous system activity before and during episodes of myocardial ischemia in patients with stable coronary artery disease during daily life. *Pacing and Clinical Electrophysiology, 23*(12), 2030–2039. https://doi.org/10.1111/j.1540-8159.2000.tb00772.x

25. Oppenheimer, S. (2006). Cerebrogenic cardiac arrhythmias: Cortical lateralization and clinical significance. *Clinical Autonomic Research, 16*(1), 6–11. https://doi.org/10.1007/s10286-006-0276-0

26. Kline, E. R., Kleinhenz, D. J., Liang, B., Dikalov, S., Guidot, D. M., Hart, C. M., . . . Sutliff, R. L. (2008). Vascular oxidative stress and nitric oxide depletion in HIV-1 transgenic rats are reversed by glutathione restoration. *American Journal of Physiology-Heart and Circulatory Physiology, 294*(6), H2792–H2804. doi:10.1152/ajpheart.91447.2007

27. Kanner, J., Harel, S., & Granit, R. (1991). Nitric oxide as an antioxidant. *Archives of Biochemistry and Biophysics, 289*(1), 130–136. https://www.sciencedirect.com/science/article/abs/pii/000398619190452O

28. Sroka, K., Peimann, C., & Seevers, H. (1997). Heart rate variability in myocardial ischemia during daily life. *Journal of Electrocardiology, 30*(1), 45–56. doi:10.1016/s0022 -0736(97)80034-9

29. Williamson, J. R., & Jamieson, D. (1966). Metabolic effects of epinephrine in the perfused rat heart I. Comparison of intracellular redox states, tissue pO_2, and force of contraction. *Molecular Pharmacology, 2*(3), 191–205. http://molpharm.aspetjournals.org /content/2/3/191.short

30. Depre, C., Ponchaut, S., Deprez, J., Maisin, L., & Hue, L. (1998). Cyclic AMP suppresses the inhibition of glycolysis by alternative oxidizable substrates in the heart. *Journal of Clinical Investigation, 101*(2), 390–397. doi:10.1172/jci1168

31. Scheuer, J., & Brachfeld, N. (1966). Coronary insufficiency: Relations between hemo-dynamic, electrical, and biochemical parameters. *Circulation Research, 18*(2), 178–189. https://doi.org/10.1161/01.res.18.2.178

32. Phypers, B., & Pierce, J. T. (2006). Lactate physiology in health and disease. *Continuing Education in Anaesthesia Critical Care & Pain, 6*(3), 128–132. https://doi.org/10.1093 /bjaceaccp/mkl018

33. Wang, Z., Ying, Z., Bosy-Westphal, A., Zhang, J., Schautz, B., Later, W., . . . Müller, M. J. (2010). Specific metabolic rates of major organs and tissues across adulthood: Evalua-tion by mechanistic model of resting energy expenditure. *The American Journal of Clinical Nutrition, 92*(6), 1369–1377. https://doi.org/10.3945/ajcn.2010.29885

34. Katz, A. M. (1973). Effects of ischemia on the contractile processes of heart muscle. *The American Journal of Cardiology, 32*(4), 456–460. doi:10.1016/s0002-9149(73)80036-0

35. George, S. A., & Poelzing, S. (2016). Cardiac conduction in isolated hearts of genetically modified mice—Connexin43 and salts. *Progress in Biophysics and Molecular Biology, 120*(1–3), 189–198. doi:10.1016/j.pbiomolbio.2015.11.004

36. Harrison, S. M., Frampton, J. E., McCall, E., Boyett, M. R., & Orchard, C. H. (1992). Contraction and intracellular Ca2+, Na+, and H+ during acidosis in rat ventricular myocytes. *American Journal of Physiology-Cell Physiology, 262*(2), C348–C357. doi:10.1152 /ajpcell.1992.262.2.c348; Spitzer, K. W., & Bridge, J. H. (1992). Relationship between intracellular pH and tension development in resting ventricular muscle and myocytes. *American Journal of Physiology-Cell Physiology, 262*(2), C316–C327. doi:10.1152/ajp-cell.1992.262.2.c316; Baroldi, G. (1974). Different morphological types of myocardial cell death in man. *Recent Advances in Studies on Cardiac Structure and Metabolism, 6*, 383–397. https://europepmc.org/article/med/1105714

37. Mohammad, M. A., Karlsson, S., Haddad, J., Cederberg, B., Jernberg, T., Lindahl, B., . . . Erlinge, D. (2018). Christmas, national holidays, sport events, and time factors as triggers of acute myocardial infarction: SWEDEHEART observational study 1998–2013. *BMJ*, k4811. doi:10.1136/bmj.k4811; Wallert, J., Held, C., Madison, G., & Olsson, E. M. (2017). Temporal changes in myocardial infarction incidence rates are associated with periods of perceived psychosocial stress: A SWEDEHEART national registry study. *American Heart Journal, 191*, 12–20. doi:10.1016/j.ahj.2017.05.015

38. Allison, T. G., Williams, D. E., Miller, T. D., Patten, C. A., Bailey, K. R., Squires, R. W., & Gau, G. T. (1995). Medical and economic costs of psychologic distress in patients with coronary artery disease. *Mayo Clinic Proceedings, 70*(8), 734–742. doi:10.4065/70.8.734

39. American College of Cardiology. More hospitalizations, deaths for U. S. heart failure patients in winter. *ScienceDaily*. ScienceDaily, March 8, 2017. www.sciencedaily.com /releases/2017/03/170308150027.htm; Kristal-Boneh, E., Froom, P., Harari, G., Malik, M., & Ribak, J. (2000). Summer-winter differences in 24 h variability of heart rate. *European Journal of Cardiovascular Risk, 7*(2), 141–146. doi:10.1177 /204748730000700209

40. Hyyti, O. M., Ledee, D., Ning, X., Ge, M., & Portman, M. A. (2010). Aging impairs myocardial fatty acid and ketone oxidation and modifies cardiac functional and meta-bolic responses to insulin in mice. *American Journal of Physiology-Heart and Circulatory Physiology, 299*(3), H868–H875. doi:10.1152/ajpheart.00931.2009; Devries, S. (2011). *Integrative cardiology*. OUP USA.

41. Bonnemeier, H., Wiegand, U. K., Brandes, A., Kluge, N., Katus, H. A., Richardt, G., & Potratz, J. (2003). Circadian profile of cardiac autonomic nervous modulation in healthy subjects. *Journal of Cardiovascular Electrophysiology, 14*(8), 791–799. doi:10.1046/j.1540-8167.2003.03078.x

42. Number of heart disease deaths per 100,000 population by sex. (2019, February 11). https://www.kff.org/other/state-indicator/heart-disease-death-rate-by-gender /?currentTimeframe=0&sortModel=%7B%22colId%22:%22Location%22,% 22sort%22:%22asc%22%7D; Yamasaki, Y., Kodama, M., Matsuhisa, M., Kishimoto, M., Ozaki, H., Tani, A., . . . Kamada, T. (1996). Diurnal heart rate variability in healthy subjects: Effects of aging and sex difference. *American Journal of Physiology-Heart and Circulatory Physiology, 271*(1), H303–H310. doi:10.1152/ajpheart.1996.271.1.h303; Heger, S. (2010). Hypothalamus und hypophyse. In O. Hiort, R. Danne, & M. Wabitsch (Eds.)., *Pädiatrische endokrinologie und diabetologie*. Berlin, Heidelberg: Springer.

43. Harvard Health Publishing. (2019, September 24). The heart attack gender gap. Author. https://www.health.harvard.edu/heart-health/the-heart-attack-gender-gap

44. Niemelä, M. J., Airaksinen, K., & Huikuri, H. V. (1994). Effect of beta-blockade on heart rate variability in patients with coronary artery disease. *Journal of the American College of Cardiology, 23*(6), 1370–1377. doi:10.1016/0735-1097(94)90379-4

45. Zhang, Y., Song, Y., Zhu, J., Hu, T., & Wan, L. (1995). Effects of enalapril on heart rate variability in patients with congestive heart failure. *The American Journal of Cardiology, 76*(14), 1045–1048. doi:10.1016/s0002-9149(99)80294-x

46. Tassorelli, C., Blandini, F., Greco, R., & Nappi, G. (2004). Nitroglycerin enhances cGMP expression in specific neuronal and cerebrovascular structures of the rat brain. *Journal of Chemical Neuroanatomy, 27*(1), 23–32. doi:10.1016/j.jchemneu.2003.08.006

47. ECG waves. (2016, September 2). The left ventricle in myocardial ischemia and infarc-tion—ECG & ECHO. Author. https://ecgwaves.com/topic/left-ventricle-ischemia -acute-myocardial-infarction-coronary-artery/

48. Neill, W. A. (1968). Myocardial hypoxia and anaerobic metabolism in coronary heart disease. *The American Journal of Cardiology, 22*(4), 507–515. doi:10.1016/0002-9149 (68)90155-0; Parker, J. O., Chiong, M. A., West, R. O., & Case, R. B. (1997). Sequential alterations in myocardial lactate metabolism, S-T segments, and left ventricular function during angina induced by atrial pacing. *Annals of Noninvasive Electrocardiology, 2*(4), 396–414. doi:10.1111/j.1542-474x.1997.tb00206.x

49. Von Känel, R., & Dimsdale, J. E. (2000). Effects of sympathetic activation by adrenergic infusions on hemostasis in vivo. *European Journal of Haematology*, 65(6), 357–369. https://doi.org/10.1034/j.1600-0609.2000.065006357.x

50. Stone, P. H. (1990). Triggers of transient myocardial ischemia: Circadian variation and relation to plaque rupture and coronary thrombosis in stable coronary artery disease. *The American Journal of Cardiology*, 66(16), G32–G36. https://doi.org/10.1016/0002-9149(90)90392-e

51. Stämpfli, S. F., Camici, G. G., Keller, S., Rozenberg, I., Arras, M., Schuler, B., . . . Tanner, F. C. (2013). Restraint stress enhances arterial thrombosis in vivo—role of the sympathetic nervous system. *Stress*, 17(1), 126–132. https://doi.org/10.3109/10253890.2013.862616

52. Miyasaka, Y., Barnes, M. E., Gersh, B. J., Cha, S. S., Bailey, K. R., Abhayaratna, W. P., . . . Tsang, T. S. (2006). Secular trends in incidence of atrial fibrillation in Olmsted County, Minnesota, 1980 to 2000, and implications on the projections for future prevalence. *Circulation*, 114(2), 119–125. https://doi.org/10.1161/circulationaha.105.595140

53. Centers for Disease Control and Prevention, National Center for Health Statistics. (2018). Underlying Cause of Death, 1999–2018. Accessed March 12, 2020. https://wonder.cdc.gov/Deaths-by-Underlying-Cause.html

54. Stavrakis, S., Humphrey, M. B., Scherlag, B. J., Hu, Y., Jackman, W. M., Nakagawa, H., . . . Po, S. S. (2015). Low-level transcutaneous electrical vagus nerve stimulation suppresses atrial fibrillation. *Journal of the American College of Cardiology*, 65(9), 867–875. https://doi.org/10.1016/j.jacc.2014.12.026

55. Stavrakis, S., Stoner, J. A., Humphrey, M. B., Morris, L., Filiberti, A., Reynolds, J. C., . . . Po, S. S. (2020). TREAT AF (Transcutaneous electrical vagus nerve stimulation to suppress atrial fibrillation). *JACC: Clinical Electrophysiology*, 6(3), 282–291. https://doi.org/10.1016/j.jacep.2019.11.008

56. Sun, J., Scherlag, B. J., & Po, S. S. (2014). Role of the autonomic nervous system in atrial fibrillation. *Cardiac Electrophysiology: From Cell to Bedside*, 469–474. https://doi.org/10.1016/b978-1-4557-2856-5.00047-9; Zhang, Y., Ilsar, I., Sabbah, H. N., Ben David, T., & Mazgalev, T. N. (2009). Relationship between right cervical vagus nerve stimulation and atrial fibrillation inducibility: Therapeutic intensities do not increase arrhythmogenesis. *Heart Rhythm*, 6(2), 244–250. https://doi.org/10.1016/j.hrthm.2008.10.043

57. Brown, S. M., Larsen, N. K., Thankam, F. G., & Agrawal, D. K. (2020). Fetal cardiomyocyte phenotype, ketone body metabolism, and mitochondrial dysfunction in the pathology of atrial fibrillation. *Molecular and Cellular Biochemistry*, 476(2), 1165–1178. https://doi.org/10.1007/s11010-020-03980-8

58. Khan, A. M., Lubitz, S. A., Sullivan, L. M., Sun, J. X., Levy, D., Vasan, R. S., . . . Wang, T. J. (2013). Low serum magnesium and the development of atrial fibrillation in the community. *Circulation*, 127(1), 33–38. https://doi.org/10.1161/circulationaha.111.082511

Chapter 9. How the Heart Evades Cancer

1. Moynihan, T. J. (2019, January 9). Heart cancer: Is there such a thing? Retrieved from https://www.mayoclinic.org/heart-cancer/expert-answers/faq-20058130

2. National Cancer Institute. (n.d.). Matters of the heart: Why are cardiac tumors so rare? Author. Retrieved from https://www.cancer.gov/types/metastatic-cancer/research/cardiac-tumors

3. Leja, M. J., Shah, D. J., & Reardon, M. J. (2011). Primary cardiac tumors. *Texas Heart Institute Journal, 38*(3), 261–262. Retrieved from https://www.ncbi.nlm.nih.gov/pmc/articles/PMC3113129/

4. Koura, M., Isaka, H., Yoshida, M. C., Tosu, M., & Sekiguchi, T. (1982). Suppression of tumorigenicity in interspecific reconstituted cells and cybrids. *Gann, 73,* 574–580. https://pubmed.ncbi.nlm.nih.gov/7152196/

5. Pedersen, P. L. (1978). Tumor mitochondria and the bioenergetics of cancer cells. *Progress in Experimental Tumor Research, 22,* 190–274. https://pubmed.ncbi.nlm.nih.gov/149996/

6. Benard, G., & Rossignol, R. (2008). Ultrastructure of the mitochondrion and its bearing on function and bioenergetics. *Antioxidants & Redox Signaling, 10*(8), 1313–1342. doi:10.1089/ars.2007.2000

7. Bhagavan, N. V. (2002). *Medical biochemistry.* Academic Press.

8. Seyfried, T. N., & Shelton, L. M. (2010). Cancer as a metabolic disease. *Nutrition and Metabolism, 27*(7), 7. doi:10.1186/1743-7075-7-7

9. Warburg, O. (1956). On the origin of cancer cells. *Science, 123*(3191), 309–314. doi:10.1126/science.123.3191.309

10. Walton, C. M., Jacobsen, S. M., Dallon, B. W., Saito, E. R., Bennett, S. L., Davidson, L. E., . . . Bikman, B. T. (2020). Ketones elicit distinct alterations in adipose mitochondrial bioenergetics. *International Journal of Molecular Sciences, 21*(17), 6255. https://doi.org/10.3390/ijms21176255

11. Gershon, N. D., Porter, K. R., & Trus, B. L. (1985). The cytoplasmic matrix: Its volume and surface area and the diffusion of molecules through it. *Proceedings of the National Academy of Sciences, 82*(15), 5030–5034. doi:10.1073/pnas.82.15.5030

12. Clegg, J. S. (2018). On the internal environment of animal cells. *Microcompartmentation,* 1–16. doi:10.1201/9781351074575-1

13. Taylor, S. R., Shlevin, H. H., & Lopez, J. R. (1979). Calcium in excitation–contraction coupling of skeletal muscle. *Biochemical Society Transactions, 7*(4), 759–764. doi:10.1042/bst0070759

14. Ling, G. N. (1962). *A physical theory of the living state: The association-induction hypothesis; with considerations of the mechanics involved in ionic specificity.* Blaisdell Publishing Company.

15. Ling, G. N. (1978). Maintenance of low sodium and high potassium levels in resting muscle cells. *The Journal of Physiology, 280*(1), 105–123. doi:10.1113/jphysiol.1978.sp012375

16. López-Beltrán, E. A., Maté, M. J., & Cerdán, S. (1996). Dynamics and environment of mitochondrial water as detected by H NMR. *Journal of Biological Chemistry, 271*(18), 10648–10653. doi:10.1074/jbc.271.18.10648

17. McCarthy, E. F. (2006). The toxins of William B. Coley and the treatment of bone and soft-tissue sarcomas. *Iowa Orthopaedic Journal, 26,* 154–158. Retrieved from https://www.ncbi.nlm.nih.gov/pmc/articles/PMC1888599/

18. Manchester, K. (1997). The quest by three giants of science for an understanding of cancer. *Endeavour, 21*(2), 72–76. doi:10.1016/s0160-9327(97)01030-2

19. Loeb, L. A. (2010). Mutator phenotype in cancer: Origin and consequences. *Seminars in Cancer Biology, 20*(5), 279–280. doi:10.1016/j.semcancer.2010.10.006; Gabor Miklos, G. L. (2005). The human cancer genome project—one more misstep in the war on cancer. *Nature Biotechnology, 23*(5), 535–537. doi:10.1038/nbt0505-535

20. Song, L. Z., Schwartz, G. E., & Russek, L. G. (1998). Heart-focused attention and heart-brain synchronization: energetic and physiological mechanisms. *Alternative Therapies in Health and Medicine, 4*(5), 44–52. Retrieved from http://europepmc.org/article /MED/9737031

21. Childre, D., & Martin, H. (2011). *The HeartMath solution: The Institute of HeartMath's revolutionary program for engaging the power of the heart's intelligence.* HarperCollins.

Chapter 10. The Ceaseless Signals of High Blood Pressure

1. Leung, T., Chen, C., Tsai, S., & Hsiao, G. (2012). Effects of far infrared rays irradiated from ceramic material (BIOCERAMIC) on psychological stress-conditioned elevated heart rate, blood pressure, and oxidative stress-suppressed cardiac contractility. *The Chinese Journal of Physiology.* https://doi.org/10.4077/cjp.2012.baa037

2. Beever, R. (2010). Do far-infrared saunas have cardiovascular benefits in people with type 2 diabetes? *Canadian Journal of Diabetes, 34*(2), 113–118. https://doi.org/10.1016 /s1499-2671(10)42007-9

3. Weller, R. B., Wang, Y., He, J., Maddux, F. W., Usvyat, L., Zhang, H., . . . Kotanko, P. (2020). Does incident solar ultraviolet radiation lower blood pressure? *Journal of the American Heart Association, 9*(5). https://doi.org/10.1161/jaha.119.013837

4. Rostand, S. G., Mcclure, L. A., Kent, S. T., Judd, S. E., & Gutierrez, O. M. (2016). Associations of blood pressure, sunlight, and vitamin D in community-dwelling adults: The reasons for geographic and racial differences in stroke (Regards) study. *Journal of Hypertension, 34*(9), 1704–1710. https://doi.org/10.1097/HJH.0000000000001018

5. Dimitriev, D. A., & Saperova, E. V. (2014). Heart rate variability and blood pressure during mental stress. *Rossiiskii Fiziologicheskii Zhurnal Imeni I.M. Sechenova, 101*(1), 98–107. https://europepmc.org/article/med/25868330; Floras, J. S., Hassan, M. O., Jones, J. V., Osikowska, B. A., Sever, P. S., & Sleight, P. (1988). Factors influencing blood pressure and heart rate variability in hypertensive humans. *Hypertension, 11*(3), 273–281. https://doi .org/10.1161/01.hyp.11.3.273

6. Pal, G. K., Ganesh, V., Karthik, S., Nanda, N., & Pal, P. (2014). The effects of short-term relaxation therapy on indices of heart rate variability and blood pressure in young adults. *American Journal of Health Promotion, 29*(1), 23–28. https://doi.org/10.4278/ajhp .130131-quan-52

7. Fuller, J. H. (1985). Epidemiology of hypertension associated with diabetes mellitus. *Hypertension, 7*(6_pt_2). https://doi.org/10.1161/01.hyp.7.6_pt_2.ii3; Saitoh, S. (2009). Insulin resistance and renin-angiotensin-aldosterone system. *Nihon rinsho, Japanese Journal of Clinical Medicine, 67*(4), 729–734. https://europepmc.org/article /med/19348235

8. Tarray, R., Saleem, S., Afroze, D., Yousuf, I., Gulnar, A., Laway, B., & Verma, S. (2014). Role of insulin resistance in essential hypertension. *Cardiovascular Endocrinology, 3*(4), 129–133. https://doi.org/10.1097/xce.0000000000000032

9. Persson, S. U. (2007). Blood pressure reactions to insulin treatment in patients with type 2 diabetes. *The International Journal of Angiology: Official Publication of the International College of Angiology, Inc, 16*(04), 135–138. https://doi.org/10.1055/s-0031-1278267

10. Fonseca, V., Bakris, G. L., Bell, D. S., McGill, J. B., Raskin, P., Messerli, F. H., Phillips, R. A., . . . Anderson, K. M. (2007). Differential effect of beta-blocker therapy on insulin resistance as a function of insulin sensitizer use: Results from GEMINI. *Diabetic Medicine, 24*(7), 759–763. https://doi.org/10.1111/j.1464-5491.2007.02151.x; Ayers, K., Byrne, L. M., DeMatteo, A., & Brown, N. J. (2012). Differential effects of nebivolol and metoprolol on insulin sensitivity and plasminogen activator inhibitor in the metabolic syndrome. *Hypertension, 59*(4), 893–898. https://doi.org/10.1161/hypertensionaha.111.189589

11. Hill, M. A., Yang, Y., Zhang, L., Sun, Z., Jia, G., Parrish, A. R., & Sowers, J. R. (2021). Insulin resistance, cardiovascular stiffening and cardiovascular disease. *Metabolism, 119*, 154766. https://doi.org/10.1016/j.metabol.2021.154766

12. Kveiborg, B., Hermann, T. S., Major-Pedersen, A., Christiansen, B., Rask-Madsen, C., Raunsø, J., . . . Dominguez, H. (2010). Metoprolol compared to carvedilol deteriorates insulin-stimulated endothelial function in patients with type 2 diabetes—a randomized study. *Cardiovascular Diabetology, 9*(1), 21. https://doi.org/10.1186/1475-2840-9-21

13. Jacob, S., Rett, K., Wicklmayr, M., Agrawal, B., Augustin, H. J., & Dietze, G. (1996). Differential effect of chronic treatment with two beta-blocking agents on insulin sensitivity. *Journal of Hypertension, 14*(4), 489–494. https://doi.org/10.1097/00004872-199604000-00012

14. Luft, F. C., Rankin, L. I., Henry, D. P., Bloch, R., Grim, C. E., Weyman, A. E., . . . Weinberger, M. H. (1979). Plasma and urinary norepinephrine values at extremes of sodium intake in normal man. *Hypertension, 1*(3), 261–266. https://doi.org/10.1161/01.hyp.1.3.261; Feldman, R. (1999). Moderate dietary salt restriction increases vascular and systemic insulin resistance. *American Journal of Hypertension, 12*(6), 643–647. https://doi.org/10.1016/s0895-7061(99)00016-3

15. Haddy, F. J., & Pamnani, M. B. (1985). The kidney in the pathogenesis of hypertension: The role of sodium. *American Journal of Kidney Diseases, 5*(4), A5–A13. https://doi.org/10.1016/s0272-6386(85)80059-7

16. Graudal, N., & Jürgens, G. (2018). Conflicting evidence on health effects associated with salt reduction calls for a redesign of the salt dietary guidelines. *Progress in Cardiovascular Diseases, 61*(1), 20–26. https://doi.org/10.1016/j.pcad.2018.04.008

17. Gandhi, S., Mosleh, W., & Myers, R. B. (2014). Hypertonic saline with furosemide for the treatment of acute congestive heart failure: A systematic review and meta-analysis. *International Journal of Cardiology, 173*(2), 139–145. https://doi.org/10.1016/j.ijcard.2014.03.020

18. Ghosh, M., & Majumdar, S. R. (2014). Antihypertensive medications, bone mineral density, and fractures: A review of old cardiac drugs that provides new insights into osteoporosis. *Endocrine, 46*(3), 397–405. https://doi.org/10.1007/s12020-014-0167-4; Suliburska, J., Bogdanski, P., Szulinska, M., & Pupek-Musialik, D. (2014). The influence of antihypertensive drugs on mineral status in hypertensive patients. *European Review for Medical and Pharmacological Sciences, 18*, 58–65. https://www.europeanreview.org/wp/wp-content/uploads/58-65.pdf

Chapter 11. The Real Heart Healthy Diet

1. Gardner, C. D., Trepanowski, J. F., Del Gobbo, L. C., Hauser, M. E., Rigdon, J., Ioannidis, J. P., . . . King, A. C. (2018). Effect of low-fat vs low-carbohydrate diet on 12-month weight loss in overweight adults and the association with genotype pattern or insulin secretion. *JAMA, 319*(7), 667. https://doi.org/10.1001/jama.2018.0245

2. Gardner, C. D., Kiazand, A., Alhassan, S., Kim, S., Stafford, R. S., Balise, R. R., . . . King, A. C. (2007). Comparison of the Atkins, zone, Ornish, and LEARN diets for change in weight and related risk factors among overweight premenopausal women. *JAMA, 297*(9), 969. https://doi.org/10.1001/jama.297.9.969

3. Hall, K. D., Guo, J., Courville, A. B., Boring, J., Brychta, R., Chen, K. Y., . . . Chung, S. T. (2020). A plant-based, low-fat diet decreases ad libitum energy intake compared to an animal-based, ketogenic diet: An inpatient randomized controlled trial. https://doi.org/10.31232/osf.io/rdjfb

4. Ungar, P. S. (2017). Evolution's bite: A story of teeth, diet, and human origins. Princeton University Press, 58.

5. Campbell, T. C., & Campbell, T. M., II. (2016). *The China Study: Revised and expanded edition: The most comprehensive study of nutrition ever conducted and the startling implications for diet, weight loss, and long-term health.* BenBella Books.

6. Minger, D. (2018, November 21). *The China Study: Fact or fallacy?* Retrieved from https://deniseminger.com/2010/07/07/the-china-study-fact-or-fallac/

7. Behrend, A. M., Harding, C. O., Shoemaker, J. D., Matern, D., Sahn, D. J., Elliot, D. L., & Gillingham, M. B. (2012). Substrate oxidation and cardiac performance during exercise in disorders of long chain fatty acid oxidation. *Molecular Genetics and Metabolism, 105*(1), 110–115. doi:10.1016/j.ymgme.2011.09.030

8. Zinman, B., Wanner, C., Lachin, J. M., Fitchett, D., Bluhmki, E., Hantel, S., . . . Inzucchi, S. E. (2016). Empagliflozin, cardiovascular outcomes, and mortality in type 2 diabetes. *New England Journal of Medicine, 374*(11), 1092–1094. doi:10.1056/nejmc1600827

9. Challoner, D., & Steinberg, D. (1966). Oxidative metabolism of myocardium as influenced by fatty acids and epinephrine. *American Journal of Physiology-Legacy Content, 211*(4), 897–902. https://doi.org/10.1152/ajplegacy.1966.211.4.897

10. Ceriello, A., Esposito, K., Piconi, L., Ihnat, M. A., Thorpe, J. E., Testa, R., . . . Giugliano, D. (2008). Oscillating glucose is more deleterious to endothelial function and oxidative stress than mean glucose in normal and type 2 diabetic patients. *Diabetes, 57*(5), 1349–1354. doi:10.2337/db08-0063

11. Shimazu, T., Hirschey, M. D., Newman, J., He, W., Shirakawa, K., Le Moan, N., . . . Verdin, E. (2012). Suppression of oxidative stress by β-hydroxybutyrate, an endogenous histone deacetylase inhibitor. *Science, 339*(6116), 211–214. doi:10.1126/science.1227166

12. Milder, J., & Patel, M. (2012). Modulation of oxidative stress and mitochondrial function by the ketogenic diet. *Epilepsy Research, 100*(3), 295–303. doi:10.1016/j.eplepsyres.2011.09.021

13. Nazarewicz, R. R., Ziolkowski, W., Vaccaro, P. S., & Ghafourifar, P. (2007). Effect of short-term ketogenic diet on redox status of human blood. *Rejuvenation Research, 10*(4), 435–440. doi:10.1089/rej.2007.0540

14. Haces, M. L., Hernández-Fonseca, K., Medina-Campos, O. N., Montiel, T., Pedra-za-Chaverri, J., & Massieu, L. (2008). Antioxidant capacity contributes to protection of ketone bodies against oxidative damage induced during hypoglycemic conditions. *Experimental Neurology, 211*(1), 85–96. doi:10.1016/j.expneurol.2007.12.029

15. Peluso, I., Raguzzini, A., Catasta, G., Cammisotto, V., Perrone, A., Tomino, C., . . . Ser-afini, M. (2018). Effects of high consumption of vegetables on clinical, immunological, and antioxidant markers in subjects at risk of cardiovascular diseases. *Oxidative Medicine and Cellular Longevity, 2018,* 1–9. https://doi.org/10.1155/2018/5417165

16. Crane, T. E., Kubota, C., West, J. L., Kroggel, M. A., Wertheim, B. C., & Thomson, C. A. (2011). Increasing the vegetable intake dose is associated with a rise in plasma carotenoids without modifying oxidative stress or inflammation in overweight or obese postmenopausal women. *The Journal of Nutrition, 141*(10), 1827–1833. https://doi.org/10.3945/jn.111.139659

17. Moller, P., Vogel, U., Pederson, A., Dragsted, L. O., Sandstrom, B., & Loft, S. (2003). No effect of 600 grams fruit and vegetables per day on oxidative DNA damage and repair in healthy nonsmokers. *Cancer Epidemiology, Biomarkers and Prevention, 12,* 1016–1022. https://pubmed.ncbi.nlm.nih.gov/14578137/

18. Sekhar, R. V., McKay, S. V., Patel, S. G., Guthikonda, A. P., Reddy, V. T., Balasubra-manyam, A., & Jahoor, F. (2010). Glutathione synthesis is diminished in patients with uncontrolled diabetes and restored by dietary supplementation with cysteine and glycine. *Diabetes Care, 34*(1), 162–167. doi:10.2337/dc10-1006

19. Ruiz-Ramírez, A., Ortiz-Balderas, E., Cardozo-Saldaña, G., Diaz-Diaz, E., & El-Hafidi, M. (2013). Glycine restores glutathione and protects against oxidative stress in vascular tissue from sucrose-fed rats. *Clinical Science, 126*(1), 19–29. doi:10.1042/cs20130164

20. Kimura, I., Inoue, D., Maeda, T., Hara, T., Ichimura, A., Miyauchi, S., . . . Tsujimoto, G. (2011). Short-chain fatty acids and ketones directly regulate sympathetic nervous system via G protein-coupled receptor 41 (GPR41). *Proceedings of the National Academy of Sciences, 108*(19), 8030–8035. doi:10.1073/pnas.1016088108

21. Millis, R. M., Austin, R. E., Bond, V., Faruque, M., Goring, K. L., Hickey, B. M., . . . DeMeersman, R. E. (2009). Effects of high-carbohydrate and high-fat dietary treatments on measures of heart rate variability and sympathovagal balance. *Life Sciences, 85*(3–4), 141–145. doi:10.1016/j.lfs.2009.05.006

22. Furness, J. B., Rivera, L. R., Cho, H., Bravo, D. M., & Callaghan, B. (2013). The gut as a sensory organ. *Nature Reviews Gastroenterology & Hepatology, 10*(12), 729–740. doi:10.1038/nrgastro.2013.180

23. Smart, H. (1987). Abnormal vagal function in irritable bowel syndrome. *The Lancet, 330*(8557), 475–478. doi:10.1016/s0140-6736(87)91792-2

24. Ames, B. N., Profet, M., & Gold, L. S. (1990). Dietary pesticides (99.99% all natural). *Proceedings of the National Academy of Sciences of the United States of America, 87*(19), 7777–7781. doi:10.1073/pnas.87.19.7777

25. Hollon, J., Puppa, E., Greenwald, B., Goldberg, E., Guerrerio, A., & Fasano, A. (2015). Effect of gliadin on permeability of intestinal biopsy explants from celiac disease patients and patients with non-celiac gluten sensitivity. *Nutrients, 7*(3), 1565–1576. doi:10.3390/nu7031565

26. Patel, B., Schutte, R., Sporns, P., Doyle, J., Jewel, L., & Fedorak, R. N. (2002). Potato glycoalkaloids adversely affect intestinal permeability and aggravate inflammatory bowel disease. *Inflammatory Bowel Diseases, 8*(5), 340–346. doi:10.1097/00054725-200209000-00005

27. Concon, J. M. (1988). *Food toxicology: Principles and concepts*. Marcel Dekker.

28. Zheng, J., Wang, M., Wei, W., Keller, J. N., Adhikari, B., King, J. F., . . . Laine, R. A. (2016). Dietary plant lectins appear to be transported from the gut to gain access to and alter dopaminergic neurons of Caenorhabditis elegans, a potential etiology of Parkinson's disease. *Frontiers in Nutrition, 3*. https://doi.org/10.3389/fnut.2016.00007

29. Wiley, R., Blessing, W., & Reis, D. (1982). Suicide transport: Destruction of neurons by retrograde transport of ricin, abrin, and modeccin. *Science, 216*(4548), 889–890. https://doi.org/10.1126/science.6177039

30. Mazurak, N., Seredyuk, N., Sauer, H., Teufel, M., & Enck, P. (2012). Heart rate variability in the irritable bowel syndrome: A review of the literature. *Neurogastroenterology & Motility, 24*(3), 206–216. https://doi.org/10.1111/j.1365-2982.2011.01866.x

31. Weingärtner, O., Lütjohann, D., Ji, S., Weisshoff, N., List, F., Sudhop, T., . . . Laufs, U. (2008). Vascular effects of diet supplementation with plant sterols. *Journal of the American College of Cardiology, 51*(16), 1553–1561. https://doi.org/10.1016/j.jacc.2007.09.074

32. Ratnayake, W. M., L'Abbé, M. R., Mueller, R., Hayward, S., Plouffe, L., Hollywood, R., & Trick, K. (2000). Vegetable oils high in phytosterols make erythrocytes less deformable and shorten the life span of stroke-prone spontaneously hypertensive rats. *The Journal of Nutrition, 130*(5), 1166–1178. https://doi.org/10.1093/jn/130.5.1166

33. Tong, T. Y., Appleby, P. N., Bradbury, K. E., Perez-Cornago, A., Travis, R. C., Clarke, R., & Key, T. J. (2019). Risks of ischaemic heart disease and stroke in meat eaters, fish eaters, and vegetarians over 18 years of follow-up: Results from the prospective EPIC-Oxford study. *BMJ*, l4897. https://doi.org/10.1136/bmj.l4897

34. Vergès, B., & Fumeron, F. (2015). Potential risks associated with increased plasma plant-sterol levels. *Diabetes & Metabolism, 41*(1), 76–81. https://doi.org/10.1016/j.diabet.2014.11.003

35. Miettinen, T. A., & Gylling, H. (2003). Synthesis and absorption markers of cholesterol in serum and lipoproteins during a large dose of statin treatment. *European Journal of Clinical Investigation, 33*(11), 976–982. https://doi.org/10.1046/j.1365-2362.2003.01229.x

36. Speijer, D. (2016). Being right on Q: Shaping eukaryotic evolution. *Biochemical Journal, 473*(22), 4103–4127. https://doi.org/10.1042/bcj20160647

37. Alvheim, A. R., Malde, M. K., Osei-Hyiaman, D., Hong Lin, Y., Pawlosky, R. J., Madsen, L., . . . Hibbeln, J. R. (2012). Dietary linoleic acid elevates endogenous 2-AG and anandamide and induces obesity. *Obesity, 20*(10), 1984–1994. https://doi.org/10.1038/oby.2012.38; Shen, M., Zhao, X., Siegal, G. P., Desmond, R., & Hardy, R. W. (2014). Dietary stearic acid leads to a reduction of visceral adipose tissue in Athymic nude mice. *PLOS ONE, 9*(9), e104083. https://doi.org/10.1371/journal.pone.0104083

38. Senyilmaz-Tiebe, D., Pfaff, D. H., Virtue, S., Schwarz, K. V., Fleming, T., Altamura, S., . . . Teleman, A. A. (2018). Dietary stearic acid regulates mitochondria in vivo in humans. *Nature Communications, 9*(1). https://doi.org/10.1038/s41467-018-05614-6

39. Cao, H., Gerhold, K., Mayers, J. R., Wiest, M. M., Watkins, S. M., & Hotamisligil, G. S. (2008). Identification of a lipokine, a lipid hormone linking adipose tissue to systemic metabolism. *Cell, 134*(6), 933–944. https://doi.org/10.1016/j.cell.2008.07.048

40. Green, H. S., & Wang, S. C. (2020). First report on quality and purity evaluations of avocado oil sold in the US. *Food Control, 116,* 107328. https://doi.org/10.1016/j.foodcont .2020.107328

41. Cortinas, L., Villaverde, C., Galobart, J., Baucells, M., Codony, R., & Barroeta, A. (2004). Fatty acid content in chicken thigh and breast as affected by dietary polyunsaturation level. *Poultry Science, 83*(7), 1155–1164. https://doi.org/10.1093/ps/83.7.1155; Gläser, K. R., Wenk, C., & Scheeder, M. R. (2002). Effect of dietary mono- and polyunsaturated fatty acids on the fatty acid composition of pigs' adipose tissues. *Archiv für Tierernaehrung, 56*(1), 51–65. https://doi.org/10.1080/00039420214178

42. Stepien, M., Gaudichon, C., Fromentin, G., Even, P., Tomé, D., & Azzout-Marniche, D. (2011). Increasing protein at the expense of carbohydrate in the diet down-regulates glucose utilization as glucose sparing effect in rats. *PLOS ONE, 6*(2), e14664. https://doi .org/10.1371/journal.pone.0014664

43. Issad, T., Pénicaud, L., Ferré, P., Kandé, J., Baudon, M. A., & Girard, J. (1987). Effects of fasting on tissue glucose utilization in conscious resting rats. Major glucose-sparing effect in working muscles. *Biochemical Journal, 246*(1), 241–244. https://doi.org/10.1042 /bj2460241

44. Jornayvaz, F. R., Jurczak, M. J., Lee, H., Birkenfeld, A. L., Frederick, D. W., Zhang, D., . . . Shulman, G. I. (2010). A high-fat, ketogenic diet causes hepatic insulin resistance in mice, despite increasing energy expenditure and preventing weight gain. *American Journal of Physiology-Endocrinology and Metabolism, 299*(5), E808–E815. https://doi.org/10.1152 /ajpendo.00361.2010

45. Tsai, S., Clemente-Casares, X., Zhou, A. C., Lei, H., Ahn, J. J., Chan, Y. T., . . . Winer, D. A. (2018). Insulin receptor-mediated stimulation boosts T cell immunity during inflammation and infection. *Cell Metabolism, 28*(6), 922–934.e4. https://doi.org/10.1016/j.cmet .2018.08.003

46. Vergari, E., Knudsen, J. G., Ramracheya, R., Salehi, A., Zhang, Q., Adam, J., . . . Rorsman, P. (2019). Insulin inhibits glucagon release by SGLT2-induced stimulation of somatostatin secretion. *Nature Communications, 10*(1). https://doi.org/10.1038/s41467 -018-08193-8

47. Dentin, R., Liu, Y., Koo, S., Hedrick, S., Vargas, T., Heredia, J., . . . Montminy, M. (2007). Insulin modulates gluconeogenesis by inhibition of the coactivator TORC2. *Nature, 449*(7160), 366–369. https://doi.org/10.1038/nature06128

48. Schade, D. S., Eaton, P. R., Pommer, I., & Temple, R. (1977). Modulation of the catabolic activity of glucagon by endogenous insulin secretion in obese man. *Acta Diabetologica Latina, 14*(1–2), 62–72. https://doi.org/10.1007/bf02624664

49. Wang, Z., Bergeron, N., Levison, B. S., Li, X. S., Chiu, S., Jia, X., . . . Hazen, S. L. (2018). Impact of chronic dietary red meat, white meat, or non-meat protein on trimethylamine N-oxide metabolism and renal excretion in healthy men and women. *European Heart Journal, 40*(7), 583–594. https://doi.org/10.1093/eurheartj/ehy799; Tang, W., Wang, Z., & Levison, B. (2013). Intestinal microbial metabolism of phosphatidylcholine and

cardiovascular risk. *Journal of Vascular Surgery, 58*(2), 549. https://doi.org/10.1016/j.jvs.2013.06.007

50. Landfald, B., Valeur, J., Berstad, A., & Raa, J. (2017). Microbial trimethylamine-N-oxide as a disease marker: something fishy? *Microbial Ecology in Health and Disease, 28*(1), 1327309. https://doi.org/10.1080/16512235.2017.1327309

51. Zaramela, L. S., Martino, C., Alisson-Silva, F., Rees, S. D., Diaz, S. L., Chuzel, L., . . . Zengler, K. (2019). Gut bacteria responding to dietary change ENCODE sialidases that exhibit preference for red meat-associated carbohydrates. *Nature Microbiology, 4*(12), 2082–2089. https://doi.org/10.1038/s41564-019-0564-9

52. Kivenson, V., & Giovannoni, S. J. (2020). An expanded genetic code enables trimethylamine metabolism in human gut bacteria. *mSystems, 5*(5). https://doi.org/10.1128/msystems.00413-20

53. Meyer, K. A., Benton, T. Z., Bennett, B. J., Jacobs, D. R., Lloyd-Jones, D. M., Gross, M. D., . . . Zeisel, S. H. (2016). Microbiota-dependent metabolite trimethylamine N-oxide and coronary artery calcium in the coronary artery risk development in young adults study (CARDIA). *Journal of the American Heart Association, 5*(10). https://doi.org/10.1161/jaha.116.003970

54. Senthong, V., Li, X. S., Hudec, T., Coughlin, J., Wu, Y., Levison, B., . . . Tang, W. W. (2016). Plasma trimethylamine N-oxide, a gut microbe–generated phosphatidylcholine metabolite, is associated with atherosclerotic burden. *Journal of the American College of Cardiology, 67*(22), 2620–2628. https://doi.org/10.1016/j.jacc.2016.03.546

55. Gran, P., & Cameron-Smith, D. (2011). The actions of exogenous leucine on mTOR signaling and amino acid transporters in human myotubes. *BMC Physiology, 11*(1), 10. https://doi.org/10.1186/1472-6793-11-10

56. Lentz, S. R. (2001). Does homocysteine promote atherosclerosis? *Arteriosclerosis, Thrombosis, and Vascular Biology, 21*(9), 1385–1386. https://doi.org/10.1161/atvb.21.9.1385

57. Mann, N., Li, D., Sinclair, A., Dudman, N., Guo, X., Elsworth, G., . . . Kelly, F. (1999). The effect of diet on plasma homocysteine concentrations in healthy male subjects. *European Journal of Clinical Nutrition, 53*(11), 895–899. https://doi.org/10.1038/sj.ejcn.1600874

58. Markova, M., Koelman, L., Hornemann, S., Pivovarova, O., Sucher, S., Machann, J., . . . Aleksandrova, K. (2020). Effects of plant and animal high protein diets on immune-inflammatory biomarkers: A 6-week intervention trial. *Clinical Nutrition, 39*(3), 862–869. https://doi.org/10.1016/j.clnu.2019.03.019

59. Hodgson, J. M., Ward, N. C., Burke, V., Beilin, L. J., & Puddey, I. B. (2007). Increased lean red meat intake does not elevate markers of oxidative stress and inflammation in humans. *The Journal of Nutrition, 137*(2), 363–367. https://doi.org/10.1093/jn/137.2.363

60. Lee, J. E., McLerran, D. F., Rolland, B., Chen, Y., Grant, E. J., Vedanthan, R., . . . Sinha, R. (2013). Meat intake and cause-specific mortality: A pooled analysis of Asian prospective cohort studies. *The American Journal of Clinical Nutrition, 98*(4), 1032–1041. https://doi.org/10.3945/ajcn.113.062638

61. Zeraatkar, D., Johnston, B. C., Bartoszko, J., Cheung, K., Bala, M. M., Valli, C., . . . El Dib, R. (2019). Effect of lower versus higher red meat intake on cardiometabolic and cancer outcomes. *Annals of Internal Medicine, 171*(10), 721. https://doi.org/10.7326/m19-0622

62. Harvard T.H. Chan School of Public Health. (2019, October 28). Fiber. *The Nutrition Source*. https://www.hsph.harvard.edu/nutritionsource/carbohydrates/fiber/

63. Scribd. (n.d.). Walter Willett, potential conflicts of interest. Author. https://www.scribd.com/document/397606854/Walter-Willett-Potential-Conflicts-of-Interest

64. Burr, M., Gilbert, J., Holliday, R., Elwood, P., Fehily, A., Rogers, S., . . . Deadman, N. (1989). Effects of changes in fat, fish, and fibre intakes on death and myocardial reinfarction: Diet and reinfarction trial (Dart). *The Lancet, 334*(8666), 757–761. https://doi.org/10.1016/s0140-6736(89)90828-3

65. Hartley, L., May, M. D., Loveman, E., Colquitt, J. L., & Rees, K. (2016). Dietary fibre for the primary prevention of cardiovascular disease. *Cochrane Database Systematic Review*, 1. https://doi.org/10.1002/14651858.CD011472.pub2

66. Kelly, S. A., Hartley, L., Loveman, E., Colquitt, J. L., Jones, H. M., Al-Khudairy, L., . . . Rees, K. (2017). Whole grain cereals for the primary or secondary prevention of cardiovascular disease. *Cochrane Database of Systematic Reviews*. https://doi.org/10.1002/14651858.cd005051.pub3

67. Depauw, S., Bosch, G., Hesta, M., Whitehouse-Tedd, K., Hendriks, W. H., Kaandorp, J., & Janssens, G. P. (2012). Fermentation of animal components in strict carnivores: A comparative study with cheetah fecal inoculum. *Journal of Animal Science, 90*(8), 2540–2548. https://doi.org/10.2527/jas.2011-4377; David, L. A., Maurice, C. F., Carmody, R. N., Gootenberg, D. B., Button, J. E., Wolfe, B. E., . . . Turnbaugh, P. J. (2013). Diet rapidly and reproducibly alters the human gut microbiome. *Nature, 505*(7484), 559–563. https://doi.org/10.1038/nature12820

68. Ho, K. (2012). Stopping or reducing dietary fiber intake reduces constipation and its associated symptoms. *World Journal of Gastroenterology, 18*(33), 4593. https://doi.org/10.3748/wjg.v18.i33.4593

69. Schatzkin, A., Lanza, E., Corle, D., Lance, P., Iber, F., Caan, B., . . . Slattery, M. (2000). Lack of effect of a low-fat, high-fiber diet on the recurrence of colorectal adenomas. *New England Journal of Medicine, 342*(16), 1149–1155. https://doi.org/10.1056/nejm200004203421601; Alberts, D. S., Martínez, M. E., Roe, D. J., Guillén-Rodríguez, J. M., Marshall, J. R., Van Leeuwen, J. B., . . . Sampliner, R. E. (2000). Lack of effect of a high-fiber cereal supplement on the recurrence of colorectal adenomas. *New England Journal of Medicine, 342*(16), 1156–1162. https://doi.org/10.1056/nejm200004203421602; Fuchs, C. S., Giovannucci, E. L., Colditz, G. A., Hunter, D. J., Stampfer, M. J., Rosner, B., . . . Willett, W. C. (1999). Dietary fiber and the risk of colorectal cancer and adenoma in women. *New England Journal of Medicine, 340*(3), 169–176. https://doi.org/10.1056/nejm199901213400301; Lanza, E., Yu, B., Murphy, G., Albert, P. S., Caan, B., Marshall, J. R., . . . Schatzkin, A. (2007). The polyp prevention trial continued follow-up study: No effect of a low-fat, high-fiber, high-fruit, and -vegetable diet on adenoma recurrence eight years after randomization. *Cancer Epidemiology Biomarkers & Prevention, 16*(9), 1745–1752. https://doi.org/10.1158/1055-9965.epi-07-0127; Peery, A. F., Sandler, R. S., Ahnen, D. J., Galanko, J. A., Holm, A. N., Shaukat, A., . . . Baron, J. A. (2013). Constipation and a low-fiber diet are not associated with diverticulosis. *Clinical Gastroenterology and Hepatology, 11*(12), 1622–1627. https://doi.org/10.1016/j.cgh.2013.06.033; Peery, A. F., Barrett, P. R., Park, D., Rogers, A. J., Galanko, J. A., Martin, C. F., & Sandler, R. S.

(2012). A high-fiber diet does not protect against asymptomatic diverticulosis. *Gastroenterology, 142*(2), 266–272.e1. https://doi.org/10.1053/j.gastro.2011.10.035

70. Moneta, G. (2006). Loss of collagen XVIII enhances neovascularization and vascular permeability in atherosclerosis. *Yearbook of Vascular Surgery, 2006*, 14. https://doi.org/10.1016/s0749-4041(08)70015-0

71. Roberts, P. R., & Zaloga, G. P. (2000). Cardiovascular effects of carnosine. *Biochemistry, 65*(7), 856–861. http://protein.bio.msu.ru/biokhimiya/contents/v65/full/65071006.html

72. Wang, Z., Liu, Y., Liu, G., Lu, H., & Mao, C. (2018). L-carnitine and heart disease. *Life Sciences, 194*, 88–97. https://www.sciencedirect.com/science/article/abs/pii/S0024320517306525

73. Hamman, B. L., Bittl, J. A., Jacobus, W. E., Allen, P. D., Spencer, R. S., Tian, R., & Ingwall, J. S. (1995). Inhibition of the creatine kinase reaction decreases the contractile reserve of isolated rat hearts. *American Journal of Physiology-Heart and Circulatory Physiology, 269*(3), H1030–H1036. https://doi.org/10.1152/ajpheart.1995.269.3.h1030

74. Milei, J., Ferreira, R., Llesuy, S., Forcada, P., Covarrubias, J., & Boveris, A. (1992). Reduction of reperfusion injury with preoperative rapid intravenous infusion of taurine during myocardial revascularization. *American Heart Journal, 123*(2), 339–345. https://doi.org/10.1016/0002-8703(92)90644-b

75. Heslop, C. L., Frohlich, J. J., & Hill, J. S. (2010). Myeloperoxidase and C-reactive protein have combined utility for long-term prediction of cardiovascular mortality after coronary angiography. *Journal of the American College of Cardiology, 55*(11), 1102–1109. https://doi.org/10.1016/j.jacc.2009.11.050; Hasegawa, T., Malle, E., Farhood, A., & Jaeschke, H. (2005). Generation of hypochlorite-modified proteins by neutrophils during ischemia-reperfusion injury in rat liver: Attenuation by ischemic preconditioning. *American Journal of Physiology-Gastrointestinal and Liver Physiology, 289*(4), G760–G767. https://doi.org/10.1152/ajpgi.00141.2005

76. McCarty, M. (1999). The reported clinical utility of taurine in ischemic disorders may reflect a down-regulation of neutrophil activation and adhesion. *Medical Hypotheses, 53*(4), 290–299. https://doi.org/10.1054/mehy.1998.0760

77. Liao, X., Zhou, X., Li, J., Yang, J., Tan, Z., Hu, Z., ... Yuan, L. (2007). Taurine inhibits osteoblastic differentiation of vascular smooth muscle cells via the ERK pathway. *Amino Acids, 34*(4), 525–530. https://doi.org/10.1007/s00726-007-0003-8; Kramer, J. H., Chovan, J. P., & Schaffer, S. W. (1981). Effect of taurine on calcium paradox and ischemic heart failure. *American Journal of Physiology-Heart and Circulatory Physiology, 240*(2), H238–H246. https://doi.org/10.1152/ajpheart.1981.240.2.h238

78. Xu, Y. J., Arneja, A. S., Tappia, P. S., & Dhalla, N. S. (2008). The potential health benefits of taurine in cardiovascular disease. *Experimental and clinical cardiology, 13*(2), 57–65. https://pubmed.ncbi.nlm.nih.gov/19343117/

79. Li, R., Xia, J., Zhang, X., Gathirua-Mwangi, W. G., Guo, J., LI, Y., McKenzie, S., & Song, Y. (2018). Associations of muscle mass and strength with all-cause mortality among US older adults. *Medicine & Science in Sports & Exercise, 50*(3), 458–467. https://doi.org/10.1249/mss.0000000000001448; Wang, H., Hai, S., Liu, Y., Liu, Y., & Dong, B. (2019). Skeletal muscle mass as a mortality predictor among nonagenarians and centenarians:

A prospective cohort study. *Scientific Reports, 9*(1). https://doi.org/10.1038/s41598-019-38893-0; Srikanthan, P., & Karlamangla, A. S. (2014). Muscle mass index as a predictor of longevity in older adults. *The American Journal of Medicine, 127*(6), 547–553. https://doi.org/10.1016/j.amjmed.2014.02.007

80. Chuang, S., Chang, H., Lee, M., Chia-Yu Chen, R., & Pan, W. (2014). Skeletal muscle mass and risk of death in an elderly population. *Nutrition, Metabolism and Cardiovascular Diseases, 24*(7), 784–791. https://doi.org/10.1016/j.numecd.2013.11.010

81. Nestares, T., Barrionuevo, M., Urbano, G., & López-Frías, M. (2001). Nutritional assessment of protein from beans (*Phaseolus vulgaris* L) processed at different pH values, in growing rats. *Journal of the Science of Food and Agriculture, 81*(15), 1522–1529. https://doi.org/10.1002/jsfa.965

82. Isanejad, M., Sirola, J., Rikkonen, T., Mursu, J., Kröger, H., Qazi, S. L., . . . Erkkilä, A. T. (2019). Higher protein intake is associated with a lower likelihood of frailty among older women, Kuopio OSTPRE-Fracture Prevention Study. *European Journal of Nutrition.* https://doi.org/10.1007/s00394-019-01978-7

83. Promislow, J. H. (2002). Protein consumption and bone mineral density in the elderly: The Rancho Bernardo study. *American Journal of Epidemiology, 155*(7), 636–644. https://doi.org/10.1093/aje/155.7.636

84. Smith, P., & Peretz, B. (1986). Hypoplasia and health status: A comparison of two lifestyles. *Human Evolution, 1*(6), 535–544. https://doi.org/10.1007/bf02437470

85. Roberts, M. N., Wallace, M. A., Tomilov, A. A., Zhou, Z., Marcotte, G. R., Tran, D., . . . Lopez-Dominguez, J. A. (2018). A ketogenic diet extends longevity and healthspan in adult mice. *Cell Metabolism, 27*(5), 1156. https://doi.org/10.1016/j.cmet.2018.04.005

86. Gottlieb, R. A., & Mentzer, R. M. (2012). Autophagy: An affair of the heart. *Heart Failure Reviews, 18*(5), 575–584. https://doi.org/10.1007/s10741-012-9367-2; Hamacher-Brady, A., Brady, N. R., & Gottlieb, R. A. (2006). Enhancing macroautophagy protects against ischemia/reperfusion injury in cardiac myocytes. *Journal of Biological Chemistry, 281*(40), 29776–29787. https://doi.org/10.1074/jbc.m603783200

87. Masiero, E., Agatea, L., Mammucari, C., Blaauw, B., Loro, E., Komatsu, M., . . . Sandri, M. (2009). Autophagy is required to maintain muscle mass. *Cell Metabolism, 10*(6), 507–515. https://doi.org/10.1016/j.cmet.2009.10.008

88. Sävendahl, L., & Underwood, L. E. (1999). Fasting increases serum total cholesterol, LDL cholesterol and apolipoprotein B in healthy, nonobese humans. *The Journal of Nutrition, 129*(11), 2005–2008. https://doi.org/10.1093/jn/129.11.2005

89. Ahmet, I., Wan, R., Mattson, M. P., Lakatta, E. G., & Talan, M. (2005). Cardioprotection by intermittent fasting in rats. *Circulation, 112*(20), 3115–3121. https://doi.org/10.1161/circulationaha.105.563817

90. Wan, R., Ahmet, I., Brown, M., Cheng, A., Kamimura, N., Talan, M., & Mattson, M. P. (2010). Cardioprotective effect of intermittent fasting is associated with an elevation of adiponectin levels in rats. *The Journal of Nutritional Biochemistry, 21*(5), 413–417. https://doi.org/10.1016/j.jnutbio.2009.01.020

91. Fontana, L., Meyer, T. E., Klein, S., & Holloszy, J. O. (2004). Long-term calorie restriction is highly effective in reducing the risk for atherosclerosis in humans. *Proceedings of the National Academy of Sciences, 101*(17), 6659–6663. https://doi.org/10.1073/pnas.0308291101

92. Safeguarding our soils. (2017). *Nature Communications, 8*(1). https://doi.org/10.1038/s41467-017-02070-6

93. U.S. Environmental Protection Agency. (2019, September 13). Sources of greenhouse gas emissions. Author. https://www.epa.gov/ghgemissions/sources-greenhouse-gas-emissions

94. U.S. Environmental Protection Agency. (2020, February 12). Inventory of U.S. greenhouse gas emissions and sinks. Author. https://www.epa.gov/ghgemissions/inventory-us-greenhouse-gas-emissions-and-sinks

95. White Oak Pastures Team. (2019, June 4). Study: White Oak Pastures beef reduces atmospheric carbon. *Around The Farm Blog.* https://blog.whiteoakpastures.com/blog/carbon-negative-grassfed-beef

96. Eschenbach, W. (2010, September 12). Animal, vegetable, or E. O. Wilson. *Watts Up With That?.* https://wattsupwiththat.com/2010/09/11/animal-vegetable-or-e-o-wilson/

97. Davis, S. L. (2003). The least harm principle may require that humans consume a diet containing large herbivores, not a vegan diet. *Journal of Agricultural and Environmental Ethics, 16,* 387–394. https://link.springer.com/article/10.1023/A:1025638030686

Chapter 12. Reducing Oxidative Stress

1. Bulur, H., Özdemirler, G., Öz, B., Toker, G., Öztürk, M., & Uysal, M. (1995). High cholesterol diet supplemented with sunflower seed oil but not olive oil stimulates lipid peroxidation in plasma, liver, and aorta of rats. *The Journal of Nutritional Biochemistry, 6*(10), 547–550. https://doi.org/10.1016/0955-2863(95)00099-l

2. Eder, E., Wacker, M., Lutz, U., Nair, J., Fang, X., Bartsch, H., . . . Lutz, W. (2006). Oxidative stress related DNA adducts in the liver of female rats fed with sunflower-, rapeseed-, olive- or coconut oil supplemented diets. *Chemico-Biological Interactions, 159*(2), 81–89. https://doi.org/10.1016/j.cbi.2005.09.004

3. Turpeinen, A., Basu, S., & Mutanen, M. (1998). A high linoleic acid diet increases oxidative stress in vivo and affects nitric oxide metabolism in humans. *Prostaglandins, Leukotrienes and Essential Fatty Acids, 59*(3), 229–233. https://doi.org/10.1016/s0952-3278(98)90067-9

4. Ng, C., Leong, X., Masbah, N., Adam, S. K., Kamisah, Y., & Jaarin, K. (2014). Heated vegetable oils and cardiovascular disease risk factors. *Vascular Pharmacology, 61*(1), 1–9. https://doi.org/10.1016/j.vph.2014.02.004

5. Crinnion, W. J. (2010). Organic foods contain higher levels of certain nutrients, lower levels of pesticides, and may provide health benefits for the consumer. *Alternative Medicine Review: A Journal of Clinical Therapeutic, 15*(1), 4–12. https://pubmed.ncbi.nlm.nih.gov/20359265/

6. Environmental Working Group. (n.d.). EWG's tap water database: Consumer resources. Author. https://www.ewg.org/tapwater/consumer-resources.php

7. Kozisek, F. (n.d.). *Health risks from drinking demineralized water.* National Institute of Public Health Czech Republic. https://www.who.int/water_sanitation_health/dwq/nutrientschap12.pdf

8. Wan, Q., Cui, X., Shao, J., Zhou, F., Jia, Y., Sun, X., . . . Zhang, L. (2014). Beijing ambient particle exposure accelerates atherosclerosis in ApoE knockout mice by upregulating visfatin expression. *Cell Stress and Chaperones, 19*(5), 715–724. https://doi.org/10.1007

/s12192-014-0499-2; Tranfield, E. M., Van Eeden, S. F., Yatera, K., Hogg, J. C., & Walker, D. C. (2010). Ultrastructural changes in atherosclerotic plaques following the instillation of airborne particulate matter into the lungs of rabbits. *Canadian Journal of Cardiology*, 26(7), e258–e269. https://doi.org/10.1016/s0828-282x(10)70422-0

9. Grabenstein, J. D. (2011). *ImmunoFacts 2012: Vaccines and immunologic drugs*. Lippincott Williams & Wilkins.

10. Albonico, H., Bräker, H., & Hüsler, J. (1998). Febrile infectious childhood diseases in the history of cancer patients and matched control. *Medical Hypotheses*, 51(4), 315–320. https://doi.org/10.1016/s0306-9877(98)90055-x; Hoption Cann, S. A., Van Netten, J., & Van Netten, C. (2006). Acute infections as a means of cancer prevention: Opposing effects to chronic infections? *Cancer Detection and Prevention*, 30(1), 83–93. https://doi.org/10.1016/j.cdp.2005.11.001

11. Kubota, Y., Iso, H., & Tamakoshi, A. (2015). Association of measles and mumps with cardiovascular disease: The Japan Collaborative Cohort (JACC) study. *Atherosclerosis*, 241(2), 682–686. https://doi.org/10.1016/j.atherosclerosis.2015.06.026

12. Chen, Q., Chen, O., Martins, I. M., Hou, H., Zhao, X., Blumberg, J. B., & Li, B. (2017). Collagen peptides ameliorate intestinal epithelial barrier dysfunction in immunostimulatory Caco-2 cell monolayers via enhancing tight junctions. *Food & Function*, 8(3), 1144–1151. https://doi.org/10.1039/c6fo01347c

13. Chen, Q., Gao, X., Zhang, H., Li, B., Yu, G., & Li, B. (2019). Collagen peptides administration in early enteral nutrition intervention attenuates burn-induced intestinal barrier disruption: Effects on tight junction structure. *Journal of Functional Foods*, 55, 167–174. https://doi.org/10.1016/j.jff.2019.02.028

14. Qiu, S., Fu, H., Zhou, R., Yang, Z., Bai, G., & Shi, B. (2020). Toxic effects of glyphosate on intestinal morphology, antioxidant capacity and barrier function in weaned piglets. *Ecotoxicology and Environmental Safety*, 187, 109846. https://doi.org/10.1016/j.ecoenv.2019.109846

15. Sharma, A., Adams, C., Cashdollar, B. D., Li, Z., Nguyen, N. V., Sai, H., . . . Pollack, G. H. (2018). Effect of health-promoting agents on exclusion-zone size. *Dose-Response*, 16(3), 155932581879693. https://doi.org/10.1177/1559325818796937

16. WHO/FAO. (2004). *Pesticide residues in food. Report of the joint meeting of the FAO panel of experts on pesticide residues in food and the environment and the WHO core assessment group. Part II: toxicology, glyphosate* [Internet]; 2004 Sep 20–29; Rome, Italy. http://www.fao.org/fileadmin/templates/agphome/documents/Pests_Pesticides/JMPR/Reports_1991-2006/report2004jmpr.pdf; Brewster, D., Jones, R. S., & Parke, D. V. (1978). The metabolism of shikimate in the rat. *Biochemical Journal*, 170(2), 257–264. https://doi.org/10.1042/bj1700257

17. Goldberg, T., Cai, W., Peppa, M., Dardaine, V., Baliga, B. S., Uribarri, J., & Vlassara, H. (2004). Advanced glycoxidation end products in commonly consumed foods. *Journal of the American Dietetic Association*, 104(8), 1287–1291. https://doi.org/10.1016/j.jada.2004.05.214

18. Urquiaga, I., Troncoso, D., Mackenna, M., Urzúa, C., Pérez, D., Dicenta, S., . . . Rigotti, A. (2018). The consumption of beef burgers prepared with wine grape pomace flour improves fasting glucose, plasma antioxidant levels, and oxidative damage markers in

humans: A controlled trial. *Nutrients*, 10(10), 1388. https://doi.org/10.3390/nu10101388; Mellor, D. D., Hamer, H., Smyth, S., Atkin, S. L., & Courts, F. L. (2010). Antioxidant-rich spice added to hamburger meat during cooking results in reduced meat, plasma, and urine malondialdehyde concentrations. *The American Journal of Clinical Nutrition*, 92(4), 996–997. https://doi.org/10.3945/ajcn.2010.29976

19. Li, Z., Henning, S. M., Zhang, Y., Rahnama, N., Zerlin, A., Thames, G., . . . Heber, D. (2013). Decrease of postprandial endothelial dysfunction by spice mix added to high-fat hamburger meat in men with type 2 diabetes mellitus. *Diabetic Medicine*, 30(5), 590–595. https://doi.org/10.1111/dme.12120

20. Vlassara, H., Cai, W., Tripp, E., Pyzik, R., Yee, K., Goldberg, L., . . . Uribarri, J. (2016). Oral AGE restriction ameliorates insulin resistance in obese individuals with the metabolic syndrome: A randomised controlled trial. *Diabetologia*, 59(10), 2181–2192. https://doi.org/10.1007/s00125-016-4053-x

Chapter 13. Achieving Autonomic Balance

1. Budge, S. E. (1967). *The book of the dead: The papyrus of ANI in the British Museum*. Courier Corporation.

2. Achanta, S., Gorky, J. M., Leung, C., Moss, A., Robbins, S., Eisenman, L., . . . Schwaber, J. S. (2020). A comprehensive integrated anatomical and molecular atlas of rodent intrinsic cardiac nervous system. *SSRN Electronic Journal*. https://doi.org/10.2139/ssrn.3526270; Wake, E., & Brack, K. (2016). Characterization of the intrinsic cardiac nervous system. *Autonomic Neuroscience*, 199, 3–16. https://doi.org/10.1016/j.autneu.2016.08.006

3. Wake, E., & Brack, K. (2016). Characterization of the intrinsic cardiac nervous system. *Autonomic Neuroscience*, 199, 3–16. https://doi.org/10.1016/j.autneu.2016.08.006

4. Grossman, P., & Kollai, M. (1993). Respiratory sinus arrhythmia, cardiac vagal tone, and respiration: Within- and between-individual relations. *Psychophysiology*, 30(5), 486–495. doi:10.1111/j.1469-8986.1993.tb02072.x

5. Porges, S. W. (2007). The polyvagal perspective. *Biological Psychology*, 74(2), 116–143. doi:10.1016/j.biopsycho.2006.06.009

6. Orwell, G. (2017). *1984*. General Press: p. 167.

7. Maegawa, Y., Itoh, T., Hosokawa, T., Yaegashi, K., & Nishi, M. (2000). Effects of near-infrared low-level laser irradiation on microcirculation. *Lasers in Surgery and Medicine*, 27(5), 427–437. https://doi.org/10.1002/1096-9101(2000)27:5<427::aid-lsm1004>3.0.co;2-a

8. Ikeda, Y., Biro, S., Kamogawa, Y., Yoshifuku, S., Eto, H., Orihara, K., . . . Tei, C. (2005). Repeated sauna therapy increases arterial endothelial nitric oxide synthase expression and nitric oxide production in cardiomyopathic hamsters. *Circulation Journal*, 69(6), 722–729. https://doi.org/10.1253/circj.69.722; Akasaki, Y., Miyata, M., Eto, H., Shirasawa, T., Hamada, N., Ikeda, Y., . . . Tei, C. (2006). Repeated thermal therapy up-regulates endothelial nitric oxide Synthase and augments angiogenesis in a mouse model of Hindlimb ischemia. *Circulation Journal*, 70(4), 463–470. https://doi.org/10.1253/circj.70.463; Miyata, M., & Tei, C. (2010). Waon therapy for cardiovascular disease: Innovative therapy for the 21st century. *Circulation Journal*, 74(4), 617–621. https://doi.org/10.1253/circj.cj-09-0939

9. Opländer, C., Volkmar, C. M., Paunel-Görgülü, A., Van Faassen, E. E., Heiss, C., Kelm, M., . . . Suschek, C. V. (2009). Whole body UVA irradiation lowers systemic blood pressure by release of nitric oxide from intracutaneous photolabile nitric oxide derivates. *Circulation Research*, 105(10), 1031–1040. https://doi.org/10.1161/circresaha.109.207019

10. Imamura, T., Kinugawa, K., Nitta, D., & Komuro, I. (2016). Real-time assessment of autonomic nerve activity during adaptive servo-ventilation support or Waon therapy. *International Heart Journal*, 57(4), 511–514. https://doi.org/10.1536/ihj.16-014

11. Spallone, V., Bernardi, L., Ricordi, L., Solda, P., Maiello, M. R., Calciati, A., . . . Menzinger, G. (1993). Relationship between the circadian rhythms of blood pressure and sympatho-vagal balance in diabetic autonomic neuropathy. *Diabetes*, 42(12), 1745–1752. https://doi.org/10.2337/diabetes.42.12.1745

12. Alvarsson, J. J., Wiens, S., & Nilsson, M. E. (2010). Stress recovery during exposure to nature sound and environmental noise. *International Journal of Environmental Research and Public Health*, 7(3), 1036–1046. https://doi.org/10.3390/ijerph7031036

13. Roe, J., Thompson, C., Aspinall, P., Brewer, M., Duff, E., Miller, D., . . . Clow, A. (2013). Green space and stress: Evidence from cortisol measures in deprived urban communities. *International Journal of Environmental Research and Public Health*, 10(9), 4086–4103. https://doi.org/10.3390/ijerph10094086

14. Passi, R., Doheny, K. K., Gordin, Y., Hinssen, H., & Palmer, C. (2017). Electrical grounding improves vagal tone in preterm infants. *Neonatology*, 112(2), 187–192. https://doi.org/10.1159/000475744

15. Chevalier, G., & Sinatra, S. T. (2011). Emotional stress, heart rate variability, grounding, and improved autonomic tone: Clinical applications. *Integrative Medicine*, 10(3), 16–21. https://www.semanticscholar.org/paper/Emotional-Stress%2C-Heart-Rate-Variability%2C-and-Tone%3A-Chevalier-Sinatra/844fa28756f93afbb1777d336bedd12cd04fdb11

16. Wang, K., Lombard, J., Rundek, T., Dong, C., Gutierrez, C. M., Byrne, M. M., . . . Brown, S. C. (2019). Relationship of neighborhood greenness to heart disease in 249 405 US Medicare beneficiaries. *Journal of the American Heart Association*, 8(6). https://doi.org/10.1161/jaha.118.010258

17. Greenspan, S. I. (1992). *Infancy and early childhood: The practice of clinical assessments and intervention with emotional and developmental challenges*. International Universities Press.

18. Porges, S. W. (2011). *The Polyvagal theory: Neurophysiological foundations of emotions, attachment, communication, and self-regulation* (Norton series on interpersonal neurobiology). W. W. Norton & Company.

19. House, J. S. (2001). Social isolation kills, but how and why? *Psychosomatic Medicine*, 63(2), 273–274. https://doi.org/10.1097/00006842-200103000-00011

20. Salyer, J., Schubert, C. M., & Chiaranai, C. (2012). Supportive relationships, self-care confidence, and heart failure self-care. *The Journal of Cardiovascular Nursing*, 27(5), 384–393. https://doi.org/10.1097/jcn.0b013e31823228cd

21. Holahan, C. J., Moos, R. H., Holahan, C. K., & Brennan, P. L. (1997). Social context, coping strategies, and depressive symptoms: An expanded model with cardiac patients. *Journal of Personality and Social Psychology*, 72(4), 918–928. https://doi.org/10.1037/0022-3514.72.4.918

22. Carey, I. M., Shah, S. M., DeWilde, S., Harris, T., Victor, C. R., & Cook, D. G. (2014). Increased risk of acute cardiovascular events after partner bereavement. *JAMA Internal Medicine, 174*(4), 598. https://doi.org/10.1001/jamainternmed.2013.14558

23. Kreitzer, M. J., & Riff, K. (2011). Spirituality and heart health. In S. Devries & J. E. Dalen (Eds.), *Integrative Cardiology.* Oxford University Press.

24. Mubanga, M., Byberg, L., Nowak, C., Egenvall, A., Magnusson, P. K., Ingelsson, E., & Fall, T. (2017). Dog ownership and the risk of cardiovascular disease and death—a nationwide cohort study. *Scientific Reports, 7*(1). https://doi.org/10.1038/s41598-017-16118-6

25. Maugeri, A., Medina-Inojosa, J. R., Kunzova, S., Barchitta, M., Agodi, A., Vinciguerra, M., & Lopez-Jimenez, F. (2019). Dog ownership and cardiovascular health: Results from the Kardiovize 2030 project. *Mayo Clinic Proceedings: Innovations, Quality & Outcomes, 3*(3), 268–275. https://doi.org/10.1016/j.mayocpiqo.2019.07.007

26. Poulin, M. J., Brown, S. L., Dillard, A. J., & Smith, D. M. (2013). Giving to others and the association between stress and mortality. *American Journal of Public Health, 103*(9), 1649–1655. https://doi.org/10.2105/ajph.2012.300876

27. Inagaki, T. K., & Eisenberger, N. I. (2015). Giving support to others reduces sympathetic nervous system-related responses to stress. *Psychophysiology, 53*(4), 427–435. https://doi.org/10.1111/psyp.12578

28. Valtorta, N. K., Kanaan, M., Gilbody, S., Ronzi, S., & Hanratty, B. (2016). Loneliness and social isolation as risk factors for coronary heart disease and stroke: Systematic review and meta-analysis of longitudinal observational studies. *Heart, 102*(13), 1009–1016. https://doi.org/10.1136/heartjnl-2015-308790

29. Wilson, E. O. (2012). *The social conquest of earth.* W. W. Norton & Company: p.17.

30. Rosenman, R. H. (1975). Coronary heart disease in Western collaborative group study. Final follow-up experience of 8 1/2 years. *JAMA: The Journal of the American Medical Association, 233*(8), 872–877. https://doi.org/10.1001/jama.233.8.872

31. Ragland, D. R., & Brand, R. J. (1988). Type A behavior and mortality from coronary heart disease. *New England Journal of Medicine, 318*(2), 65–69. https://doi.org/10.1056/nejm198801143180201; Barefoot, J. C., Peterson, B. L., Harrell, F. E., Hlatky, M. A., Pryor, D. B., Haney, T. L., . . . Williams, R. B. (1989). Type A behavior and survival: A follow-up study of 1,467 patients with coronary artery disease. *The American Journal of Cardiology, 64*(8), 427–432. https://doi.org/10.1016/0002-9149(89)90416-5

32. Hardy, J. D., & Smith, T. W. (1988). Cynical hostility and vulnerability to disease: Social support, life stress, and physiological response to conflict. *Health Psychology, 7*(5), 447–459. https://doi.org/10.1037/0278-6133.7.5.447

33. Kivimäki, M., Nyberg, S. T., Batty, G. D., Fransson, E. I., Heikkilä, K., Alfredsson, L., . . . IPD-Work Consortium (2012). Job strain as a risk factor for coronary heart disease: A collaborative meta-analysis of individual participant data. *Lancet (London, England), 380*(9852), 1491–1497. https://doi.org/10.1016/S0140-6736(12)60994-5; Väänänen, A., Koskinen, A., Joensuu, M., Kivimäki, M., Vahtera, J., Kouvonen, A., & Jäppinen, P. (2008). Lack of predictability at work and risk of acute myocardial infarction: An 18-Year prospective study of industrial employees. *American Journal of Public Health, 98*(12), 2264–2271. https://doi.org/10.2105/ajph.2007.122382

34. Kawachi, I., Sparrow, D., Spiro, A., Vokonas, P., & Weiss, S. T. (1996). A prospective study of anger and coronary heart disease. *Circulation, 94*(9), 2090–2095. https://doi .org/10.1161/01.cir.94.9.2090; Houston, B. K., Babyak, M. A., Chesney, M. A., Black, G., & Ragland, D. R. (1997). Social dominance and 22-Year all-cause mortality in men. *Psychosomatic Medicine, 59*(1), 5–12. https://doi.org/10.1097/00006842-199701000-00002; Siegman, A. W. (1993). Cardiovascular consequences of expressing, experiencing, and repressing anger. *Journal of Behavioral Medicine, 16*(6), 539–569. https://doi.org/10.1007 /bf00844719; Glass, D. C., Krakoff, L. R., Contrada, R., Hilton, W. F., Kehoe, K., Mannucci, E. G., . . . Elting, E. (1980). Effect of harassment and competition upon cardiovascular and plasma catecholamine responses in type a and type B individuals. *Psychophysiology, 17*(5), 453–463. https://doi.org/10.1111/j.1469-8986.1980.tb00183.x

35. Leedham, B., Meyerowitz, B. E., Muirhead, J., & Frist, W. H. (1995). Positive expectations predict health after heart transplantation. *Health Psychology, 14*(1), 74–79. https://doi.org /10.1037/0278-6133.14.1.74

36. Helgeson, V. S. (1999). Applicability of cognitive adaptation theory to predicting adjustment to heart disease after coronary angioplasty. *Health Psychology, 18*(6), 561–569. https://doi.org/10.1037/0278-6133.18.6.561

37. Nadarajah, S. R., Buchholz, S. W., Wiegand, D. L., & Berger, A. (2016). The lived experience of individuals in cardiac rehabilitation who have a positive outlook on their cardiac recovery: A phenomenological inquiry. *European Journal of Cardiovascular Nursing, 16*(3), 230–239. https://doi.org/10.1177/1474515116651977

38. Redwine, L. S., Henry, B. L., Pung, M. A., Wilson, K., Chinh, K., Knight, B., . . . Mills, P. J. (2016). Pilot randomized study of a gratitude journaling intervention on heart rate variability and inflammatory biomarkers in patients with stage B heart failure. *Psychosomatic Medicine, 78*(6), 667–676. https://doi.org/10.1097/psy.0000000000000316

39. Mills, P. J., Redwine, L., Wilson, K., Pung, M. A., Chinh, K., Greenberg, B. H., . . . Chopra, D. (2015). The role of gratitude in spiritual well-being in asymptomatic heart failure patients. *Spirituality in Clinical Practice, 2*(1), 5–17. https://doi.org/10.1037 /scp0000050

40. McCraty, R., Atkinson, M., Tomasino, D., & Bradley, R. T. (2009). The coherent heart: Heart–brain interactions, psychophysiological coherence, and the emergence of system-wide order. *Integral Review, 5*(2), 10–115. https://doaj.org/article/dcb4d5cc482 b42998d4fec2e0d64d6f2

41. Cameron, O. G. (2002). *Visceral sensory neuroscience: Interoception.* Oxford University Press.

42. Liester, M. B. (2020). Personality changes following heart transplantation: The role of cellular memory. *Medical Hypotheses, 135*, 109468. https://doi.org/10.1016/j.mehy .2019.109468

43. Bunzel, B., Schmidl-Mohl, B., Grundböck, A., & Wollenek, G. (1992). Does changing the heart mean changing personality? A retrospective inquiry on 47 heart transplant patients. *Quality of Life Research, 1*(4), 251–256. https://doi.org/10.1007/bf00435634

44. Pearsall, P., Schwartz, G. E., & Russek, L. G. (2000). Changes in heart transplant recipients that parallel the personalities of their donors. *Integrative Medicine, 2*(2-3), 65–72. https:// doi.org/10.1016/s1096-2190(00)00013-5

45. Pert, C. (2012). *Molecules of emotion: Why you feel the way you feel.* Simon & Schuster.

46. Lipton, B. H. (2016). *The biology of belief: Unleashing the power of consciousness, matter & miracles*. Hay House.

47. Elliot, S. (2011, January 23). Diaphragm mediates action of autonomic and enteric nervous systems. *BMED Report*. https://www.bmedreport.com/archives/8309

48. Lin, I., Tai, L., & Fan, S. (2014). Breathing at a rate of 5.5 breaths per minute with equal inhalation-to-exhalation ratio increases heart rate variability. *International Journal of Psychophysiology, 91*(3), 206–211. https://doi.org/10.1016/j.ijpsycho.2013.12.006

49. Wu, S., & Lo, P. (2008). Inward-attention meditation increases parasympathetic activity: A study based on heart rate variability. *Biomedical Research, 29*(5), 245–250. https://doi.org/10.2220/biomedres.29.245

50. Paul-Labrador, M., Polk, D., Dwyer, J. H., Velasquez, I., Nidich, S., Rainforth, M., . . . Merz, C. N. (2006). Effects of a randomized controlled trial of transcendental meditation on components of the metabolic syndrome in subjects with coronary heart disease. *Archives of Internal Medicine, 166*(11), 1218. https://doi.org/10.1001/archinte.166.11.1218

51. Bachurin, V. I. (1979). Effect of low doses of electromagnetic waves on some human organs and systems. *Vrachebnoye Delo, 7*, 95–97. https://pubmed.ncbi.nlm.nih.gov/473758/

52. Dumanskiy, Y. D., & Rudichenko, V. F. (1976). Dependence of the functional activity of the liver mitochondria on UHF irradiation. *Gigiyena i Sanitariya, 4*, 16–19. https://pubmed.ncbi.nlm.nih.gov/955436/; Chernysheva, O. N., & Kolodub, F. A. (1975). Influence of a variable magnetic field of industrial frequency (50 Hz) on metabolic processes in the organs of rats. *Gigiyena truda i professional'nyye zabolevaniya, 11*, 20–23. https://pubmed.ncbi.nlm.nih.gov/1205186/

53. Pall, M. L. (2013). Electromagnetic fields activation of voltage-gated calcium channels to produce beneficial or adverse effects. *Journal of Cellular and Molecular Medicine, 17*(8), 958–965. https://doi.org/10.1111/jcmm.12088

54. Pall, M. L. (2014). Microwave electromagnetic fields act by activating voltage-gated calcium channels: why the current international safety standards do not predict biological hazard. *Recent Research and Development in Molecular and Cellular Biology, 7*, 1–15. https://rfreduce.com/robertsblog/dl/Microwave-electromagnetic-fields-act-by-activating_Pallmicrow-vgccnoheat.pdf

55. Al-Nimer, M., Majeed, A., & Alhusseiny, A. (2012). Electromagnetic energy radiated from mobile phone alters electrocardiographic records of patients with ischemic heart disease. *Annals of Medical and Health Sciences Research, 2*(2), 146. https://doi.org/10.4103/2141-9248.105662

56. Derkacz, A., Gawrys, J., Gawrys, K., Podgorski, M., Magott-Derkacz, A., Poreba, R., & Doroszko, A. (2017). Effect of electromagnetic field accompanying the magnetic resonance imaging on human heart rate variability—a pilot study. *International Journal of Injury Control and Safety Promotion, 25*(2), 229–231. https://doi.org/10.1080/17457300.2017.1363783

57. Bortkiewicz, A., Gadzicka, E., & Zmyślony, M. (1996). Heart rate variability in workers exposed to medium-frequency electromagnetic fields. *Journal of the Autonomic Nervous System, 59*(3), 91–97. https://doi.org/10.1016/0165-1838(96)00009-4

58. Li, Z. (2020, July 31). [Personal communication].

59. Azab, A. E. (2017). Exposure to electromagnetic fields induces oxidative stress and Pathophysiological changes in the cardiovascular system. *Journal of Applied Biotechnology & Bioengineering, 4*(2). https://doi.org/10.15406/jabb.2017.04.00096

Chapter 14. Heart Healthy Exercise

1. Wilson, M., O'Hanlon, R., Prasad, S., Deighan, A., MacMillan, P., Oxborough, D., . . . Whyte, G. (2011). Diverse patterns of myocardial fibrosis in lifelong, veteran endurance athletes. *Journal of Applied Physiology, 110*(6), 1622–1626. https://doi.org/10.1152/jappl physiol.01280.2010

2. La Gerche, A., Burns, A. T., Mooney, D. J., Inder, W. J., Taylor, A. J., Bogaert, J., . . . Prior, D. L. (2011). Exercise-induced right ventricular dysfunction and structural remodelling in endurance athletes. *European Heart Journal, 33*(8), 998–1006. https://doi.org/10.1093/eurheartj/ehr397

3. Kroger, K., Lehmann, N., Rappaport, L., Perrey, M., Sorokin, A., Budde, T., . . . Mohlenkamp, S. (2011). Carotid and peripheral atherosclerosis in male marathon runners. *Medicine & Science in Sports & Exercise, 43*(7), 1142–1147. https://doi.org/10.1249/mss.0b013e3182098a51

4. Siegel, A. J., Stec, J. J., Lipinska, I., Van Cott, E. M., Lewandrowski, K. B., Ridker, P. M., & Tofler, G. H. (2001). Effect of marathon running on inflammatory and hemostatic markers. *The American Journal of Cardiology, 88*(8), 918–920. https://doi.org/10.1016/s0002-9149(01)01909-9

5. Noakes, T. D., Opie, L. H., Rose, A. G., Kleynhans, P. H., Schepers, N. J., & Dowdeswell, R. (1979). Autopsy-proved coronary atherosclerosis in marathon runners. *New England Journal of Medicine, 301*(2), 86–89. https://doi.org/10.1056/nejm197907123010205

6. Trivax, J. E., & McCullough, P. A. (2012). Phidippides cardiomyopathy: A review and case illustration. *Clinical Cardiology, 35*(2), 69–73. https://doi.org/10.1002/clc.20994

7. McDougall, C. (2011). *Born to run: A hidden tribe, superathletes, and the greatest race the world has never seen.* Vintage.

8. Franco, V., Callaway, C., Salcido, D., McEntire, S., Roth, R., & Hostler, D. (2014). Characterization of electrocardiogram changes throughout a marathon. *European Journal of Applied Physiology, 114*(8), 1725–1735. https://doi.org/10.1007/s00421-014-2898-6

9. Baldesberger, S., Bauersfeld, U., Candinas, R., Seifert, B., Zuber, M., Ritter, M., . . . Attenhofer Jost, C. H. (2007). Sinus node disease and arrhythmias in the long-term follow-up of former professional cyclists. *European Heart Journal, 29*(1), 71–78. https://doi.org/10.1093/eurheartj/ehm555

10. Volek, J. S., Freidenreich, D. J., Saenz, C., Kunces, L. J., Creighton, B. C., Bartley, J. M., . . . Phinney, S. D. (2016). Metabolic characteristics of keto-adapted ultra-endurance runners. *Metabolism, 65*(3), 100–110. https://doi.org/10.1016/j.metabol.2015.10.028

11. Dessypris, A., Kuoppasalmi, K., & Adlercreutz, H. (1976). Plasma cortisol, testosterone, androstenedione and luteinizing hormone (LH) in a non-competitive marathon run. *Journal of Steroid Biochemistry, 7*(1), 33–37. https://doi.org/10.1016/0022-4731(76)90161-8

12. MacConnie, S., Barkan, A., Lampman, R., Schork, M., & Beitins, I. (1987). Decreased hypothalamic gonadotropin-releasing hormone secretion in male marathon runners. *Journal of Urology, 137*(5), 1076–1077. https://doi.org/10.1016/s0022-5347(17)44405-3

13. De Souza, M., Arce, J., Pescatello, L., Scherzer, H., & Luciano, A. (1994). Gonadal hormones and semen quality in male runners. *International Journal of Sports Medicine*, 15(07), 383–391. https://doi.org/10.1055/s-2007-1021075

14. Barrow, G. W., & Saha, S. (1988). Menstrual irregularity and stress fractures in collegiate female distance runners. *The American Journal of Sports Medicine*, 16(3), 209–216. https://doi.org/10.1177/036354658801600302

15. Mathews, S. C., Narotsky, D. L., Bernholt, D. L., Vogt, M., Hsieh, Y., Pronovost, P. J., & Pham, J. C. (2012). Mortality among marathon runners in the United States, 2000–2009. *The American Journal of Sports Medicine*, 40(7), 1495–1500. https://doi.org/10.1177/0363546512444555

16. Gaudreault, V., Tizon-Marcos, H., Poirier, P., Pibarot, P., Gilbert, P., Amyot, M., . . . Larose, E. (2013). Transient myocardial tissue and function changes during a marathon in less fit marathon runners. *Canadian Journal of Cardiology*, 29(10), 1269–1276. https://doi.org/10.1016/j.cjca.2013.04.022

17. Lee, D., Pate, R. R., Lavie, C. J., Sui, X., Church, T. S., & Blair, S. N. (2014). Leisure-time running reduces all-cause and cardiovascular mortality risk. *Journal of the American College of Cardiology*, 64(5), 472–481. https://doi.org/10.1016/j.jacc.2014.04.058

18. Seifert, T., Brassard, P., Wissenberg, M., Rasmussen, P., Nordby, P., Stallknecht, B., . . . Secher, N. H. (2010). Endurance training enhances BDNF release from the human brain. *American Journal of Physiology-Regulatory, Integrative and Comparative Physiology*, 298(2), R372–R377. https://doi.org/10.1152/ajpregu.00525.2009; Shephard, R. J. (2001). Absolute versus relative intensity of physical activity in a dose-response context. *Medicine and Science in Sports and Exercise*, 33(Supplement), S400–S418. https://doi.org/10.1097/00005768-200106001-00008; Steinberg, H., Sykes, E. A., Moss, T., Lowery, S., LeBoutillier, N., & Dewey, A. (1997). Exercise enhances creativity independently of mood. *British Journal of Sports Medicine*, 31(3), 240–245. https://doi.org/10.1136/bjsm.31.3.240; Jones, A. M., & Carter, H. (2000). The effect of endurance training on parameters of aerobic fitness. *Sports Medicine*, 29(6), 373–386. https://doi.org/10.2165/00007256-200029060-00001

19. Aagaard, P., Simonsen, E. B., Andersen, J. L., Magnusson, P., & Dyhre-Poulsen, P. (2002). Increased rate of force development and neural drive of human skeletal muscle following resistance training. *Journal of Applied Physiology*, 93(4), 1318–1326. https://doi.org/10.1152/japplphysiol.00283.2002; Havas, E., Parviainen, T., Vuorela, J., Toivanen, J., Nikula, T., & Vihko, V. (1997). Lymph flow dynamics in exercising human skeletal muscle as detected by scintography. *The Journal of Physiology*, 504(1), 233–239. https://doi.org/10.1111/j.1469-7793.1997.233bf.x; O'Connor, P. J., Herring, M. P., & Caravalho, A. (2010). Mental health benefits of strength training in adults. *American Journal of Lifestyle Medicine*, 4(5), 377–396. https://doi.org/10.1177/1559827610368771; McNeely, E. (2013). Training to improve bone density in adults: A review and recommendations. *The Sport Journal*, 21. https://www.cabdirect.org/cabdirect/abstract/20103228588

20. Dolezal, B. A., & Potteiger, J. A. (1998). Concurrent resistance and endurance training influence basal metabolic rate in nondieting individuals. *Journal of Applied Physiology*, 85(2), 695–700. https://doi.org/10.1152/jappl.1998.85.2.695; Zurlo, F., Larson, K., Bogardus, C., & Ravussin, E. (1990). Skeletal muscle metabolism is a major determinant

of resting energy expenditure. *Journal of Clinical Investigation, 86*(5), 1423–1427. https://doi.org/10.1172/jci114857

21. Rani, M., Singh, U., Agrawal, G. G., Natu, S. M., Kala, S., Ghildiyal, A., & Srivastava, N. (2013). Impact of yoga nidra on menstrual abnormalities in females of reproductive age. *The Journal of Alternative and Complementary Medicine, 19*(12), 925–929. https://doi.org/10.1089/acm.2010.0676; Rani, K., Tiwari, S., Kumar, S., Singh, U., Prakash, J., & Srivastava, N. (2016). The effect of yoga nidra on psychological problems of woman with menstrual disorders: A randomized clinical trial. *Journal of Caring Sciences, 5*(1), 1–9. https://doi.org/10.15171/jcs.2016.001; Chimkode, S. M. (2015). Effect of yoga on blood glucose levels in patients with type 2 diabetes mellitus. *Journal of Clinical and Diagnostic Research.* https://doi.org/10.7860/jcdr/2015/12666.5744

22. Kraemer, W., Gordon, S., Fleck, S., Marchitelli, L., Mello, R., Dziados, J., . . . Fry, A. (1991). Endogenous anabolic hormonal and growth factor responses to heavy resistance exercise in males and females. *International Journal of Sports Medicine, 12*(02), 228–235. https://doi.org/10.1055/s-2007-1024673

Chapter 15. The Dental Health–Heart Health Connection

1. Price, W. A. (1923). *Dental infections: Oral and systemic: Being a contribution to the pathology of dental infections, focal infections and the degenerative diseases.* Forgotten Books.

2. Slavkin, H. C. (2000). Relationship of dental and oral pathology to systemic illness. *JAMA, 284*(10), 1215. https://doi.org/10.1001/jama.284.10.1215; Casamassimo, P. S. (2000). Relationships between oral and systemic health. *Pediatric Clinics of North America, 47*(5), 1149–1157. https://doi.org/10.1016/s0031-3955(05)70261-3

3. Joshipura, K., Ritchie, C., & Douglass, C. (1999). Strength of evidence linking oral conditions and systemic disease. *Compendium of Continuing Education in Dentistry, 30,* 12–23. https://europepmc.org/article/med/11908384

4. Szeto, C., Kwan, B. C., Chow, K., Lai, K., Chung, K., Leung, C., & Li, P. K. (2008). Endotoxemia is related to systemic inflammation and atherosclerosis in peritoneal dialysis patients. *Clinical Journal of the American Society of Nephrology, 3*(2), 431–436. https://doi.org/10.2215/cjn.03600807; Wiedermann, C. J., Kiechl, S., Dunzendorfer, S., Schratzberger, P., Egger, G., Oberhollenzer, F., & Willeit, J. (1999). Association of endotoxemia with carotid atherosclerosis and cardiovascular disease. *Journal of the American College of Cardiology, 34*(7), 1975–1981. https://doi.org/10.1016/s0735-1097(99)00448-9

5. Stoll, L. L., Denning, G. M., & Weintraub, N. L. (2004). Potential role of endotoxin as a proinflammatory mediator of atherosclerosis. *Arteriosclerosis, Thrombosis, and Vascular Biology, 24*(12), 2227–2236. https://doi.org/10.1161/01.atv.0000147534.69062.dc

6. Mayr, F., Spiel, A., Leitner, J., Firbas, C., Sieghart, W., & Jilma, B. (2007). Effects of low dose endotoxemia on endothelial progenitor cells in humans. *Atherosclerosis, 195*(1), e202–e206. https://doi.org/10.1016/j.atherosclerosis.2007.04.003

7. Ruane, L., Buckley, T., Soo Hoo, S., Hansen, P., McCormac, C., Shaw, E., & Tofler, G. (2016). Triggering of acute myocardial infarction by respiratory infection. *Heart, Lung and Circulation, 25,* S70. https://doi.org/10.1016/j.hlc.2016.06.160

8. Håheim, L. L. (2011). *Oral infections and cardiovascular disease.* Bentham Science Publishers.

9. Hamasaki, T., Kitamura, M., Kawashita, Y., Ando, Y., & Saito, T. (2016). Periodontal disease and percentage of calories from fat using national data. *Journal of Periodontal Research*, *52*(1), 114–121. https://doi.org/10.1111/jre.12375

10. Drago, S., El Asmar, R., Di Pierro, M., Grazia Clemente, M., Sapone, A. T., Thakar, M., . . . Fasano, A. (2006). Gliadin, zonulin and gut permeability: Effects on celiac and non-celiac intestinal mucosa and intestinal cell lines. *Scandinavian Journal of Gastroenterology*, *41*(4), 408–419. https://doi.org/10.1080/00365520500235334

11. Caplan, D. J., Pankow, J. S., Cai, J., Offenbacher, S., & Beck, J. D. (2009). The relationship between self-reported history of endodontic therapy and coronary heart disease in the atherosclerosis risk in communities study. *The Journal of the American Dental Association*, *140*(8), 1004–1012. https://doi.org/10.14219/jada.archive.2009.0311

12. Netea, M. G., Demacker, P. N., Kullberg, B. J., Jacobs, L. E., Verver-Jansen, T. J., Boerman, O. C., . . . Van der Meer, J. W. (1998). Bacterial lipopolysaccharide binds and stimulates cytokine-producing cells before neutralization by endogenous lipoproteins can occur. *Cytokine*, *10*(10), 766–772. https://doi.org/10.1006/cyto.1998.0364

13. Brune, D. (1986). Metal release from dental biomaterials. *Biomaterials*, *7*(3), 163–175. https://doi.org/10.1016/0142-9612(86)90097-9

14. Zhuang, P., McBride, M. B., Xia, H., Li, N., & Li, Z. (2009). Health risk from heavy metals via consumption of food crops in the vicinity of Dabaoshan mine, South China. *Science of The Total Environment*, *407*(5), 1551–1561. https://doi.org/10.1016/j.scitotenv .2008.10.061; Jaishankar, M., Tseten, T., Anbalagan, N., Mathew, B. B., & Beeregowda, K. N. (2014). Toxicity, mechanism and health effects of some heavy metals. *Interdisciplinary Toxicology*, *7*(2), 60–72. https://doi.org/10.2478/intox-2014-0009

Chapter 16. Chiropractic and Heart Health

1. Lyons, D. D. (2003). Response to Gonstead chiropractic care in a 27 year old athletic female with a 5 year history of infertility. *Journal of Vertebral Subluxation Research*. https:// drjuliewellness.com/wp-content/uploads/2015/05/Chiropractic-for-Fertlity.pdf; Vilan, R. (2004). The role of chiropractic care in the resolution of migraine headaches and infertility. *Journal of Clinical Chiropractic Pediatrics*, *6*(1). https://www.researchgate.net/profile /Sharon_Vallone/publication/291023374_Chiropractic_evaluation_and_treatment_of _musculoskeletal_dysfunction_in_infants_demonstrating_difficulty_breastfeeding/links /5e1b312c299bf10bc3a8f9e1/Chiropractic-evaluation-and-treatment-of-musculoskeletal -dysfunction-in-infants-demonstrating-difficulty-breastfeeding.pdf#page=12; Murphy, J. T. (2010). A review of complementary and alternative care for infertility issues. *Journal of Clinical Chiropractic Pediatrics*, *11*(2). http://jccponline.com/jccp_v11_n2.pdf#page=43

2. Anderson, R. (1992). Spinal manipulation before chiropractic. In S. Haldeman (Ed.), *Principles and practice of chiropractic* (2nd ed., pp. 3–14). Appleton & Lange.

3. Agocs, S. (2011, June). Chiropractic's fight for survival. *Journal of Ethics*, American Medical Association. https://journalofethics.ama-assn.org/article/chiropractics-fight-survival /2011-06

4. Kimbrough, M. L. (1998). Jailed chiropractors: Those who blazed the trail. *Chiropractic History: The Archives and Journal of the Association for the History of Chiropractic*, *18*(1), 79–100. https://pubmed.ncbi.nlm.nih.gov/11620299/

5. Wilk v. American Medical Association, 671 FSupp 1465 (N D Ill 1987).

6. Trever, W. (1972). *In the public interest*. Scriptures Unlimited.

7. Wilk v. American Medical Association, 895 F2d 352 (7th Cir), cert denied, 111 S Ct 513 (1990).

8. Getzendanner, S. (1988). Permanent injunction order against AMA. *JAMA: The Journal of the American Medical Association, 259*(1), 81–82. https://doi.org/10.1001/jama.259.1.81

9. Herzog, W., Leonard, T., Symons, B., Tang, C., & Wuest, S. (2012). Vertebral artery strains during high-speed, low amplitude cervical spinal manipulation. *Journal of Electromyography and Kinesiology, 22*(5), 740–746. https://doi.org/10.1016/j.jelekin.2012.03.005

10. Cassidy, J. D., Boyle, E., Côté, P., He, Y., Hogg-Johnson, S., Silver, F. L., & Bondy, S. J. (2008). Risk of vertebrobasilar stroke and chiropractic care. *European Spine Journal, 17*(S1), 176–183. https://doi.org/10.1007/s00586-008-0634-9

11. Kosloff, T. M., Elton, D., Tao, J., & Bannister, W. M. (2015). Chiropractic care and the risk of vertebrobasilar stroke: Results of a case–control study in U.S. commercial and Medicare Advantage populations. *Chiropractic & Manual Therapies, 23*(1). https://doi.org/10.1186/s12998-015-0063-x

12. Whedon, J. M., Song, Y., Mackenzie, T. A., Phillips, R. B., Lukovits, T. G., & Lurie, J. D. (2015). Risk of stroke after chiropractic spinal manipulation in Medicare B beneficiaries aged 66 to 99 years with neck pain. *Journal of Manipulative and Physiological Therapeutics, 38*(2), 93–101. https://doi.org/10.1016/j.jmpt.2014.12.001

13. Church, E. W., Sieg, E. P., Zalatimo, O., Hussain, N. S., Glantz, M., & Harbaugh, R. E. (2016). Systematic review and meta-analysis of chiropractic care and cervical artery dissection: No evidence for causation. *Cureus.* https://doi.org/10.7759/cureus.498

14. Meade, T. W., Dyer, S., Browne, W., Townsend, J., & Frank, A. O. (1990). Low back pain of mechanical origin: Randomised comparison of chiropractic and hospital outpatient treatment. *BMJ, 300*(6737), 1431–1437. https://doi.org/10.1136/bmj.300.6737.1431; Palmgren, P. J., Sandström, P. J., Lundqvist, F. J., & Heikkilä, H. (2006). Improvement after chiropractic care in cervicocephalic kinesthetic sensibility and subjective pain intensity in patients with nontraumatic chronic neck pain. *Journal of Manipulative and Physiological Therapeutics, 29*(2), 100–106. https://doi.org/10.1016/j.jmpt.2005.12.002; Tuchin, P. J., Pollard, H., & Bonello, R. (2000). A randomized controlled trial of chiropractic spinal manipulative therapy for migraine. *Journal of Manipulative and Physiological Therapeutics, 23*(2), 91–95. https://doi.org/10.1016/s0161-4754(00)90073-3

15. Haavik-Taylor, H., & Murphy, B. (2007). Cervical spine manipulation alters sensorimotor integration: A somatosensory evoked potential study. *Clinical Neurophysiology, 118*, 391–402. https://pubmed.ncbi.nlm.nih.gov/17137836/

16. Kunert, W. (1965). Functional disorders of internal organs due to vertebral lesions. *CIBA Symposium, 13*(3), 85–96.

17. Lewit, K. (1985). *Manipulative therapy in rehabilitation of the locomotor system*. Butterworth-Heinemann.

18. Jarmel, M. E. (1989). Possible role of spinal joint dysfunction in the genesis of sudden cardiac death. *Journal of Manipulative and Physiological Therapeutics, 12*(6), 469–477. https://pubmed.ncbi.nlm.nih.gov/2697737/

19. Treadwell, B. V., & Mankin, H. J. (1986). The synthetic processes of articular cartilage. *Clinical Orthopaedics and Related Research, 213*, 50–61. https://doi.org/10.1097/00003086-198612000-00007

20. Stokes, I. A., & Iatridis, J. C. (2004). Mechanical conditions that accelerate intervertebral disc degeneration: Overload versus immobilization. *Spine, 29*(23), 2724–2732. https://doi.org/10.1097/01.brs.0000146049.52152.da

21. Sugiura, Y., Lee, C., & Perl, E. (1986). Central projections of identified, unmyelinated (C) afferent fibers innervating mammalian skin. *Science, 234*(4774), 358–361. https://doi.org/10.1126/science.3764416

22. Craig, A. D. (1995). Distribution of brainstem projections from spinal lamina I neurons in the cat and the monkey. *The Journal of Comparative Neurology, 361*(2), 225–248. https://doi.org/10.1002/cne.903610204

23. Grassi, G., Arenare, F., Pieruzzi, F., Brambilla, G., & Mancia, G. (2009). Sympathetic activation in cardiovascular and renal disease. *Journal of Nephrology, 22*(2), 190–195. https://pubmed.ncbi.nlm.nih.gov/19384835/

24. Budgell, B., & Hirano, F. (2001). Innocuous mechanical stimulation of the neck and alterations in heart-rate variability in healthy young adults. *Autonomic Neuroscience, 91*(1-2), 96–99. https://doi.org/10.1016/s1566-0702(01)00306-x

25. Win, N. N., Jorgensen, A. M., Chen, Y. S., & Haneline, M. T. (2015). Effects of upper and lower cervical spinal manipulative therapy on blood pressure and heart rate variability in volunteers and patients with neck pain: A randomized controlled, cross-over, preliminary study. *Journal of Chiropractic Medicine, 14*(1), 1–9. https://doi.org/10.1016/j.jcm.2014.12.005

26. Kolberg, C., Horst, A., Moraes, M. S., Duarte, F. C., Riffel, A. P., Scheid, T., . . . Partata, W. A. (2015). Peripheral oxidative stress blood markers in patients with chronic back or neck pain treated with high-velocity, low-amplitude manipulation. *Journal of Manipulative and Physiological Therapeutics, 38*(2), 119–129. https://doi.org/10.1016/j.jmpt.2014.11.003

27. Ogura, T., Tashiro, M., Masud, M., Watanuki, S., Shibuya, K., Yamaguchi, K., . . . Yanai, K. (2011). Cerebral metabolic changes in men after chiropractic spinal manipulation for neck pain. *Alternative Therapies in Health and Medicine, 17*(6), 12–17. https://pubmed.ncbi.nlm.nih.gov/22314714/

28. Inami, A., Ogura, T., Watanuki, S., Masud, M. M., Shibuya, K., Miyake, M., . . . Tashiro, M. (2017). Glucose metabolic changes in the brain and muscles of patients with nonspecific neck pain treated by spinal manipulation therapy: A [18F] FDG PET study. *Evidence-Based Complementary and Alternative Medicine, 2017*, 1–9. https://doi.org/10.1155/2017/4345703

Chapter 17. Aspirin and Ouabain

1. Crichton, M. (1988). *Travels.* The Ballantine Publishing Group: p. 385.

2. Crichton, M. (1988). *Travels.* The Ballantine Publishing Group: p. 385.

3. Plaisance, K. I., Kudaravalli, S., Wasserman, S. S., Levine, M. M., & Mackowiak, P. A. (2000). Effect of antipyretic therapy on the duration of illness in experimental influenza A, *Shigella sonnei*, and *Rickettsia rickettsii* infections. *Pharmacotherapy, 20*(12), 1417–1422. https://doi.org/10.1592/phco.20.19.1417.34865

4. Ford, E. S. (1999). Serum magnesium and ischaemic heart disease: Findings from a national sample of US adults. *International Journal of Epidemiology, 28*(4), 645–651. https://doi.org/10.1093/ije/28.4.645

5. Williams, R. J. (1972). Nutrition against disease. *Perspectives in Biology and Medicine, 15*(3), 481–481. https://doi.org/10.1353/pbm.1972.0055

6. Ravn, H. B., Kristensen, S. D., Hjortdal, V. E., Thygesen, K., & Husted, S. E. (1997). Early administration of intravenous magnesium inhibits arterial thrombus formation. *Arteriosclerosis, Thrombosis, and Vascular Biology, 17*(12), 3620–3625. https://doi.org/10.1161/01.atv.17.12.3620; Rukshin, V., Shah, P. K., Cercek, B., Finkelstein, A., Tsang, V., & Kaul, S. (2002). Comparative antithrombotic effects of magnesium sulfate and the platelet glycoprotein IIb/IIIa inhibitors tirofiban and eptifibatide in a canine model of stent thrombosis. *Circulation, 105*(16), 1970–1975. https://doi.org/10.1161/01.cir.0000014612.88433.62; Rukshin, V., Azarbal, B., Shah, P. K., Tsang, V. T., Shechter, M., Finkelstein, A., . . . Kaul, S. (2001). Intravenous magnesium in experimental stent thrombosis in swine. *Arteriosclerosis, Thrombosis, and Vascular Biology, 21*(9), 1544–1549. https://doi.org/10.1161/hq0901.094493

7. Fowkes, F., Price, J., & Stewart, M. (2011). Aspirin for prevention of cardiovascular events in a general population screened for a low ankle brachial index: A randomized controlled trial. *Journal of Vascular Surgery, 53*(4), 1158. https://doi.org/10.1016/j.jvs.2011.02.038

8. Gensenway, D. (2002) Do your patients need aspirin therapy?. *ACP-ASIM Annals of Internal Medicine.*

9. Strom, B. L., & Carson, J. L. (2018). Nonsteroidal antiinflammatory drugs and upper gastrointestinal bleeding. *Pharmacoepidemiology*, 229–241. https://doi.org/10.1201/9780203743669-22; Wilcox, C. M., Alexander, L. N., Cotsonis, G. A., & Clark, W. S. (1997). Nonsteroidal antiinflammatory drugs are associated with both upper and lower gastrointestinal bleeding. *Digestive Diseases and Sciences, 42*, 990–997. https://link.springer.com/article/10.1023/A:1018832902287

10. Mellemkjaer, L., Blot, W. J., Sørensen, H. T., Thomassen, L., McLaughlin, J. K., Nielsen, G. L., & Olsen, J. H. (2002). Upper gastrointestinal bleeding among users of NSAIDs: A population-based cohort study in Denmark. *British Journal of Clinical Pharmacology, 53*(2), 173–181. https://doi.org/10.1046/j.0306-5251.2001.01220.x

11. Wolfe, M. M., Lichtenstein, D. R., & Singh, G. (2000). Gastrointestinal toxicity of nonsteroidal antiinflammatory drugs. *Survey of Anesthesiology, 44*(3), 180–181. https://doi.org/10.1097/00132586-200006000-00057; Cryer, B. (2005). NSAID-associated deaths: The rise and fall of NSAID-associated GI mortality. *The American Journal of Gastroenterology, 100*(8), 1694–1695. https://doi.org/10.1111/j.1572-0241.2005.50565.x

12. Fored, C. M., Ejerblad, E., Lindblad, P., Fryzek, J. P., Dickman, P. W., Signorello, L. B., . . . Nyrén, O. (2001). Acetaminophen, aspirin, and chronic renal failure. *New England Journal of Medicine, 345*(25), 1801–1808. https://doi.org/10.1056/nejmoa010323

13. Kim, J. K., Kim, Y., Fillmore, J. J., Chen, Y., Moore, I., Lee, J., . . . Shulman, G. I. (2001). Prevention of fat-induced insulin resistance by salicylate. *Journal of Clinical Investigation, 108*(3), 437–446. https://doi.org/10.1172/jci11559; Yuan, M. (2001). Reversal of obesity- and diet-induced insulin resistance with salicylates or targeted disruption of Ikkbeta.

Science, 293(5535), 1673–1677. https://doi.org/10.1126/science.1061620; Hundal, R. S., Petersen, K. F., Mayerson, A. B., Randhawa, P. S., Inzucchi, S., Shoelson, S. E., & Shulman, G. I. (2002). Mechanism by which high-dose aspirin improves glucose metabolism in type 2 diabetes. *Journal of Clinical Investigation, 109*(10), 1321–1326. https://doi.org/10.1172/jci0214955

14. Jardine, M. J., Ninomiya, T., Perkovic, V., Cass, A., Turnbull, F., Gallagher, M. P., . . . Zanchetti, A. (2010). Aspirin is beneficial in hypertensive patients with chronic kidney disease: A post-hoc subgroup analysis of a randomized controlled trial. *Journal of the American College of Cardiology, 56*(12), 956–965. https://www.jacc.org/doi/full/10.1016/j.jacc.2010.02.068

15. Kauffman, J. M. (2000). Should you take aspirin to prevent heart attack? *Journal of Scientific Explorations, 14*(4), 623–641. http://citeseerx.ist.psu.edu/viewdoc/download?doi=10.1.1.558.6115&rep=rep1&type=pdf

16. Satoh, E., & Nakazato, Y. (1992). On the mechanism of ouabain-induced release of acetylcholine from Synaptosomes. *Journal of Neurochemistry, 58*(3), 1038–1044. https://doi.org/10.1111/j.1471-4159.1992.tb09359.x; Blasi, J. M., Cena, V., Gonzalez-Garcia, C., Marsal, J., & Solsona, C. (1988). Ouabain induces acetylcholine release from pure cholinergic synaptosomes independently of extracellular calcium concentration. *Neurochemical Research, 13*(11), 1035–1041. https://doi.org/10.1007/bf00973147

17. Manunta, P., Ferrandi, M., Bianchi, G., & Hamlyn, J. M. (2009). Endogenous ouabain in cardiovascular function and disease. *Journal of Hypertension, 27*(1), 9–18. https://doi.org/10.1097/hjh.0b013e32831cf2c6

18. Gremels, H. (1937). Uber den Einfluß von Digitalisglykosiden auf die energetischen Vorgänge am Säugetierherzen. *Naunyn-Schmiedebergs Archiv für Experimentelle Pathologie und Pharmakologie, 186*(6), 625–660. https://doi.org/10.1007/bf01865162

19. Dohrmann, R. E., & Dohrmann, M. (1984). Neuere therapie der instabilen Angina pectoris bei koronarer herzerkrankung. *Erfahrungsheilkunde—Acta Medica Empirica, 33*, 183–190.

20. Salz, H., & Schneider, B. (1985). Perlinguales g-Strophanthin bei stabiler Angina pectoris. *Z f Allgemeinmedizin, 61*, 1223–1228.

21. Sarre, H. (1952/53). Strophanthinbehandlung bei Angina pectoris. *Therapiewoche, 3*, 311–314.

22. Sroka, K. S. (2013). "Ouabain": The wasted opportunity to save heart patients. Heart Attack | Facts | Alternatives | Prevention | Well-Being | Eine weitere WordPress-Seite. https://heartattacknew.com/faq/what-can-be-done-to-prevent-a-heart-attack/ouabain-the-wasted-opportunity/

23. Cowan, T. (2014). What causes heart attacks? Townsend Letter. https://jeffreydachmd.com/wp-content/uploads/2014/08/Thomas_Cowan_What_Causes_Heart_Attacks_Townsend_Letter_2014.pdf

24. Ren, Y., Zhang, M., Zhang, T., & Huang, R. (2013). Effect of ouabain on myocardial remodeling in rats. *Experimental and Therapeutic Medicine, 6*(1), 65–70. https://doi.org/10.3892/etm.2013.1098

25. Wu, J., Li, D., Du, L., Baldawi, M., Gable, M. E., Askari, A., & Liu, L. (2015). Ouabain prevents pathological cardiac hypertrophy and heart failure through activation of phosphoinositide 3-kinase α in mouse. *Cell & Bioscience, 5*(1). https://doi.org/10.1186/s13578-015-0053-7

Chapter 18. Biometrics: Tracking Your Risk

1. Ceriello, A., Esposito, K., Piconi, L., Ihnat, M. A., Thorpe, J. E., Testa, R., . . . Giugliano, D. (2008). Oscillating glucose is more deleterious to endothelial function and oxidative stress than mean glucose in normal and type 2 diabetic patients. *Diabetes, 57*(5), 1349–1354. https://doi.org/10.2337/db08-0063

2. Vincent, H., Innes, K. E., & Taylor, A. G. (2007). Chronic stress and insulin-resistance--related indices of cardiovascular disease risk. Part I. Neurophysiological responses and pathological sequelae. *Alternative Therapies in Health and Medicine, 13*(4). https://www.researchgate.net/publication/322754701_Chronic_stress_and_insulin-resistance-related_indices_of_cardiovascular_disease_risk_Part_I_Neurophysiological_responses_and_pathological_sequelae

3. National Institutes of Health. (1984). *The National Institutes of Health (NIH) consensus development program: Lowering blood cholesterol to prevent heart disease.* https://consensus.nih.gov/1984/1984Cholesterol047html.htm

4. Kolata, G. (1985). Heart panel's conclusions questioned. *Science, 227*(4682), 40–41. https://doi.org/10.1126/science.3880617

5. Zhou, L., Wu, Y., Yu, S., Shen, Y., & Ke, C. (2020). Low-density lipoprotein cholesterol and all-cause mortality: Findings from the China health and retirement longitudinal study. *BMJ Open, 10*(8), e036976. https://doi.org/10.1136/bmjopen-2020-036976

6. *Hypertension.* (2018). Correction to: 2017 ACC/AHA/Aapa/Abc/Acpm/Ags/Apha/Ash/Aspc/Nma/Pcna guideline for the prevention, detection, evaluation, and management of high blood pressure in adults: A report of the American College of Cardiology/American Heart Association task force on clinical practice guidelines. *Hypertension, 71*(6). https://doi.org/10.1161/hyp.0000000000000076

7. Vernon, S. T., Coffey, S., Bhindi, R., Soo Hoo, S. Y., Nelson, G. I., Ward, M. R., . . . Figtree, G. A. (2017). Increasing proportion of ST elevation myocardial infarction patients with coronary atherosclerosis poorly explained by standard modifiable risk factors. *European Journal of Preventive Cardiology, 24*(17), 1824–1830. https://doi.org/10.1177/2047487317720287; Vernon, S. T., Coffey, S., D'Souza, M., Chow, C. K., Kilian, J., Hyun, K., . . . Figtree, G. A. (2019). ST-segment–elevation myocardial infarction (STEMI) patients without standard modifiable cardiovascular risk factors—How common are they, and what are their outcomes? *Journal of the American Heart Association, 8*(21). https://doi.org/10.1161/jaha.119.013296

8. Hoevenaar-Blom, M. P., Spijkerman, A. M., Kromhout, D., Van den Berg, J. F., & Verschuren, W. M. (2011). Sleep duration and sleep quality in relation to 12-Year cardiovascular disease incidence: The MORGEN study. *Sleep, 34*(11), 1487–1492. https://doi.org/10.5665/sleep.1382

9. Jiddou, M. R., Pica, M., Boura, J., Qu, L., & Franklin, B. A. (2013). Incidence of myocardial infarction with shifts to and from daylight savings time. *The American Journal of Cardiology, 111*(5), 631–635. https://doi.org/10.1016/j.amjcard.2012.11.010

10. Simpson, N. S., Banks, S., Arroyo, S., & Dinges, D. F. (2010). Effects of sleep restriction on adiponectin levels in healthy men and women. *Physiology & Behavior, 101*(5), 693–698. https://doi.org/10.1016/j.physbeh.2010.08.006

11. Morishita, E., Asakura, H., Jokaji, H., Saito, M., Uotani, C., Kumabashiri, I., . . . Matsuda, T. (1996). Hypercoagulability and high lipoprotein(a) levels in patients with type II

diabetes mellitus. *Atherosclerosis*, *120*(1-2), 7–14. https://doi.org/10.1016/0021
-9150(95)05647-5; Pawlak, K., Mysliwiec, M., & Pawlak, D. (2014). OxLDL—the
molecule linking hypercoagulability with the presence of cardiovascular disease in
hemodialyzed uraemic patients. *Thrombosis Research*, *134*(3), 711–716. https://doi.
org/10.1016/j.thromres.2014.07.007; Nomura, S., Shouzu, A., Omoto, S., Nishikawa,
M., Iwasaka, T., & Fukuhara, S. (2004). Activated platelet and oxidized LDL induce
endothelial membrane vesiculation: Clinical significance of endothelial cell-derived
Microparticles in patients with type 2 diabetes. *Clinical and Applied Thrombosis/Hemosta-
sis*, *10*(3), 205–215. https://doi.org/10.1177/107602960401000302

12. Simpson, H., Meade, T., Stirling, Y., Mann, J., Chakrabarti, R., & Woolf, L. (1983). Hypertri-
glyceridaemia and hypercoagulability. *The Lancet*, *321*(8328), 786–790. https://doi
.org/10.1016/s0140-6736(83)91849-4; Domingueti, C. P., Dusse, L. M., Carvalho, M. D.,
De Sousa, L. P., Gomes, K. B., & Fernandes, A. P. (2016). Diabetes mellitus: The linkage
between oxidative stress, inflammation, hypercoagulability and vascular complications.
Journal of Diabetes and Its Complications, *30*(4), 738–745. https://doi.org/10.1016/j.jdia
comp.2015.12.018; Kakafika, A., Liberopoulos, E., Karagiannis, A., Athyros, V., & Mikha-
ilidis, D. (2006). Dyslipidaemia, Hypercoagulability and the metabolic syndrome. *Current
Vascular Pharmacology*, *4*(3), 175–183. https://doi.org/10.2174/157016106777698432

13. Jeppesen, J., Hein, H. O., Suadicani, P., & Gyntelberg, F. (2001). Low triglycerides–high
high-density lipoprotein cholesterol and risk of ischemic heart disease. *Archives of Internal Medicine*, *161*(3), 361. https://doi.org/10.1001/archinte.161.3.361; Kurl, S., Zaccardi,
F., Onaemo, V. N., Jae, S. Y., Kauhanen, J., Ronkainen, K., & Laukkanen, J. A. (2014).
Association between HOMA-IR, fasting insulin and fasting glucose with coronary heart
disease mortality in nondiabetic men: A 20-year observational study. *Acta Diabetologica*,
52(1), 183–186. https://doi.org/10.1007/s00592-014-0615-x

14. Yip, J., Facchini, F. S., & Reaven, G. M. (1998). Resistance to insulin-mediated glucose
disposal as a predictor of cardiovascular disease. *The Journal of Clinical Endocrinology &
Metabolism*, *83*(8), 2773–2776. https://doi.org/10.1210/jcem.83.8.5005

15. Eddy, D., Schlessinger, L., Kahn, R., Peskin, B., & Schiebinger, R. (2008). Relationship of
insulin resistance and related metabolic variables to coronary artery disease: A mathe-
matical analysis. *Diabetes Care*, *32*(2), 361–366. https://doi.org/10.2337/dc08-0854

16. Hegele, R. A. (2001). Premature atherosclerosis associated with monogenic insulin
resistance. *Circulation*, *103*(18), 2225–2229. https://doi.org/10.1161/01.cir.103.18.2225

Conclusion

1. Angell M. Drug Companies & Doctors: A Story of Corruption. *The New York Review of
Books magazine*. [Last accessed August 5, 2015]. Available from: http://www.nybooks.
com/articles/archives/2009/jan/15/drug-companies-doctorsa-story-of-corruption/

2. Every-Palmer, S., & Howick, J. (2014). How evidence-based medicine is failing due to
biased trials and selective publication. *Journal of Evaluation in Clinical Practice*, *20*(6),
908–914. https://doi.org/10.1111/jep.12147

3. Horwitz, R. I., & Singer, B. H. (2017). Why evidence-based medicine failed in patient care
and medicine-based evidence will succeed. *Journal of Clinical Epidemiology*, *84*, 14–17.
https://doi.org/10.1016/j.jclinepi.2017.02.003

Index

About the Author

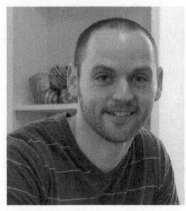

Tricia Louque

Dr. Stephen Hussey is a board-certified chiropractor and functional medicine practitioner. He has a bachelor's degree in health and wellness promotion from the University of North Carolina Asheville as well as a doctorate of chiropractic and masters in human nutrition and functional medicine from the University of Western States. In addition to working as a chiropractor in clinical practice, Dr. Hussey has worked with people all over the world, coaching them back to health, and sees the power of food, lifestyle change, and personal environment modification to change lives every day. He can be found on his website, www.resourceyourhealth.com, or on social media @drstephenhussey. When he is not working, he enjoys time outdoors as well as reading, researching, playing sports, and spending time with his wife and their pets. *Understanding the Heart* is Dr. Hussey's second book, his first book is *The Health Evolution: Why Understanding Evolution Is the Key to Vibrant Health*.